T0259307

Forensic Psychiatry

Editor

CHARLES L. SCOTT

PSYCHIATRIC CLINICS OF NORTH AMERICA

www.psych.theclinics.com

December 2012 • Volume 35 • Number 4

ELSEVIER

1600 John F. Kennedy Boulevard • Suite 1800 • Philadelphia, PA 19103-2899

http://www.theclinics.com

PSYCHIATRIC CLINICS OF NORTH AMERICA Volume 35, Number 4
December 2012 ISSN 0193-953X, ISBN-13: 978-1-4557-4929-4

Editor: Joanne Husovski
Developmental Editor: Donald Mumford

Psychiatric Clinics of North America (ISSN 0193-953X) is published quarterly by Elsevier Inc., 360 Park Avenue South, New York, NY 10010-1710. Months of issue are March, June, September, and December. Business and Editorial Offices: 1600 John F. Kennedy Blvd., Suite 1800, Philadelphia, PA 19103-2899. Periodicals postage paid at New York, NY and additional mailing offices. Subscription prices are $265.00 per year (US individuals), $473.00 per year (US institutions), $131.00 per year (US students/residents), $321.00 per year (Canadian individuals), $589.00 per year (Canadian Institutions), $399.00 per year (foreign individuals), $589.00 per year (foreign institutions), and $194.00 per year (international & Canadian students/residents). Foreign air speed delivery is included in all *Clinics'* subscription prices. All prices are subject to change without notice. **POSTMASTER:** Send address changes to *Psychiatric Clinics of North America*, Elsevier Health Sciences Division, Subscription Customer Service, 3251 Riverport Lane, Maryland Heights, MO 63043. Customer Service: 1-800-654-2452 (US). From outside the United States, call 1-314-447-8871. Fax: 1-314-447-8029. E-mail: journalscustomerservice-usa@elsevier.com (for print support) and journalsonlinesupport-usa@elsevier.com (for online support).

Reprints. For copies of 100 or more, of articles in this publication, please contact the Commercial Reprints Department, Elsevier Inc., 360 Park Avenue South, New York, New York 10010-1710. Tel.: (212) 633-3813, Fax: (212) 462-1935, E-mail: reprints@elsevier.com.

Psychiatric Clinics of North America is covered in *MEDLINE/PubMed (Index Medicus)*, *Current Contents/Social and Behavioral Sciences, Social Science Citation Index, Embase/Excerpta Medica,* and PsycINFO.

Printed and bound by CPI Group (UK) Ltd, Croydon, CR0 4YY

Transferred to digital print 2012

Contributors

GUEST EDITOR

CHARLES L. SCOTT, MD
Chief, Division of Psychiatry and the Law, Training Director of the Forensic Psychiatry Fellowship Program and Clinical Professor of Psychiatry, Department of Psychiatry and Behavioral Sciences, University of California, Davis Medical Center, Sacramento, California

AUTHORS

MADELON BARANOSKI, PhD
Associate Professor, Department of Psychiatry, Yale University School of Medicine, New Haven, Connecticut

JAMES CAVNEY, MBChB, FRANZCP
Honorary Lecturer of Mason Clinic Regional Forensic Psychiatry Services, University of Auckland, Auckland, New Zealand

BRADLEY W. FREEMAN, MD
Assistant Professor of Psychiatry, Child Adolescent Division, Department of Psychiatry, Vanderbilt University School of Medicine, Nashville, Tennessee

SUSAN HATTERS FRIEDMAN, MD
Associate Professor of Psychiatry and Pediatrics, Case Western Reserve University School of Medicine, Connections Mental Health Center, Beachwood, Ohio

THOMAS G. GUTHEIL, MD
Professor of Psychiatry, Department of Psychiatry, Beth Israel-Deaconess Medical Center and the Massachusetts Mental Health Center, Harvard Medical School, Brookline, Massachusetts

CORY JAQUES, MD
Psychiatry Resident, Department of Psychiatry, UCLA Semel Institute for Neuroscience and Human Behavior, Los Angeles, California

JAMES L. KNOLL IV, MD
Director of Forensic Psychiatry, Associate Professor of Psychiatry, Division of Forensic Psychiatry, Department of Psychiatry, SUNY Upstate Medical University, Syracuse, New York; and Forensic Fellowship Director, Central New York Psychiatric Center, New York

BARBARA E. McDERMOTT, PhD
Professor of Clinical Psychiatry, Division of Psychiatry and the Law, Department of Psychiatry and Behavioral Sciences, University of California, Davis Medical Center, Sacramento, California

WILLIAM J. NEWMAN, MD
Assistant Clinical Professor of Psychiatry and Associate Training Director of the Forensic Psychiatry Fellowship Program, Division of Psychiatry and the Law, Department of Psychiatry and Behavioral Sciences, University of California, Davis Medical Center, Sacramento, California

MAYA PRABHU, MD, LLB
Assistant Professor, Department of Psychiatry, Yale University School of Medicine, New Haven, Connecticut

PHILLIP J. RESNICK, MD
Director, Division of Forensic Psychiatry, Professor of Psychiatry, Case Western Reserve University School of Medicine, Cleveland, Ohio

JASON G. ROOF, MD
Assistant Clinical Professor of Psychiatry, Division of Psychiatry and the Law, Department of Psychiatry and Behavioral Sciences, University of California, Davis Medical Center, Sacramento, California

RONALD SCHOUTEN, MD, JD
Director, Law and Psychiatry Service, Associate Professor of Psychiatry, Massachusetts General Hospital, Harvard Medical School, Boston, Massachusetts

CHARLES L. SCOTT, MD
Chief, Division of Psychiatry and the Law, Training Director of the Forensic Psychiatry Fellowship Program and Clinical Professor of Psychiatry, Department of Psychiatry and Behavioral Sciences, University of California, Davis Medical Center, Sacramento, California

MATTHEW SOULIER, MD
Assistant Clinical Professor of Psychiatry, Division of Psychiatry and the Law, Training Director of the Child Psychiatry Residency, Department of Psychiatry and Behavioral Sciences, University of California, Davis Medical Center, Sacramento, California

HUMBERTO TEMPORINI, MD
Department of Psychiatry, Kaiser Permanente South Sacramento Medical Center, Sacramento, California

CHRISTOPHER THOMPSON, MD
Assistant Clinical Professor of Psychiatry, Child & Adolescent Division, Department of Psychiatry and Biobehavioral Sciences, David Geffen School of Medicine at UCLA, Los Angeles, California

Contents

Child pornography can be found on the Web, in newsgroups, and on peer-to-peer networks (the most common source at present). Offenders are a heterogeneous group, with different motivations and levels of risk. The possibility of crossover to a contact sexual offense exists, depending on the presence of other risk factors. Possession of child pornography without a history of contact offenses does not appear to increase the risk of future contact reoffending.

conflict between an employee and the employer or coworkers. It summarizes key principles and observations that are common to psychiatric consultations in the workplace and then offers case examples that are representative of such consultations and highlights those principles. Although the focus is on psychiatric consultation to employers, an employee may seek consultation himself or herself, especially when prospects for adversarial proceedings arise. The principles described here apply in both sets of circumstances.

This article discusses the ever-increasing opportunity for forensic mental health evaluators to provide assistance to the legal system in the areas of testamentary capacity and guardianship assessments. These areas of evaluation are defined, and a discussion of preparation and execution of effective evaluations is provided. The legal concepts of undue influence and insane delusion are defined and applied to the evaluator's interview. Common cognitive concerns such as dementia and delirium may affect an evaluee's capacity, and their presence and effect on the evaluee are considered. Evaluators are encouraged to carefully consider specific capacities related to the relevant legal questions posed.

This article adds to the existing literature on the role of mental health professionals in assisting attorneys in the asylum and refugee determination process primarily in the United States. The authors describe the legal context for asylum and refugee processing, challenges in conducting evaluations, diagnostic considerations, and specific competencies needed for mental health evaluators. Various cases are presented to illustrate key points. These cases purposely do not include any identifying information of any specific client, yet they are representative of the range and scope of issues that arise in this context.

The deposition is an important stage in the legal process, which poses special challenges for the deponent. This article reviews those challenges from the standpoint of the expert witness, addressing the stages of the deposition, the deposing attorney's strategies, the role and goals of the expert witness serving as the deponent, the approach to answering the attorney's questions, strategies for clarifying or reframing those questions, and the approaches to reviewing the deposition after the transcript has been printed. The article emphasizes tricks and traps used by the deposing attorney and how to avoid them.

This article is designed to provide an overview of the existing literature on pharmacologically managing aggression, with a specific focus on psychiatric diagnoses commonly associated with increased aggression. Self-injurious behaviors and suicide are sometimes classified as forms of aggression, but information presented here focuses primarily on aggression toward others (physical and/or verbal).

PSYCHIATRIC CLINICS OF NORTH AMERICA

FORTHCOMING ISSUES

Integrative Therapies in Psychiatry
Philip Muskin, MD, Robert Brown, MD,
and Patricia Gerbarg, MD, *Guest Editors*

Disaster Psychiatry
Craig Katz, MD, and Anand Pandya, MD,
Guest Editors

RECENT ISSUES

September 2012
Schizophrenia
Peter F. Buckley, MD, *Guest Editor*

June 2012
Addiction
Itai Danovitch, MD, and
John J. Mariani, MD, *Guest Editors*

March 2012
Depression
David L. Mintz, MD, *Guest Editor*

RELATED INTEREST

International Journal of Law and Psychiatry,
January–February 2010 (Vol. 33, No. 1)
The Concept of Free Will and Forensic Psychiatry
Niklas Juth and Frank Lorentzon

Preface

Mental Health and Legal Systems Inextricably Intertwined

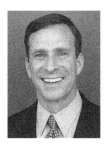

Charles L. Scott, MD
Guest Editor

Forensic psychiatry focuses on mental health issues that interface with the law. This fascinating field, however, is not an esoteric isolated subspecialty. Quite the contrary! In fact, mental health evaluators and experts are increasingly confronted with complex and often frightening issues that mirror our evolving society. These issues range from an aging population with declining competencies to mass shooters whose violence shocks our conscience.

The articles in this volume were specifically chosen to address topics current and relevant in criminal and civil mental health contexts. Five of the articles review important areas in the criminal justice system. These include the assessment of individuals who commit mass shootings on innocent civilians, evaluation of criminal defendants who claim amnesia for their alleged crimes, adults who kill children, and adults who are charged with child pornography possession. These 4 topics are both tragic and timely.

Important subjects that arise during the civil context are also highlighted. These 3 topics include assessment of an individual's testamentary capacity and need for guardianship, evaluation of asylum seekers related to immigration and potential deportation, and consultation with employers and evaluation of employees on mental health issues in the workplace.

Two important issues relevant to children and adolescents are reviewed in the articles on bullying and a juvenile's competence to stand trial. The final 3 articles overlap with many of the areas above and include important factors to consider when giving a deposition, psychological testing strategies and assessments important to consider during the evaluation process, and psychopharmacologic approaches to managing aggressive behaviors.

This particular volume offers specific topics useful for general psychiatrists and nearly every psychiatric subspecialty, including child and adolescent psychiatry, geriatric psychiatry, psychosomatic medicine, and forensic psychiatry. As our mental

Psychiatr Clin N Am 35 (2012) xi–xii
http://dx.doi.org/10.1016/j.psc.2012.08.013
0193-953X/12/$ – see front matter © 2012 Elsevier Inc. All rights reserved.

health and legal systems become increasingly and inextricably intertwined, mental health providers need to maintain an updated understanding of important fundamental principles that govern their assessments and treatment. The goal of this volume is to assist the reader in achieving that goal.

A very special thanks to David Spagnolo, who served as the editorial assistant on this project, and whose wisdom, professionalism, and amazingly positive attitude always makes the impossible possible.

Charles L. Scott, MD
Division of Psychiatry and the Law
Forensic Psychiatry Fellowship Program
Department of Psychiatry and Behavioral Sciences
University of California
Davis Medical Center
2516 Stockton Blvd
Sacramento, CA 95817, USA

E-mail address:
charles.scott@ucdmc.ucdavis.edu

Mass Murder
Causes, Classification, and Prevention

James L. Knoll IV, MD[a,b],*

KEYWORDS

- Mass murder • Revenge • Classification • Psycholinguistics • Prevention

KEY POINTS

- Mass murder is the killing of four or more victims at one location within one event.
- Common factors include offenders killing in public during the daytime, planning the offense, coming prepared with powerful firearms, and often expecting to be killed.
- Psychosocial factors common to mass murder include extreme feelings of anger, social alienation, rumination on violent revenge, psychiatric illness, and precipitating social stressors.
- Understanding motives and psychopathology requires an understanding of the psychology of revenge, feelings of persecution, and destructive envy.
- The final communications of mass murderers can be analyzed to provide an enhanced understanding of their motives, psychopathology, and classification.
- Prevention must rely on various methods, including enhanced social responsibility, psychiatric efforts, research, cultural considerations, and media responsibility.

OVERVIEW

Mass murder, the killing of four or more victims at one location within one event, is a rare and catastrophic phenomenon.[1] The prevalence of firearms, media coverage, and increasing awareness of the subject has led to speculations about the influence of a western cultural script being played out.[2,3] In the case of mass murder, the play is an appalling tragedy in which the main themes are a wounded ego, revenge, and infamy. Western influences aside, mass killings are not new. News media tend to suggest that the era of mass public killings was ushered in by Charles Whitman atop the University of Texas at Austin tower, and thereafter became "a part of American life" in subsequent decades.[4] In contrast, research indicates that the news media

Disclosures: Dr Knoll has nothing to disclose.
a Division of Forensic Psychiatry, Department of Psychiatry, SUNY Upstate Medical University, 750 East Adams Street, Syracuse, NY 13210, USA; b Central New York Psychiatric Center, NY, USA
* Corresponding author. Division of Forensic Psychiatry, Department of Psychiatry, SUNY Upstate Medical University, 750 East Adams Street, Syracuse, NY 13210, USA.
E-mail address: knollj@upstate.edu

Psychiatr Clin N Am 35 (2012) 757–780
http://dx.doi.org/10.1016/j.psc.2012.08.001

have heavily influenced public perception of mass murder, particularly the question-able speculation that its incidence is increasing.[5] It is typically the high-profile cases that are most heavily covered by the media, yet these are the least representative mass killings.

An example of mass murder existing long before Whitman is the tragic case of the Bath School disaster of 1927, now long forgotten.[6] The perpetrator, Andrew Kehoe, lived in Michigan where he encountered serious stressors of financial problems and a wife who was seriously ill with tuberculosis. Kehoe seemed to displace and focus his substantial anger and despair on a local town conflict over property taxes levied on a school building. After becoming utterly overwhelmed with resentment, Kehoe killed his wife, set his farm ablaze, and killed some 45 individuals by setting off a bomb. Kehoe was killed in the blast and, like many modern-day mass murderers, left a final communication. His message, inscribed on a plaque outside his property read "criminals are made, not born," a statement suggestive of externalization of blame and a long-held grievance.

MASS MURDER COMMONALITIES

The challenges involved in researching mass murder include its low base rate and the fact that few perpetrators survive to be interviewed. In cases where the perpetrator does survive to face prosecution, he may be likely to "redefine" the act by "omitting and minimizing" certain aspects for the purpose of mitigating responsibility.[7] From a definitional standpoint, there seems to be a consensus that at least four to five victims should be used to define mass murder. However, in many cases the precise number of victims may be arbitrary, so that one is left with a common theme of "a number of victims at one time and in one space."[7]

Factors common to mass murder include extreme feelings of anger and revenge; lack of an accomplice (in adult mass murder); feelings of social alienation; and plan-ning and organizing the offense. In a detailed case study of five mass murderers who were caught before they were killed, several common traits and historical factors were found.[2] The subjects had all been bullied or isolated as children, turning into loners who felt despair over being socially excluded. They were suspicious, resentful, grudge holders, who demonstrated obsessional or rigid traits. Narcissistic and gran-diose traits were present, along with the heavy use of externalization as a way of coping. They held a worldview of others being rejecting and uncaring. As a result, they spent a great deal of time feeling resentful, and ruminating on past humiliations. These ruminations invariably evolved into fantasies of violent revenge. Offenders seemed to "welcome death," even perceiving it as bringing them fame with an aura of power.

Careful study of individual cases of mass murder often reveals that the offender felt compelled to leave a final message for others.[8,9] These messages may be written or verbal, and at least one case has described the use of YouTube to transmit a final message.[10] The examination of these messages using forensic psycholinguistic anal-ysis is addressed later in this article. Individual case analysis also demonstrates that the offender often engages in various forms of "private ritual" in preparation for the offense.[7] Rituals may take the form of selecting and purchasing special weapons, ammunition, clothing, and related provisions. Ritual preparations may also include modification of appearance, modeling the special clothing and weapons, and taking pictures of oneself, as was seen in the Seung-Hui Cho (Virginia Tech) case. Ultimately, Cho sent his ritualistic modeling pictures to the media shortly before his offense. It is possible that the process of engaging in this private ritual, in addition to the practical purpose of preparation, may briefly alleviate tension and enhance feelings of control until the time the offender is ready to commit mass murder.[7]

From an etiologic standpoint, the factors contributing to mass murder are broad and must be approached by the biopsychosocial model.[10] Biologic factors include possible brain pathology, and psychiatric illnesses, such as depression and psychosis. Psychological factors include negative or fragile self-image, strong sense of entitlement, and vulnerability to humiliation. Social factors include social isolation or alienation, being bullied, and marital or financial loss. **Box 1** gives a list of putative contributing factors. Given the paucity of research seen clarifying the spectrum of mass murder, it is difficult to draw conclusions beyond the hypothesis that it is caused by a "complex interaction" between axis I and II disorders, traumatic life events, and precipitating factors.[7]

MASS MURDER: TOWARD CLASSIFICATION

Research has previously developed a classification system for the phenomenon known as homicide-suicide (H-S). H-S is an event in which an individual commits a homicide and subsequently (usually within 24 hours) commits suicide.[11,12] H-S is a distinct category of homicide that has features that differ from other forms of killing. It is a rare event, estimated to occur between 0.2 and 0.38 per 100,000 persons

---

Box 1
Mass murder: contributing factors

Biologic

- Psychosis
- Depression
- Brain pathology
- Personality disorders

Psychological

- Problems with self-esteem
- Persecutory or paranoid outlook
- Entitlement
- Antisocial traits
- Obsessional or rigid traits
- Narcissistic, grandiose traits
- Externalization, unable to take responsibility
- World seen as rejecting, uncaring
- Resentful with rumination on past humiliations
- Fantasize about violent revenge

Social

- Social alienation
- Being bullied
- Life stressors: marital, financial
- Access to and familiarity with firearms

annually.[12,13] Most H-S are carefully planned by the perpetrator as a two-stage sequential act. Marzuk and coworkers[14] proposed classifying H-S by the relationship the perpetrator had to the victim (spousal, familial, and so forth), along with the perpetrator's motive (jealousy, altruism, revenge, and so forth). Their five proposed H-S types are summarized in **Box 2**.

Of the five major H-S types, it is the consortial-possessive type involving an estranged intimate partner that accounts for most (50%–75%) H-S. Much less common is the adversarial (also called extrafamilial) type of H-S. The pseudocommando type mass murderer, as described by Dietz,[15] and the analogous "autogenic massacre" described by Mullen[2] best fit into this category. Other variants of this

---

Box 2
Homicide-suicide classification

Classification

- Relationship plus motive

  - Relationship between victim and perpetrator (spousal, familial, and so forth)

  - Motivation of perpetrator (jealousy, altruism, revenge, and so forth)

Major Patterns

I. Consortial-possessive

Most common type, accounting for 50% to 75% of all homicide-suicides. Involves a male in his 30s or 40s, recently estranged from his partner. Relationship often characterized by domestic abuse and multiple separations and reunions.

II. Consortial–physically ailing

Committed by one spouse with a chronic medical condition leading to pain and suffering. The perpetrator is usually an elderly man with poor health, an ailing spouse, or both. The failing health has typically resulted in financial difficulties. Depression is frequent, and the motive may involve altruism or despair about the future. Suicide notes are often left and describe an inability to cope with poor health, finances, and loneliness.

III. Filicide-suicide

About 40% to 60% of fathers and 16% to 29% of mothers commit suicide immediately after murdering their children. Infants, however, are more likely to be killed by the mother. A mother killing a neonate is unlikely to suicide. There are further subtypes of filicide-suicide based on motives, such as psychosis, altruism, and revenge.

IV. Familicide-suicide

Men are more likely than women to kill their entire family. Most commonly involves a depressed man who is experiencing precipitating stressors of marital problems, custody disputes, or financial problems.

V. Adversarial homicide–suicide (extrafamilial)

This type usually involves a disgruntled ex-employee, a bullied student, or resentful paranoid loner. He externalizes blame onto others, and feels wronged in some way. He is very likely to have depression and paranoid or narcissistic traits. Actual persecutory delusions may sometimes be seen. Other variants of this type include disgruntled litigants or clients. This perpetrator often uses a powerful arsenal of weapons, and has no escape planned. The event may involve a "suicide by cop" in that he forces police to kill him in a last stand "blaze of glory."

Adapted from Marzuk P, Tardiff K, Hirsch C. The epidemiology of murder-suicide. JAMA 1992;267:3179–83.

type of H-S include disgruntled ex-employees and "school shooters." These types of mass murder can be considered an H-S in many cases, because the perpetrator goes to the offense expecting not only to kill, but also to be killed. He often has no escape planned, and may either kill himself, or force police to kill him.[16]

To date, the phenomenon of mass murder has eluded a broadly accepted classification system. The literature contains descriptors, such as family annihilator, school shooter, pseudocommando, disgruntled employee, and so forth. However, these terms and their vague boundaries may run the risk of impeding future research. Given the concept that mass murder often ends in the suicide of the perpetrator, and that it has been described as "suicide with hostile intent,"[3] a classification system similar to that used for H-S seems to make sense. **Box 3** gives a proposed classification system for mass murder that is based on the H-S classification system of Marzuk and coworkers.

Box 3
Mass murder classification

Classification Scheme:

- Relationship/Linkage + Motive

- *Relationship or link* between victims and perpetrator (work, school, family, specific community, pseudocommunity, etc.)

- *Motive* of perpetrator (resentful, psychotic, depressed, etc.)

Pattern Examples:

Familial-Depressed

A depressed senior man of a household. There are often associated precipitating stressors of marital problems, finances, or work related problems. He may view his action as an altruistic "delivery" of his family from continued hardships. He may also suspect marital infidelity and be misusing substances. There is evidence of depression or depressive cognitions distorting judgment.

Specific Community-Resentful

Includes disgruntled clients or others harboring deep resentment toward an identifiable group, culture or political movement.

Pseudocommunity-Psychotic

Includes individuals experiencing paranoid or persecutory delusions flowing from a psychotic disorder. They target a group which they delusionally believe is persecuting them. Paranoid psychoses and/or strong paranoid cognitions are common diagnoses.

Indiscriminate-Resentful

Generally rageful, depressed and often paranoid individual who releases his anger arbitrarily in some public place. The victim group may be chosen randomly, or on the basis of convenience or ease of access to large numbers of victims.

Workplace-Resentful

Disgruntled ex-employee, or resentful employee who is upset with a supervisor, co-worker(s), or some aspect of the work environment. He externalizes blame onto others, and feels wronged in some way. He is very likely to have depression, as well as paranoid and/or narcissistic traits. Actual persecutory delusions may sometimes be seen.

From Marzuk P, Tardiff K, Hirsch C. The epidemiology of murder-suicide. JAMA 1992;267: 3179–83; with permission.

Marzuk, Tardiff, and Hirsch H-S Classification System

The term "linkage" is added to the "relationship" descriptor to emphasize that some perpetrators may have no meaningful interpersonal relationship with their victims, but may have only a connection by some mutually shared activity, such as work or school.

In this proposed system, the school-resentful type of mass murderer includes offenders who target schoolmates and have the motive of hostile revenge. Examples include Seung-Hui Cho and Columbine offenders Harris and Klebold.[17] The workplace-resentful type describes the disgruntled employee who feels aggrieved in some way. An example is Atlanta day trader Mark Barton, who shot and killed 9 people and injured 13 more in 1999.[18] Barton was motivated by depression and anger, and serious financial and marital troubles. Barton had developed a highly resentful, hopeless attitude about his life and career. His suicide note stated, "I don't plan to live very much longer, just long enough to kill as many of the people that greedily sought my destruction."[19] He entered two adjacent Atlanta day trading firms, first stating, "I hope this doesn't ruin your trading day" before carrying out the shootings. Shortly afterward, Barton committed suicide by shooting himself.

The indiscriminate-resentful type describes the generally rageful, depressed, and often paranoid individual who releases his anger arbitrarily in some public place. An example is James Huberty, who shot and killed 22 and injured 19 others at a San Diego McDonalds in 1984.[20] A rageful and nonpsychotic Huberty told his wife immediately before the offense that "society had their chance," and that he was going "hunting humans." There was no evidence that Huberty felt particularly aggrieved by that specific McDonalds. Rather, there was evidence that Huberty chose the McDonald's out of familiarity and his knowledge that there were likely to be large numbers of potential victims at the location.

In a seminal paper on mass, serial, and sensational homicides, Dietz[15] described a type of mass murderer he termed the "pseudocommando." This type of mass murderer is driven by strong feelings of anger and resentment, in addition to having a paranoid character. He plans out the offense ritualistically, and comes prepared with a powerful arsenal of weapons. In terms of the relationship to the victims, Dietz[15] noted that the pseudocommando may focus his resentment on a specific community based in reality, or a "pseudocommunity" that was the product of psychosis or strong paranoid cognitions. Thus, the proposed classification system captures these types as a specific community–resentful type and a pseudocommunity-psychotic type, respectively. The specific community–resentful type includes disgruntled clients or others harboring deep resentment toward an identifiable group, culture, or political movement. The pseudocommunity-psychotic type includes only those experiencing paranoid or persecutory delusions flowing from a psychotic disorder. As suggested in **Box 3**, the relationship/linkage–motive classification scheme allows for multiple permutations that can be applied to best classify each individual case.

THE PSEUDOCOMMANDO

To investigate a more detailed method of studying mass murder, this article now focuses on a single type of mass murderer, the pseudocommando, and what forensic psycholinguistic analysis can provide in terms of understanding his motives and psychopathology. A forensic psycholinguistic analysis begins with the assumption that the offender would not have bothered to communicate his message unless it had great personal meaning. The final communications of two pseudocommando-type mass murderers, Seung-Hui Cho (Virginia Tech) and Jiverly Wong (Binghamton, NY), are analyzed to show that their final communications reveal important similarities and differences in terms of their motives and psychopathology.

As noted, the term "pseudocommando" was used to describe a type of mass murderer who plans his actions "after long deliberation."[15] He most often kills in public during the daytime, comes prepared with a powerful arsenal of weapons, and has no escape planned. Pseudocommandos are "collectors of injustice" who nurture their wounded narcissism and ultimately retreat into a fantasy life of violence and revenge. Mullen[2] described the results of his detailed personal evaluation of five pseudocommando type mass murderers who, by chance, were caught before they could kill themselves or be killed. Mullen[2] noted that the massacres were often well planned out (ie, not impulsive, the offender did not "snap"), with the offender arriving at the crime scene well-armed, often in camouflage or "warrior" gear, and seemed to be pursuing a highly personal agenda of "payback." Mullen and Dietz described this type of offender as a suspicious grudge holder who is preoccupied with firearms. It should be noted that the pseudocommando as described by Dietz and Mullen could be classified by the proposed classification system as either a specific community–resentful type, a pseudocommunity-psychotic type, or an indiscriminate-resentful type.

Ego Survival and Revenge

The threatened ego model explaining pseudocommando psychology is consistent with Menninger's perspective on the cause of explosions of rage. According to Menninger, there are five critical elements prompting an explosion of violent behavior[21]:

1. Narcissistic injury perceived as grossly unfair
2. Hopelessness about a reasonable resolution
3. Perception that the limits of toleration have been exceeded and some action must be taken
4. Access to weapons
5. Disregard for the consequences, combined with a sense of "potent" rage

To clarify this process, Menninger uses the example of when a child suffers some type of pain. Immediately, the child "wants to let others know about it… to know exactly how he or she hurts."[21] The internal dialogue may be represented as: "When I am hurt by you, I want you to hurt like I hurt; therefore if you hit me, I will hit you back."[21] But in the case of the pseudocommando, the drive for revenge does not abide by principle of functional symmetry. The type of severe narcissistic rage they experience "serves the purpose of the preservation of the self"[21] that has exceeded its limit of aversive self-awareness, and demands excessive retaliation, and transfer of a disproportionate amount of pain to others.[21] The very public and arguably theatrical nature of mass murder as revenge speaks clearly to the offender's "need for recognition from an audience."[22] Thus, the offender's dramatic act of revenge can also be seen as an attempt to "reestablish the sense of an audience" that had been lost by virtue of his social alienation.[22]

The pseudocommando has been aptly described as a "collector of injustice" who holds onto perceived insults, amassing a pile of "evidence" that they have been grossly mistreated.[15] In addition to justifying his vengeful act, his collection helps sustain a revenge "romance." He collects the unwanted, hated, or feared aspects of himself, and then reassembles the collection into the form of an "enemy" who "deserves" to be the target of a merciless, incendiary rage. Thus, the pseudocommando maintains object relations based heavily on envy and splitting. The more intense desire for revenge is likely to signal a more intense idealization of the hated objects. Targets of a very intense revenge desire must be made out to be worthy of their fate and portrayed as barely worthy of being considered human beings, much as Seung-Hui Cho portrayed other students (whom he hardly knew) as "hedonistic," selfish "brats" who had "crucified" him and "raped" his soul.[21] Yet at the same time, he must view himself as blame free, thereby completing the other half of the splitting and projection dynamic.

The pseudocommando's revenge fantasy serves to obliterate an intolerable reality and aversive self-awareness. His rumination "dominates thought and impels action much as an addiction or erotomania does."[23] He not only denies his powerlessness, but goes further, gaining "virtually limitless power. An eye for an eye soon gives way to a life for an eye."[23] In this way, revenge "is an attempt to restore the grandiose self."[23] It allows the pseudocommando's "omnipotence" to rise triumphantly from the ashes of shame, loss, and vulnerability. But the revenge fantasy and primitive defenses cannot protect him indefinitely, particularly where strong feelings of persecution and envy lead him down the path of cognitive deconstruction, nihilism, and willingness to sacrifice himself.

Pseudocommando Mindset: Persecution, Envy, Obliteration

The study of violent offenders suggests that they often demonstrate an impaired ability to trust and have a persecutory worldview, leaving them with a strong self-centered, paranoid character style.[24] This is analogous to the mental construct described by Klein, known as the "paranoid-schizoid position," in which the individual's worldview is based on feelings of mistreatment and frustration at what is perceived as "intentional" harm, or purposeful deprivation.[23,25] This parallels the observation of Dietz,[15] who noted that most if not all men in the United States who have killed 10 or more victims in a single incident have demonstrated "paranoid symptoms of some kind." The paranoid-schizoid offender demonstrates the use of more primitive defense mechanisms, such as splitting, externalization, and projective identification.[24]

Envy

Consistent with their feelings of being persecuted, paranoid-schizoid offenders also suffer from strong feelings of destructive envy. This type of offender is not simply envious of the Other's possessions or social status, but the way in which the Other is able to enjoy these things. The term "Other" is used here to signify another person and the projection of the offender's own ego onto the other person. His true goal is to destroy the Other's capacity to enjoy the prized object or status.[25] For example, Seung-Hui Cho provides an excellent example of this in his manifesto when he rebukes other students as a result of his perception that they possessed "everything" they ever wanted, such as "Mercedes.... golden necklaces.... trust funds.... vodka and cognac."[26] Yet, in the very same manifesto, he reveals his powerfully destructive envy, by stating: "Oh the happiness I could have had mingling among you hedonists, being counted as one of you, if only you didn't ***** the living ***** out of me."[26] By projection, such individuals perceive others as persecutory not only as a result of paranoid cognitions, but also because of their views of others as withholding the "goodness" and happiness to which they feel entitled.

Nihilism

Clinical observations suggest that some of these offenders who remain fixed in the persecutory position ultimately develop an entrenched nihilistic attitude.[27] This nihilism then pervades their worldview, attitudes toward treatment, and life in general. Their feelings of hopelessness may result in suicidality and other self-defeating actions.[28] The observations of the adverse effects of social rejection and nihilistic beliefs in incarcerated offenders are consistent with research findings in nonincarcerated populations. For example, social rejection has been found in normal subjects to increase feelings of meaninglessness, decrease self-awareness, and impair the ability to self-regulate behavior.[29,30]

Research in social psychology has shown that when nihilism and the drive to avoid painful or aversive self-awareness becomes strong enough, there is a significantly increased risk of suicide or self-destructive behaviors.[31] This theory has been called the "escape theory" of suicide to denote the suicidal individual's motivation to escape aversive self-awareness. According to escape theory, when the individual is unable to avoid negative affect and aversive self-awareness, a process of "cognitive deconstruction" occurs in which there is a rejection of meaning (nihilism, hopelessness); increased irrationality; and disinhibition. In applying this theory to the psychology of the pseudocommando, the stage of cognitive deconstruction seems to signal a potentially deadly turning point. Having tried, but failed, to place his aversive self-awareness outside of himself, he redoubles his efforts to externalize. These efforts inevitably return to him as more powerful persecutory attacks from the outside. In select individuals, this may culminate in a real-life physical attack directed outward to avoid what is within.

Shakespeare's Richard III is a classic example of a mind committed to revenge and driven by powerful grievance. His state of mind may be regarded as a nihilistic and obliterative state of mind, in that it functions to spread more grievance, destruction, and ultimately annihilation.[32] Such individuals may come to embrace a self-styled image based on unhealthy self-perceptions that may be tinged with an ominous or threatening undertone. In effect, they embrace their dark, negative cognitions, and fashion them into a recognizable suit of "black" armor. Just as Richard III defined himself by his own deformity, so Seung-Hui Cho defined himself by his "outcast" status and dubbing himself the "question mark kid." Such individuals who are driven by envy and destruction often see others "as in the light and [choose] to stay in the dark."[33]

Entitlement

In the case of the pseudocommando bent on annihilation, there is more at work than envy alone. He must hold fast to his "hatred of anything such as growth, beauty, or humanity which is an advance over a bleak, static interior landscape."[33] He must also maintain a feeling of being an "exception" to the rules, of being entitled to harm others, because in his view "Nature has done me a grievous wrong.... Life owes me reparation.... I have a right to be an exception, to disregard the scruples by which others let themselves be held back. I may do wrong myself, since wrong has been done to me."[34] Once he has embraced this mindset, he condemns himself to a mental space in which "he cannot envision rescue from this commitment to a killing field externally or internally."[33]

Heroic Revenge Fantasy

To halt the death march toward obliteration, such individuals require mental "sanctuary" from the oppressive, relentless nihilism that assails them. It is only from such a sanctuary that he has a hope of achieving greater mental clarity, freedom from persecution, and relinquishing his pseudoempowering revenge fantasies. Sadly, it is the case that some individuals may never be able to relinquish the obliterative mindset, because all attempts at empathy may be met with suspicion, defensiveness, and contempt. It could be said that such individuals' destructive revenge fantasies and refusal to compromise can progress to a fatal, malignant stage. He becomes unable or unwilling to re-emerge from the "heroic" fantasy of revenge. As he comes closer to turning fantasy into reality, he must undergo a process in which he increasingly comes to accept that he will be sacrificing his own life. It may be that this obstacle is easier for him to overcome where his catastrophic thinking leads him to believe violent H-S is his only option; and his obliterative mindset has caused him to feel that his "self" is already dead and that his physical death is of little consequence.

These dynamics have the effect of distorting his judgment and undermining his ability to find meaning in life or sublimate aggression. Now he is able to override his survival instinct and reach the point of "willingness to sacrifice one's body."[35] It is also at this point that he begins to formulate his final communications. These communications have great meaning to him, because he realizes they will be the only "living" testament to his motivations, struggle, and "heroic sacrifice."

FORENSIC PSYCHOLINGUISTICS AND MASS MURDER

On July 22, 2011, Norway experienced the immeasurable fallout from a pseudocommando who obliterated more than 70 innocent people. Anders Behring Breivik, a 32-year-old Norwegian extremist, perpetrated a dual attack in Norway: the bombing of government buildings in Oslo that resulted in eight deaths, and the mass shooting at a camp of the Workers' Youth League of the Labor Party on the island of Utoya where he killed 69, most of whom were teenagers.[36] Breivik composed a 1492-page manifesto he published on the Internet hours before his attack.[37] Hempel and coworkers[8] were among the first to note that mass murderers with a "warrior mentality" often "convey their central motivation in a psychological abstract."

To date, the actual communications of the mass murder have received little analysis, despite the fact that "the words people use … can reveal important aspects of their social and psychological worlds."[38] Beyond basic demographic data, the use of language may provide a wealth of information, such as diagnostic considerations and the subject's overall level of psychological distress. An offender's use of language may lend clues about his past experience, ethnic background, and primary motivations. The pseudocommando may go to significant lengths to ensure that his final communications are transmitted to and read by others. In the two case examples examined later (Seung Hui Cho and Jiverly Wong), both men made special efforts to deliver their messages to the news media shortly before committing their mass murders. It is possible to examine such communications for what they reveal about the important aspects of the offenders' "social and psychological worlds."[39] Forensic psycholinguistic analysis allows the examiner to discern subtleties of linguistic style, personality variables, cognitive styles, and the presence of certain types of mental illness.[40]

Psycholinguistic Method

Forensic psycholinguistic analysis is best done as a part of a team approach, which may include law enforcement, private investigators, forensic computer specialists, and forensic document examiners.[41] From the outset, the forensic evaluator should pay careful attention to the quality of the evidence examined. The best possible sample of the writing or communication should be obtained. If copies are used, one must make sure they are high quality and complete. It may be helpful to make multiple copies of single documents so that highlighting, notes, and so forth can take place, yet one still retains a clean, unaltered copy. Reviewing the documents and other materials carefully, slowly, and multiple times is necessary. Each review may be done with a different primary purpose. For example, the first review may simply be to obtain a general first impression. Subsequent reviews may be done for the following reasons:

- Identification of themes, motives
- Identification of evidence of mental illness
- Identification of idiosyncratic language or symbol use
- Identification of basic features, such as type of medium, style of handwriting, dates, drawings, postage markings, and so forth
- Identification of threatening language, types of threats
- Identification of general fund of knowledge and intelligence
- Comparison with other related documents
- Analysis of communication delivery method
- Identification of intended audience

After multiple, careful examinations, the investigator may be able to determine important basic information, such as educational level, religious orientation, and other valuable data.[42] The use of language may also suggest different types of mental illness, such as schizophrenia,[43] depression,[44] or general emotional turmoil. For example, research has found that the excessive use of pronouns has been associated with high levels of psychological distress.[45] The use of metaphor may also lend clues about an individual's past experience, ethnic background, primary motivations, and level of distress.[33] Even a piece of data as seemingly unimportant as an e-mail address may suggest clues about the subject's personality structure.[46] One psycholinguistic study of threateners from the Federal Bureau of Investigation's National Center for the Analysis of Violent Crimes database found that "higher conceptual complexity" and "lower ambivalent hostility/paranoia" were more strongly associated with predatory violence.[47] While keeping such research findings in mind during the analysis, one should also consider paying close attention to the following:

- Changes in tone, affect, organization, and so forth over time in the case of serial communications
- Evidence of persecutory delusions coexisting with organized thought processes
- Severity of mental disorder as suggested by communications
- Overall personality structure suggestive of an "externalizing" style of coping
- Statements demonstrating a forceful sense of entitlement (eg, "I'm not going to ask for my dignity, I'm going to take it back.")
- Frequency and intensity of relevant cognitive distortions (eg, minimization, denial, and projection)

The forensic psycholinguistic analysis begins with the assumption that the offender would not have bothered to write down or otherwise communicate his "manifesto" unless it had great personal meaning. In both cases examined next, the offenders took the time and effort to deliver their communications to the television news media, suggesting that it was highly important to them that their "message" be disseminated to the public. This analysis does not constitute an "expert" legal opinion. Rather, it is a linguistic exercise aimed at trying to better understand the offenders' motives and psychology. As such, the psycholinguistic analyses that follow should be viewed as working hypotheses. The analyses are limited by the lack of a personal evaluation of the offender.

Case Example: Seung Hui Cho

On April 16, 2007, Seung Hui Cho, a student at Virginia Tech, shot to death 33 students and faculty.[48] He wounded 24 more and then committed suicide by shooting himself.

The incident was an unfathomable tragedy for surviving college students, families of the deceased, Virginians, and the entire country. The Virginia Office of the Inspector General for Mental Health, Mental Retardation and Substance Abuse Services conducted an investigation, finding that Cho did not significantly raise any concerns until approximately December of 2005.[49] At that time, he was perceived as threatening and odd to peers and faculty. He was seen several times by the campus police for complaints by other students of harassment. On December 13, 2005, campus police told him that his continued harassment could lead to criminal charges. That same day, Cho sent an instant message to a roommate stating, "I might as well kill myself or something." Cho was evaluated by a social work clinician, which led to his temporary detention in a behavioral health unit. The following day, Cho was evaluated by a psychologist who found him mentally ill, but not an imminent danger to himself or others. Several hours later, he was released with an appointment at a counseling center for later that day. It is unclear whether or not Cho kept the appointment. There were no further incidents reported until the shootings on April 16, 2007. Before his evaluation, and after, it has been theorized that he began to have violent revenge fantasies. This is deduced primarily by his writings, which consisted of "plays" about violence and revenge.[39]

The Office of the Inspector General for Mental Health, Mental Retardation and Substance Abuse Services investigation reported that after his psychiatric evaluation, his peers described him as rarely making eye contact. He kept isolated and would usually not respond if spoken to, or would give an occasional one-word answer. He was known for never showing much emotion, but peers reported not observing any evidence of confused thinking, odd behavior, or agitation. He appeared mildly sad, but not significantly depressed. Most of his peers concluded that they did not know much about him. On the day of the shootings, NBC reported receiving a package containing a 1800-word video manifesto on CD, plus 43 photos, 11 of them showing Cho aiming handguns at the camera.[42] In one dramatic photo, Cho holds a handgun in each hand, with his arms spread out on either side. He wears a military style vest for carrying ammunition and a large knife strapped to his belt as he stares menacingly into the camera. In two other photos, Cho seems to be mimicking suicidal behaviors. In one photo, he points a handgun at his right temple, again staring menacingly into the camera. In the second photo, he holds what seems to be a 6-in hunting knife to the left side of his neck with his right hand. He is shown in other photos aiming handguns directly at the camera, while wearing several handgun holsters and black gloves.

Cho's ritual preparatory stage included the crafting of his manifesto. What follows is an analysis of some of the more revelatory excerpts from his manifesto, beginning with this:

"You had a hundred billion chances and ways to have avoided today."

The word "chances" suggests that until the day of the shooting, Cho viewed himself as keeping a running tally of mistreatments and failed opportunities on the part of others to set things right. The strong element of externalization of blame is self-evident. The theme of externalization of blame and projection continues with the phrase:

"But you decided to spill my blood. You forced me into a corner and gave me only one option. The decision was yours. Now you have blood on your hands that will never wash off…"

Here, Cho assigns every bit of blame to others, seeing himself as blame free, and even giving innumerable "chances" to victims. His reference to "blood on your hands" suggests the fantasy that others will remain tormented by guilt that will "never" be alleviated. But for Cho, externalization of blame was not enough. His ego was so fragile it required that he be a "heroic" sacrifice to "save" the weak. Thus, he transforms himself in fantasy into not just all good, but God-like:

"Thanks to you, I die like Jesus Christ, to inspire generations of the weak and the defenseless people… If not for me, for my children and my brothers and sisters that you [expletive]. I did it for them."

In contrast to his fantasy of being an inspirational, "all good" hero, the "others" are portrayed as having committed acts of a most heinous and unforgivable nature

"You have vandalized my heart, raped my soul and torched my conscience. You thought it was one pathetic boy's life you were extinguishing."

The metaphors Cho uses here are extremely powerful, describing a sadistic persecutor who purposely selected him for torture followed by execution. His use of the term "pathetic boy" exposes his own threadbare self-esteem. He did not need to include this descriptor, and this is one of the only points in his manifesto in which he reveals his own fragility and fear about his own self-worth.[50] The following two excerpts represent strong evidence of Cho's paranoid-schizoid dynamics:

"You had everything you wanted. Your Mercedes wasn't enough, you brats. Your golden necklaces weren't enough, you snobs. Your trust fund wasn't enough. Your vodka and cognac wasn't enough. All your debaucheries weren't enough. Those weren't enough to fulfill your hedonistic needs. You had everything…"

In Cho's persecutory mindset, all of life's "goodness" and pleasure were in the possession of the others. He proclaims this with derision and disdain because they had access to an unlimited supply of pleasure (debaucheries, hedonistic fulfillments, and so forth), and yet it still was not "enough" for them. Here we see the extreme nature of Cho's splitting: the others had access to a paradise of enjoyment, whereas he was "raped" and "torched." This attempt to disparage the others' access to goodness must be contrasted with the following statement, which reveals his overwhelming feelings of envy:

"Oh the happiness I could have had mingling among you hedonists, being counted as one of you, if only you didn't [expletive] the living [expletive] out of me."

This rueful statement exposes Cho's true desire, to be accepted socially, which also had the meaning to him of gaining access to "hedonistic" levels of enjoyment from life. But the very group of "others" who seemed to him to possess such goodness were the very ones persecuting him to an extreme degree. Returning to Kleinian theory and paranoid-schizoid dynamics, the subject may take the view that if the wished for goodness is not forthcoming, it must necessarily be the case that it is being purposely withheld, resulting in sadistic, persecutory deprivation.

Case Example: Jiverly Wong

JiverlyAntares Wong was a 41-year-old Vietnamese immigrant living in Johnson City, New York, in early 2009. He had no recognized psychiatric history before April 3, 2009, when he burst into the Binghamton, New York, American Civic Association carrying two handguns and wearing body armor. Before entering the Civic Association, he used his father's car to block off the back door, which was the only other way out of the building. In the very place where he had been taking English classes, he proceeded to kill 13 people before shooting himself. He was equipped with large amounts of ammunition, and he had held permits since approximately 1996 for the two guns he used (J. Zikuski, Binghamton Police Chief, personal communication, 2009).[52] Media coverage of the mass tragedy gave rise to speculations about Wong's motives ranging from a "mystery," to there having been "hints" before the killings. However, local law enforcement investigation quickly uncovered that the mass murder was not at all surprising to those who were close to Wong.[51]

Wong immigrated to New York with his family in 1990. He was the second of four children, and was ethnically Chinese, but had lived with his family in Vietnam. His father reported that not long after they had moved, when Mr. Wong was approximately 22 years old, Mr. Wong "told his father someone was trying to kill him."[52] He had also complained of visual hallucinations of someone trying to harm him. He willingly went to a local hospital with his father, but was evaluated briefly and released without treatment or follow-up. Retrospectively, Mr. Wong's father wondered if his son's lack of treatment may have been partly because of a language barrier, because he and his son spoke little English. Wong became an American citizen in 1995, but left the country shortly thereafter. He returned in 1999 to California, where he was married and divorced. He kept in poor contact with his family during his 15 years in California and, notably, refused to share his mailing address with them.

After losing his job as a truck driver in California, Wong moved back to New York to live with his parents in 2007. By this time, he was approximately 39 years old. His parents noticed significant changes; he did not care to have friends, and barely spoke to anyone.[53] There were other, more peculiar changes. Despite the summer heat he never failed to wear long sleeve shirts and pants, and there were several uncharacteristic incidents of aggression directed toward his family. For example, in 2008, Wong slapped his younger sister across the face during an argument and raised his voice inappropriately to his father over a minor household issue, behaviors that were distinctly uncharacteristic for Wong.

Wong was laid off from his 3 PM to midnight job at a vacuum cleaner plant in November of 2008, the day before Thanksgiving. He began attending classes at the American Civic Association, the site of the mass shooting, to improve his English. His family described him as isolating himself from others in the year leading up to the tragedy. He was also noted to be a gun enthusiast who would spend weekends target shooting at a gun range.[54] A coworker at the vacuum cleaner plant reported that Wong sometimes "joked" about shooting politicians.[55] Retrospectively, people in his local community recalled that he was upset about not being able to obtain work. In the 2 weeks leading up to the tragedy, his father reported that he stopped eating dinner, stopped watching television, and became even more isolative.[53] This period was about the time he composed the letter that he sent to "News 10 Now" (Syracuse, NY, television station), as evidenced by his having dated the letter March 18, 2009.

According to survivors of the shooting, Wong did not speak before opening fire. Several days after the tragedy, his letter was received by the television station. The package he sent contained a two-page handwritten letter, photographs of himself holding handguns pointed upward while seated and smiling modestly, a gun permit, and his driver's license. Although the written letter was dated March 18, 2009, it was postmarked April 3, 2009, suggesting that he had been planning the shootings for a significant period of time.

The letter was written in all capital letters, and contained numerous errors in spelling and grammar. What follows is an analysis of selected excerpts.

"I am Jiverly Wong shooting the people."

This is the opening sentence of Wong's letter and its purpose is clear: to make sure that the news media give him credit. Throughout the letter, there are sentences that seem perplexing in that their tone and intent are incongruent with the overall theme and purpose of the letter. For example, Wong's letter is explaining why he will be killing people and how he believed he was severely persecuted, yet he makes such statements as:

"The first I want to say sorry I know a little English I hope you understand all of this."

"Please continue second page thank you."

"And you have a nice day."

These statements are strikingly courteous and incongruent with the emotional tone of the rest of the letter, and there are several possible explanations. The courteousness may represent a cultural phenomenon carried through his limited English writing skills. The incongruousness or inappropriateness may also suggest the inappropriate affect sometimes seen in major psychotic disorders. Finally, it may represent simple sarcasm and mockery, as when Atlanta day trader and mass murderer Mark Barton stated: "I hope this doesn't ruin your trading day." However, given Wong's cultural background and the sincere tone observed in the rest of his letter, this possibility seems less likely. Wong's note gets quickly to the point, contains no "last goodbyes," instructions, or apologies. It simply begins:

"Of course you need to know why I shooting? Because undercover cop gave me a lot of ass during eighteen years."

Wong bluntly answers the question he knew would be on everyone's mind: Why? His answer: he felt severely persecuted for almost two decades. Of special note is that he repeatedly refers to his persecutors as "undercover" cops. In real life, undercover police are difficult to identify, and pursue the suspect using subterfuge. In addition, note that the time period of 18 years places the beginning of Wong's perceived persecution at about the same time he first told his father he feared for his life and seemed to experience visual hallucinations. The early twenties are commonly observed to be the age at which major psychotic disorders begin to express themselves, and particularly the time associated with a "first break" in schizophrenia.[56] As the letter continues, it becomes more apparent that Wong was suffering from severe paranoia and persecutory delusions:

"Let talk about when I live in California…. Cop used 24 hours the technique of ultramodern and camera for burn the chemical in my house. For switch the channel Ti Vi. For adjust the fan. For made me unbreathable. For made me vomit. For connect the music into my ear."

Wong seems to describe classic persecutory delusions of technology. Such delusions of a technical content have been reported to occur with greater frequency in men compared with women.[57] One also wonders about olfactory hallucinations because his complaint of burning chemicals in his house. The possibility of auditory hallucinations is clearly raised by his complaint that his persecutor caused him to hear "music" in his "ear." Although such hallucinations are typically seen in such illnesses as schizophrenia, the phenomenon of olfactory hallucinations and auditory hallucinations of music may sometimes be seen in certain seizure disorders, such as temporal lobe epilepsy.[58,59]

It is difficult to say whether his perceptions of his fan and television being affected represented hallucinations, illusions, or paranoid delusions of reference. His statement about being "unbreathable" is curious and raises the question of anxiety and panic-like symptoms possibly resulting from his delusions of being poisoned by "burning chemicals." Regardless, Wong clearly felt he was under "24-hour" surveillance and was being persecuted. The same delusional theme (persecution by an "undercover cop") evinces itself after Wong left California to live in New York again:

> "[When I lived in Johnson City, NY]... it terrible...Cop wait until midnight when I off the light and went to the bed. Cop unlock my door and came in take a sit in my room <<cop did it thirteen time on the year 1994>> on the thirteen time had three time touch me when I sleeping."

It seems that Wong's persecutory delusions, on returning to New York, became more threatening and invasive. His persecutors are no longer harassing him from a distance, but have actually invaded his personal space. In psychodynamic terms, this may represent a more severe breakdown in Wong's ego functioning, allowing his persecutors to break through his remaining fragile defenses and enter his private space where he can no longer distinguish reality from delusional beliefs. Because of his limited English, it is difficult to tell whether Wong meant to say that the "cop" entered his room (invading his private space) and "sat" down, or whether he meant to say that the "cop" defecated ("take a sit") in his room. Of significant concern is that his persecutor advances to the level of actually touching him.

These more invasive and threatening delusions suggest a possible worsening of his illness that continues over time. For example, he writes: "One time [cop] stolen 20 dollar in my wallet. One time used electric gun shoot at the behind my neck." These sentences indicate that Wong's invasive persecutory delusions continued, and his delusions of a technical nature. It also seems as though Wong believed that there was some type of conspiracy between the "undercover cop" in California and the one in New York: "Many time from 1990 to 1997.... Spread a rumor nasty like the California Cop." Wong makes other statements suggesting that he believed such rumors caused him terrible hardship, such as losing his job and others treating him poorly. Feelings of cultural persecution also seem to have played a role. For example, Wong states, "...one time Cop leave a massage in my voice mail and said <<come back your country>>" This statement may be a combination of culturally tinged paranoia, in addition to auditory hallucination.

It becomes clear that Wong has descended into the obliterative state of mind, as evidenced by the last lines of his letter:

> "...I cannot accepted my poor life. Before I cut my poor life I must oneself get a judge job for make an impartial with undercover Cop by at least two people with me go to return to the dust of Earth. Already impartial now... Cop bring about this shooting. Cop must responsible."

Like Cho, Wong reveals briefly his own decimated self-esteem. However, unlike Cho, Wong does not portray his plans and actions as a "heroic" revenge fantasy. Rather, Wong simply puts forth his nihilistic state of mind and his inability to "accept" his circumstances. He has endured more persecution than his ego can tolerate and cannot envision his life ever being different. He believed his life was a "poor" one, suggesting aversive self-awareness, and the only escape from this situation he is able to formulate is suicide. But because he believes he has been relentlessly persecuted, he must have justice (revenge). Or in his words, his undercover persecutor "must" be held "respon-sible." For Wong, there is no heroic story line, nor are there any overt statements suggestive of envy as there are in Cho's communication. Wong simply leaves a forth-right message, albeit a product of his psychosis, which may be reformulated as: "I want others to hurt like I do – maybe then my persecutors will be held responsible."

There are two noteworthy questions in the case of Wong: why did he choose the American Civic Center for the shooting, and (2) why did he go on to kill 13 people when he gave the more modest number of "at least two" in his letter. His choice of the American Civic Center may be the missing expression of envy, one which he simply failed to allude to in his letter. The immigrants learning at the Civic Center may have represented to him future hope and opportunity in the United States. His envy of others achieving what he had wanted may have been a driving force in his choice to "destroy" others he saw as achieving this goal.

Finally, it may be that because of his language skills and cultural background, his letter may not have communicated the full extent of the rage and hostility he had been harboring. Although he writes about killing "at least two" people, according to police, he brought with him more than enough ammunition.[51] He went on to kill 13 people, yet shot himself on hearing the police sirens. It is also possible that from the time he authored his letter until he carried out the shooting 2 weeks later, his revenge fantasies and anger intensified during a period of isolative rumination. Thus, two began to grow in number, and the phrasing "at least" seems to foreshadow this outcome.

Discussion of Forensic Psycholinguistic Analysis

The two cases discussed seem, on the surface, very similar. Both offenders committed mass murder as defined by the present-day, accepted Bureau of Justice definition. Both followed the pattern of the pseudocommando in terms of being heavily armed, wearing "warrior" gear, committing the act during the day, planning for the act, and expecting to be killed. The final communications of both men also revealed that they harbored extremely strong emotions of anger, feelings of persecution, severely damaged self-esteem, and the desire for revenge. Both had reached the obliterative mindset in which nothing matters, and violent destruction is viewed as the only final outcome.

In contrast, the forensic psycholinguistic analysis of their communications reveals their motivations, psychopathology, and classification to be remarkably dissimilar. Wong's final letter provides clear evidence that he suffered from a major psychotic disorder. Although Wong was resentful about the status of his "poor life," he attributed all of his misfortunes to a bizarre persecution by "undercover cops." He suffered from a delusional belief that secret persecutors destroyed his chances of assimilating and working successfully in the country to which he and his family had immigrated. In reality, it is likely that his undetected, untreated severe mental illness prevented him from achieving his goals in his new country. In the case of Wong, much less overt envy is expressed in his final communication. Rather, his letter dwells mainly on his persecutory delusions, and his plan to commit H-S because of his aversive self-awareness and strong feelings of resentment.

Conversely, Cho's final communications more clearly portray the psychology of envy and social exclusion. He acknowledges his fantasy of being part of the "hedonistic" crowd, who he imagined had unlimited access to all of the pleasurable things in life. Cho's manifesto does not contain any overtly delusional material, although it could be argued that his feelings of persecution might have reached delusional or near delusional levels. However, with Cho there is no evidence of bizarre delusions as with Wong. Cho's communications provide evidence of heavy reliance on external-ization, splitting, and rage caused by feelings of social exclusion. Another significant difference is Cho's portrayal of his act as a heroic, grandiose sacrifice.

A final contrast between the two offenders is plainly seen in the photographs they sent to the media. Whereas the photographs sent by Wong consisted mainly of him sitting down holding a gun pointing upward, Cho's photos were more numerous and clearly posed for dramatic effect. For example, Cho aims his gun directly at the camera. In another, he holds two guns with his arms outspread reminiscent of an action movie star. In sum, Cho's photos suggest substantially more drama, grandiosity, and narcissism. These data, taken together with their writings, suggest that Wong primarily suffered from a major psychotic disorder, whereas Cho's primary psychopathology was likely characterologic. This is not meant to exclude the possibility that Cho had begun to suffer from a thought disorder; however, the evidence for this is far less striking than with Wong. Under the proposed classification system, Cho could be classified as a school-resentful type, whereas Wong could be classified as a school-psychotic type mass murderer.

PREVENTION OF MASS MURDER AND FUTURE DIRECTIONS

Mass murder is a multidetermined event with no simple preventive solution. The reality is that such events are exceptionally hard to anticipate and avert.[60] Thus, prevention must rely on various approaches acting together to provide a widely cast safety net. Such approaches might include enhanced social responsibility, psychiatric efforts, cultural considerations, and media responsibility.

Social Responsibility in Mass Murders

Social responsibility may take the form of greater public awareness, willingness to contact authorities when appropriate. and reconsidering societal gun control laws. Third parties often have preoffense knowledge, yet remain quiet for various reasons.[61] Nevertheless "prevention may only be possible when somebody warns that such behavior may occur.... Acquaintances often acknowledge concerns prior to the incident."[10] Preoffense messages may be communicated in various forms including verbally, or by Internet pages or YouTube. It may be the case that family members or social contacts are the only ones who could reasonably take steps to have the potential offender evaluated and treated.[62]

Efforts to educate the public about when to notify authorities of danger seem important. Yet, society must ultimately decide how and when to take responsibility in the face of concerning signs. When an individual gives a preoffense message of intent, or there is some type of "leakage" where threats are made known to third parties,[63] at what point does society's interest in averting a potential risk of public harm supersede the confidentiality and privacy rights of the individual? Society has currently addressed these concerns in the form of emergency psychiatric detentions and civil commitment statutes and it is likely the case that many mass murderers were in need of psychiatric treatment before their offense. However, in the case of an isolative potential mass murderer who has not clearly revealed overt signs of danger, the burden of reporting to law enforcement and mental health authorities may be noticeably greater. Regarding cases of school or workplace linked offenders, coworkers, teachers, or classmates may consider notifying authorities or human resource staff once they become reasonably concerned. Education in these venues is not difficult to achieve and can be folded into already existing outreach programs, such as antibullying and domestic violence awareness efforts.

Another subject that society has to consider is what it wishes to do about gun control. By the Brady Handgun Violence Prevention Act of 1993 (Brady Act),[51] the US Attorney General established the National Instant Criminal Background Check

System (NICS) for Federal Firearms Licensees to transmit information immediately as to whether the transfer of a firearm would violate Section 922 (g) or (n) of Title 18, United States Code, or state law. All states have the option to implement a state-based NICS program. However, the use of the NICS system remains controversial, particularly when it comes to individuals with mental illness who have a history of involuntary treatment. One of the problems with the NICS system is that it captures only individuals who attempt to purchase firearms legally. It does nothing to address the problem of those who purchase firearms either illegally or through the gun show loophole. Further, state-based NICS programs and their relevant statutes are not uniform.[53] In addition, prohibited persons in various states can range from those who received outpatient psychiatric treatment, to persons who have been civilly committed or found not guilty by reason of insanity.

Countries with less stringent gun control laws have been observed to have a higher risk of mass murder than countries with stricter laws.[55] Although it is clear that gun control in the United States remains a tenacious and controversial issue, other countries have had some success pursuing this area. For example, an Australian observational study compared mass murders before and after 1996, the year of a widely publicized mass murder in Tasmania.[64] Australia quickly enacted gun law reforms that included removing semiautomatic firearms, pump-action shotguns, and rifles from civilian possession. Results of the study revealed that in the 18 years before the gun laws, there were 13 mass shootings in Australia. In the 10.5 years after the gun law reforms, there were none. Although comparing firearm laws among countries may make drawing firm conclusions difficult, currently available data suggest that mass tragedies occur with less frequency in countries with stricter gun control laws.[65]

Psychiatric Efforts in Mass Murder Risk

Given the extremely low base rate of mass murder, psychiatric efforts are best spent in directions other than prediction.[66] Thus, the role of mental health professionals should be reframed as it pertains to mass murder. Rather than prediction, clinical risk assessment and management may be emphasized as a part of an overall competent and quality psychiatric patient care effort.[29,67–69] Although future research will undoubtedly enhance awareness of the presence of "identification warning behaviors,"[70] mental health clinicians will best serve patients at risk by crafting a risk-management plan at clinically relevant or critical times.

There has been very little psychiatric research into the problem of mass murder that would serve to better inform mental health professionals. In a clinical study of 144 threateners, eight were found to have threatened mass homicide.[71] All of these eight subjects said they intended to kill as many people as possible and all cases involved targeting a specific group the threatener had held a grievance against. Over the 12-month study period, none of the eight subjects enacted or attempted to enact their plans. However, two of the eight assaulted a person unrelated to the targeted group. Authors recommended a thorough assessment of such individuals, with particular attention to "availability of means, planning, preparation, and the acknowledged commitment to put the words into action irrespective of consequences." Finally, it was noted that such threateners are likely to have "complex mental health needs and equally complicated personal lives." Thus, in addition to treating the threatener's mental illness, psychotherapy interventions should target coping skills and effective, prosocial methods of managing anger.

To date, the actual communications of mass murderers have received little detailed analysis. The study of preoffense "leakage" (threats made to third parties) and after the fact communications may assist in gaining insight and informing preventive efforts.[9,71,72] Risk assessments of individuals with strong revenge fantasies have to consider the intensity and quality of the revenge fantasies, "vulnerability to ego threats,"[73] and the relevant biopsychosocial variables. Finally, support for nationwide research efforts improving the ability to prevent such tragedies is essential.

Cultural Considerations in Mass Murder

Cultural concerns must be taken into consideration, especially when there is the potential for an immigrant to develop strong feelings of social exclusion. In vulnerable individuals, intense "acculturative stress" may result in strong feelings of "marginaliza-tion."[74] In transcultural psychiatry, the concept of marginalization is not dissimilar from the psychological construct of social exclusion. There is the potential for the margin-alized individual to develop feelings of rejection and alienation, and in some instances, to form a hostile, negative identity. Improving mental health access in immigrant communities to clinicians with competence in transcultural psychiatry may serve a preventive role in select cases. Other steps may involve identifying communities with poor access to or inadequate mental health services so that this part of the safety net remains intact. Communities with significant immigrant populations would be well served to employ culturally competent mental health professionals.

Media Responsibility in Reporting Mass Murder

News media and journalists may be disinclined to admit that they are often in the busi-ness of searching for "the right sort of madness" to capture the public's imagination.[75] This commonly involves exploiting violent and tragic acts carried out by mentally or emotionally disturbed individuals. However, the reality is that it is a difficult task to report the occurrence of a mass murder in such a way that the public is adequately informed, yet certain details (eg, numbers of victims, whether the offender was killed, and so forth) are not reported. Efforts to develop a universal reporting code have been recommended that would appropriately cover the tragedy and reduce the impact of the copycat effect.[3,76] Most recommendations involve ensuring that the perpetrator is neither glorified nor demonized. For example, it has been suggested that news media should avoid too much emphasis on the perpetrator.[3] Instead, media should emphasize victim and community recovery efforts, and deflect attention away from the perpetrator.

SUMMARY

Mass murder is not a recent phenomenon, having occurred since well before the Charles Whitman shooting in 1966. Access to powerful, automatic firearms, media attention, and a possible glorification of the phenomenon among certain vulnerable, disaffected individuals are factors making present-day mass murders unique.[2] The existing research base suggests that factors common to mass murder include extreme feelings of anger and revenge, social alienation, rumination on violent revenge fantasies, variable psychiatric illness, precipitating social stressors, and significant planning before the offense. This article has outlined a proposed classification system for mass murder, to coordinate future research efforts, based on the system used in classifying H-S. The system uses the relationship/linkage–motive descriptors to assist in classification efforts.

Understanding the motives and psychopathology of the mass murder requires an in-depth understanding of the psychology of revenge, and how these individuals nurture feelings of persecution, resentment, and destructive envy. Before carrying out their offenses, mass murderers often communicate some final message or "manifesto" to the public or news media. Such communications are rich sources of data that may assist in understanding the motives, psychopathology, and classification of mass murderers, whose offenses can seem similar from a purely behavioral perspective. Mass murder is a complex and multidetermined event and there are no current evidence-based methods of reliable prediction. Prevention must rely on various methods, including enhanced social responsibility, psychiatric efforts, cultural considerations, and media responsibility.

ACKNOWLEDGMENTS

The author acknowledges the assistance and compassion of Joseph Zikuski (Binghamton, NY, Chief of Police), and Gerald Mollen (Binghamton, NY, District Attorney) for their insights into the Binghamton, New York, American Civic Association tragedy.

REFERENCES

1. Burgess AW. Mass, spree and serial homicide. In: Douglas J, Burgess AW, Burgess AG, et al, editors. Crime classification manual. 2nd edition. San Francisco (CA): Jossey-Bass; 2006. p. 438–71.
2. Mullen P. The autogenic (self-generated) massacre. Behav Sci Law 2004;22: 311–23.
3. Preti A. School shooting as a culturally enforced way of expressing suicidal hostile intentions. J Am Acad Psychiatry Law 2008;36:544–50.
4. Why are mass shootings on the rise? While some see connection to guns, others blame erosion of community. The Associated Press; 2007. Available at: http://www.msnbc.msn.com/id/18249724/. Accessed May 25, 2009.
5. Duwe G. A circle of distortion: the social construction of mass murder in the United States. West Criminol Rev 2005;6:59–78.
6. Bernstein A. Bath massacre: America's first school bombing. Ann Arbor (MI): The University of Michigan Press; 2009.
7. Declercq F, Audenaert K. Predatory violence aiming at relief in a case of mass murder: Meloy's criteria for applied forensic practice. Behav Sci Law 2011;29: 578–91.
8. Hempel A, Meloy J, Richards T. Offender and offense characteristics of a non-random sample of mass murderers. J Am Acad Psychiatry Law 1999;27(2):13–225.
9. Knoll J. The pseudocommando mass murder: part II, the language of revenge. J Am Acad Psychiatry Law 2010;38:263–72.
10. Aitken L, Oosthuizen P, Emsley R, et al. Mass murders: implications for mental health professionals. Int J Psychiatry Med 2008;38(3):261–9.
11. Felthous A, Hempel A. Combined homicide-suicides: a review. J Forensic Sci 1995;40:846–57.
12. Bossarte R, Simon T, Barker L. Characteristics of homicide followed by suicide incidents in multiple states, 2003-04. Inj Prev 2006;12:ii33–8.
13. Coid J. The epidemiology of abnormal homicide and murder followed by suicide. Psychol Med 1983;13:855–60.
14. Marzuk P, Tardiff K, Hirsch C. The epidemiology of murder-suicide. JAMA 1992; 267:3179–83.
15. Dietz P. Mass, serial and sensational homicides. Bull N Y Acad Med 1986;62: 477–91.
16. Mohandie K, Meloy J. Clinical and forensic indicators of "suicide by cop". J Forensic Sci 2000;45:384–9.

17. Cullen D. Columbine. Twelve. New York (NY): Hachette Book Group; 2009.
18. Cohen A. A portrait of the killer. Time, 1999. Available at: http://www.time.com/time/magazine/article/0,00.html?promoid=googlep,9171,991676. Accessed May 25, 2009.
19. otes. The New York Times; 1999. Available at: http://www.nytimes.com/1999/07/31/us/shootings-in-atlanta-the-notes-there-is-no-reason-for-me-to-lie-now.html. Accessed May 25, 2009.
20. Mitchell R. Dancing at Armageddon: survivalism and chaos in modern times. Chicago: University of Chicago Press; 2002.
21. Menninger W. Uncontained rage: a psychoanalytic perspective on violence. Bulletin of the Menninger Clinic 2007;71:115–31.
22. Neuman Y. On revenge. J Psychoanal Cult Soc 2012;17:1–15.
23. Klein M. Envy and gratitude, and other works, 1946-1963. New York: The Free Press; 1975.
24. Kaylor L. Antisocial personality disorder: diagnostic, ethical and treatment issues. Issues Ment Health Nurs 1999;20:247–58.
25. Hyatt-Williams A. Cruelty, violence and murder: understanding the criminal mind. Northvale (NJ): Jason Aronson; 1998.
26. Alfano S. Gunman: Now you have blood on your hands. April 18, 2007. Available at: CBS News.com, http://www.cbsnews.com/stories/2007/04/18/virginiatechshooting/main2697827.shtml. Accessed December 12, 2009.
27. Knoll J. Treating the morally objectionable. In: Andrade J, editor. Handbook of violence risk assessment and treatment: new approaches for mental health professionals. New York: Springer Publishing Company; 2009. p. 311–45.
28. Edwards M, Holden R. Coping, meaning in life, and suicidal manifestations: examining gender differences. J Clin Psychol 2001;57:1517–34.
29. Baumeister R, DeWall CN, Ciarocco NJ, et al. Social exclusion impairs self-regulation. J Pers Soc Psychol 2005;88:589–604.
30. Twenge J, Catanese K, Baumeister R. Social exclusion and the deconstructed state: time perception, meaninglessness, lethargy, lack of emotion, and self-awareness. J Pers Soc Psychol 2005;85:409–23.
31. Baumeister R. Suicide as escape from self. Psychol Rev 1990;97:90–113.
32. Anderson M. The death of a mind: a study of Shakespeare's Richard III. J Anal Psychol 2006;51:701–16.
33. Eynon T. Cognitive linguistics. Adv Psychiatr Treat 2002;8:399–407.
34. Freud S. The standard edition of the complete psychological works of Sigmund Freud, vol. 14. Toronto: The Hogarth Press; 1981. p. 314–5.
35. Gilligan J. Preventing violence. New York: Thames & Hudson; 2001.
36. Available at: http://www.minnpost.com/worldcsm/2011/08/03/30524norway_attacks_what_happens_if_breivik_is_deemed_insane. Accessed May 31, 2012.
37. 2083: A European Declaration of Independence. Available at: https://docs.google.com/viewer?a=v&pid=explorer&chrome=true&srcid=0BwZX2bK7Uc5dY2ExYzc4YjctMDJIZC00M2QzLTk5NDUtNDhiMDhmMzhkZWQ4&hl=en_US. Accessed May 31, 2012.
38. Pennebaker J, Mehl M, Niederhoffer K. Psychological aspects of natural language use: our words, our selves. Annu Rev Psychol 2003;54:547–77.
39. Cho S. Richard McBeef. Available at: http://www.thesmokinggun.com/archive/years/2007/0417071vtech1.html. Accessed September 14, 2012.
40. Smith S, Shuy R. Forensic psycholinguistics: using language analysis for identifying and assessing offenders. FBI Law Enforcement Bulletin 2002;16–21.

41. Morris R. Forensic handwriting identification: fundamental concepts and principles. San Diego (CA): Academic Press; 2000.
42. Available at: http://web.archive.org/web/20080113013401/http://www.msnbc.msn.com/id/18185859/. Accessed July 23, 2009.
43. Stephane M, Pellizzer G, Fletcher CR, et al. Empirical evaluation of language disorder in schizophrenia. J Psychiatry Neurosci 2007;32:250–8.
44. Pennebaker J, Stone L. Katie's diary: unlocking the mystery of a suicide. New York (NY): Brunner-Routledge; 2004.
45. Henken V. Banality reinvestigated: a computer-based content analysis of suicidal and forced death documents. Suicide 1976,6:36–43.
46. Back M, Schmukle S, Egloff B. How extraverted is honey.bunny77@hotmail.de?: inferring personality from e-mail addresses. Not Found In Database 2008;42: 1116–22.
47. Smith S. From violent words to violent deeds: assessing risk from FBI threatening communication cases. In: Meloy J, Sheridan L, Hoffman J, editors. Stalking, threatening, and attacking public figures: a psychological and behavioral analysis. New York: Oxford Press; 2008. p. 435–55.
48. Summary of Key Findings. In: Mass shooting at Virginia Tech: Report of the review panel. 2007. Available at: http://www.governor.virginia.gov/TempContent/techPanelReport-docs/4%20SUMMARY%20OF%20KEY%20FINDINGS.pdf. Accessed June 2, 2009.
49. Stewart J. Investigation of April 17, 2007 critical incident at Virginia Tech. Office of the Inspector General For Mental Health, Mental Retardation & Substance Abuse Services, Report No. 140–07. Available at: http://www.oig.virginia.gov/documents/VATechRpt140-07.pdf. Accessed July 23, 2009.
50. DePue R. A theoretical profile of Seung Hui Cho: from the perspective of a forensic behavioral scientist, Appendix N. In: Mass shooting at Virginia Tech: report of the Review Panel. August, 2007. Available at: http://www.governor.virginia.gov/TempContent/techPanelReport.cfm. Accessed June 2, 2009.
51. Brady Act 18 USC § 922 (s1–s6). See: http://www.law.cornell.edu/uscode/text/18/922 [Federal Statute].
52. Chen P. Jiverly Wong's father: what prompted mass killing in Binghamton remains a mystery. The Post Standard; 2009. Available at: http://www.syracuse.com/news/index.ssf/2009/04/jiverly_wongs_father_our_son_w.html. Accessed April 5, 2010.
53. Norris D, Price M, Gutheil T, et al. Firearm laws, patients, and the roles of psychiatrists. Am J Psychiatry 2006;163:1392–6.
54. Rivera R. Before killings, hints of plans and grievance. The New York Times; 2009. Available at: http://www.nytimes.com/2009/04/05/nyregion/05suspect.html?ref=jiverlywong. Accessed September 14, 2012.
55. Lee J, Lee T, Ng B. Reflections on a mass homicide. Ann Acad Med Singapore 2007;36:444–7.
56. Minzenberg M, Yoon J, Carter C. Schizophrenia. In: Hales R, Yudofsky S, Gabbard G, editors. The American Psychiatric Publishing textbook of psychiatry. 5th edition. Arlington (VA): American Psychiatric Publishing; 2008. p. 407–56.
57. Kraus A. Phenomenology of the technical delusion in schizophrenia. Not Found In Database 1994;25:51–69.
58. Taber K, Hurley R. Neuroanatomy for the psychiatrist. In: Hales R, Yudofsky S, Gabbard G, editors. The American Psychiatric Publishing textbook of psychiatry. 5th edition. Arlington (VA): American Psychiatric Publishing; 2008. p. 157–90.

59. Adams R, Victor M. Neurologic disorders caused by lesions in particular parts of the cerebrum. In: Principles of Neurology. 5th edition. New York: McGraw-Hill; 1993. p. 378–410.

60. Saleva O, Putkonen H, Kiviruusu O, et al. Homicide-suicide: an event hard to prevent and separate from homicide or suicide. Forensic Sci Int 2007;166:204–8.

61. Kluger J. Inside a mass murderer's mind. Time, 2007. Available at: http://www.time.com/time/magazine/article/0,9171,1612694,00.html. Accessed on March 19, 2012.

62. Anders Behring Breivik's sister warned mother about his behaviour two years ago. Available at: http://www.telegraph.co.uk/news/worldnews/europe/norway/8934136/Anders-Behring-Breiviks-sister-warned-mother-about-his-behaviour-two-years-ago.html. Accessed March 19, 2012.

63. O'Toole M. The school shooter: a threat assessment perspective. Quantico (VA): Critical Incident Response Group, National Center for the Analysis of Violent Crime; 2000.

64. Chapman S, Alpers P, Agho K, et al. Australia's 1996 gun law reforms: faster falls in firearm deaths, firearm suicides, and a decade without mass shootings. Inj Prev 2006;12:365–72.

65. Rosenbaum J. Gun utopias? Firearm access and ownership in Israel and Switzerland. J Public Health Policy 2012;33:46–58.

66. Dressing H, Meyer-Lindenberg A. Risk assessment of threatened amok: new responsibilities for psychiatry? Nervenarzt 2010;81:594–601.

67. Swanson J. Preventing the unpredicted: managing violence risk in mental health care. Psychiatr Serv 2008;59:191–3.

68. Swanson J. Explaining rare acts of violence: the limits of evidence from population research. Psychiatr Serv 2011;62:1369–71.

69. Knoll J. Violence risk assessment for mental health professionals. In: Jamieson A, Moenssens A, editors. Wiley encyclopedia of forensic science. Chichester (United Kingdom): John Wiley & Sons; 2009. p. 2597–602.

70. Meloy R, Hoffman J, Guldimann A, et al. The role of warning behaviors in threat assessment: an exploration and suggested typology. Behav Sci Law 2011;30:256–79.

71. Warren LJ, Mullen PE, Ogloff JR. A clinical study of those who utter threats to kill. Behav Sci Law 2011;29:141–54.

72. Knoll J. The pseudocommando mass murder: part I, the psychology of revenge & obliteration. J Am Acad Psychiatry Law 2010;38:87–94.

73. Baumeister R, Smart L, Boden J. Relation of threatened egotism to violence and aggression: the dark side of high self-esteem. Psychol Rev 1996;103:5–33.

74. Kohn R, Wintrob R, Alarcon R. Transcultural psychiatry. In: Sadock B, Sadock V, Ruiz P, editors. Kaplan and Sadock's comprehensive textbook of psychiatry. 9th edition. Philadelphia: Lippincott Williams & Wilkins; 2009. p. 734–53.

75. Ronson J. The psychopath test: a journey through the madness industry. New York: Riverhead Books; 2011.

76. Etzerdorfer E, Sonneck G. Preventing suicide by influencing the mass media reporting: the Viennese experience, 1980-1996. Arch Suicide Res 1998;4:67–74.

Child Murder by Parents and Evolutionary Psychology

Susan Hatters Friedman, MD[a],*, James Cavney, MBChB[b],
Phillip J. Resnick, MD[c]

KEYWORDS

- Child homicide • Infanticide • Filicide • Neonaticide • Parenting • Evolution

KEY POINTS

- Most child homicides are perpetrated by their parents. Mothers and fathers are responsible for similar numbers of deaths.
- The highest risk of child homicide victimization is on the first day of life, known as "neonaticide"; these perpetrators are most often mothers.
- Stepparents kill at much higher rates than genetic parents.
- Evolutionary psychology helps explain some filicides as rational acts.
- The most common motive for child murder by parents is fatal child maltreatment related to chronic abuse or neglect. Other motives include altruistic, acutely psychotic, unwanted child, and partner revenge.
- Mothers found insane for killing their children often have altruistic or acutely psychotic motivations.
- Two dozen nations outside the United States, including the United Kingdom and Australia, have infanticide statutes that provide decreased penalties for mothers who kill their child within the first year of life.

INTRODUCTION

The act of filicide, a parent killing their child, is perhaps one of the most emotive and tragic acts in the human behavioral repertoire. It is also one of the oldest human

Disclosures: None.
Portions of this paper were presented at the Royal Australia New Zealand College of Psychiatry (Forensic Section)/Australia New Zealand Academy of Psychiatry, Psychology and the Law meeting, Wellington, New Zealand, November 2011.
[a] Departments of Psychiatry and Pediatrics, Case Western Reserve University School of Medicine, Connections Mental Health Center, 24200 Chagrin Boulevard, Beachwood, OH 44122, USA; [b] Department of Psychiatry, Mason Clinic Regional Forensic Psychiatry Services, University of Auckland, Private Bag 19986 Avondale, Auckland 1746, New Zealand; [c] Division of Forensic Psychiatry, Department of Psychiatry, Case Western Reserve University School of Medicine, W.O. Walker Center, 10524 Euclid Avenue, Cleveland, OH 44106, USA
* Corresponding author.
E-mail address: susanhfmd@hotmail.com

behaviors; early oral and written records from many cultures and civilizations include archetypal stories about filicide in religion and mythology. Examples include Abraham and Medea.

Modern anthropologic studies have reported evidence of filicides in "primitive" contemporary societies, which has been interpreted to represent enduring human behavior patterns extending back into human prehistory.[1] In modern society, filicide cases often have a high public profile and media attention. The forensic clinician is tasked with the assessment of parents alleged to have committed filicide for issues of legal culpability and mitigation of sentence.

The question of whether mental impairment is a mitigating factor is often the key question for assessment. It is therefore imperative that forensic clinicians are well informed about the subtleties of causation and the heterogeneity of filicide events. To develop a conceptual understanding of what are abnormal parental motivations for filicide, one must consider the uncomfortable corollary: that there are normal parental motivations for filicide.

Relatively small but in-depth psychological analyses of psychiatric samples of filicide offenders assist the understanding of abnormal parental motives resulting from psychopathology.[2] However, low prevalence rates have made research and the scientific analysis of filicide difficult. There has been a gradual development of larger longitudinal national and cross-cultural data sets that have enhanced analyses of causes for filicide.

Multiple classification systems of filicidal motives have emerged that allow comparison of different types of filicide. Yet, the scientific analysis of filicide has continued to be largely descriptive without a unifying theory. Theoretical contributions to the understanding have nevertheless arisen from multiple academic disciplines including criminology, law, sociology, anthropology, psychology, and psychiatry. Each has offered a useful but only partial contribution to understanding the complex process that leads to a parent killing their own child. Without a unifying theoretical approach to the topic of filicide, contributions from one field have often had little direct influence on another. As a result, the literature has arguably been of limited assistance for clinicians in the assessment of parental culpability.

The social science literature has seen the increasing influence of evolutionary theory in the analysis of filicide.[1] Hrdy[3] suggested that infanticide was a primate reproductive strategy, and observed that if a victim was defective or born at a bad time, they would require extra cost and effort in child-rearing.[4] The mismatch paradigm (also referred to as dancing with ghosts[5]) helps to explain how human behavior evolved over the course of 10,000 years, since humans lived in bands of hunter-gatherers. Thus, some traits that were adaptive then, would no longer be adaptive. For example, the taste for alcohol was previously adaptive, because there were nutritional rewards. Similarly, the taste for food developed in a climate of scarce resources, but obesity is no longer adaptive.

The contemporary discipline of evolutionary psychology has advanced some theoretically grounded explanations for filicide. Evolutionary psychology has enabled the generation of several testable hypotheses in relation to filicide. However, evolutionary psychology is less well described in the clinical literature and has not yet been conveyed in a useful manner to assist forensic clinicians in the assessment of parental culpability for filicide.

This article proposes evolutionary theory as a framework theory[6] to meaningfully understand research about filicide. Using evolutionary psychology as a theoretical lens, this article reviews the research on filicide over the past 40 years, and describes epidemiologic and typologic studies of filicide and theoretical analyses from a range of disciplines. Forensic clinicians may find evolutionary psychology to be a useful heuristic to approach the assessment of filicide offenders.

EVOLUTIONARY PSYCHOLOGY AND FILICIDE

In *The Origin of Species*, Darwin[7] outlined a theory of evolution by "natural selection." Natural selection acts to preserve and accumulate minor advantageous trait mutations within a given species, thus enabling that species to compete better in its ecologic habitat. Spencer[8] later coined the term "survival of the fittest" to describe this process. Evolutionary theory has five underlying principles (**Table 1**): (1) variation, (2) competition, (3) offspring, (4) genetics, and (5) natural selection.

In applying evolutionary theory to the study of filicide, we explore the hypothesis that killing one's own children has somehow served as an adaptive reproductive strategy for human beings, that has survived as part of the human behavioral repertoire.[9] At first this may seem counterintuitive. However, it is well known that many species kill their offspring and some even eat them.[10] The development of evolutionary theory over the twentieth century has led to several hypotheses of particular relevance to whether filicides may have conveyed some adaptive advantage for parental perpetrators in our evolutionary past.

Parental Investment Theory and Parent Offspring Conflict

Fisher[11] introduced parental investment theory. He observed that the human sex ratio in offspring is close to 1:1, and predicted that parental expenditure of effort on both sexes should be equal. The preservation of this ratio in the human species has thus become an evolutionarily stable strategy.[12] Parental investment theory was further developed by Trivers[9] as an evolutionary-based theory of parent offspring conflict whereby the currency of cost and benefit was considered regarding passing on one's genes to one's offspring. Parental investment theory explains that individuals invest in their kin because of their shared genes. Women have about 400 ova during their lifetime, whereas men may have 250 million sperm with each ejaculation. As such, women may be more invested in their individual offspring than men. Physiologically, one must consider the costs of gestation, lactation, and previously high maternal mortality rates.

Kin Selection Theory

Hamilton[13,14] introduced kin selection theory to explain the evolution of altruistic behavior. Using the formula $rB>C$, Hamilton's rule proposed that altruistic behavior would be selected when the evolutionary benefit of altruistic behavior to the recipient (B) multiplied by the genetic relatedness of the recipient to the performer (r) is greater than the evolutionary cost to the performer of the altruistic act (C). Nonaltruistic (selfish) behavior would only evolve when Hamilton's inequality was not satisfied.

Table 1	
Principles of evolutionary theory	
Variation	There is variation in every population
Competition	Organisms compete for limited resources
Offspring	Organisms produce more offspring than can survive
Genetics	Organisms pass genetic traits on to their offspring
Natural selection	Those organisms with the most beneficial traits are more likely to survive and reproduce

Filicide Hypotheses

In relation to filicide, these observations lead to preliminary hypotheses that parents would be less likely to kill their own children compared with stepchildren. Furthermore, there should not be any inherent bias in killing children of one gender. However, one could also expect filicide to be more prevalent toward children who represent a potential reproductive disadvantage to the parent (eg, children who prevent the raising of other children, and factors suggesting the child would not reach reproductive maturity). Implicit is an assumption that parents must somehow evaluate various environmental stimuli in relation to their own reproductive fitness to manifest the appropriate functional responses, potentially including filicide.

Evolutionary psychology argues that cognitive mechanisms have evolved to enable the processing of environmental stimuli to adaptive advantage that results in predictable expressions of behavior.[15] Importantly, however, these cognitive programs are hypothesized to have been selected to enhance fitness by solving adaptive problems in our phylogenetic past. Yet, cognitive programs that were adaptively selected for, in response to distal selection pressures, may not remain adaptive in a modern environment. Behaviors that exist across different cultures, times, and places are likely to represent cognitive programs that were adaptive in our evolutionary past. Current-day proximal selection pressures are considered less important influences in the expression of the associated behaviors.

From an evolutionary psychology perspective, culture becomes critically important in understanding the contemporary circumstances that elicit biologic propensities.[16] Moreover, other sociologic, biologic, and psychological theories of human behavior can be articulated with reference to the different parameters that might feed into these cognitive programs, present to some extent in all humans as the result of a common evolutionary heritage. Daly and Wilson[1] provided the earliest analysis of filicide within an evolutionary psychology framework. They reviewed an extensive anthropologic database and identified reports of filicide in most cultures. They divided these into four broad categories of motive: (1) scarce resources, (2) poor quality child, (3) paternal uncertainty, and (4) coercion by others.

To conceptualize filicidal motive as an evolved adaptive human behavior offers a starting point for a forensic clinician to consider issues of culpability, mental impairment, and disposition. Filicide is a cross-cultural phenomenon that has been an adaptive reproductive strategy in the evolutionary past for optimizing parental genetic investment. One might expect a convergence of modern parental filicidal motive with stressors comparable with past adaptive pressures. The greater the divergence away from such adaptive motivations for filicide, the more probable it is that mental illness is involved.

Evolutionary theory thus offers clinicians a variety of hypotheses: (1) stepparents would be more likely to kill children than biologic parents; (2) younger children would be more at risk; (3) younger mothers' motives are more likely to reflect past adaptive reproductive pressures; (4) older mothers' motives are more likely to be maladaptive and suggestive of mental impairment. Furthermore, parents would be more likely to kill offspring when there are scarce resources to raise the child; (1) when the quality of the child is poor; (2) when there is parental uncertainty; or (3) when there is external coercion.

NATURE OF THE PROBLEM: EPIDEMIOLOGY

The United States has the highest rate of child murder among developed nations. It is the fourth leading cause of death from ages 1 to 11 in the United States. The most common perpetrator of child homicide is a parent. The highest risk to the child is on the first day of life.[17,18] In a North Carolina study, 2.1 per 100,000 infants were killed on the first day of life.[19] In infancy, the US rate of homicide is 8 per 100,000, several times higher than Canada at 2.9 per 100,000.[20] The rates of child homicide decrease with the child's age, consistent with evolutionary explanations of the amount of required parental investment by the child's age. Specifically, the younger is the child, the more resources that are required for the child to reach reproductive maturity. During the preschool years, rates are 2.5 per 100,000; in the school years, they decrease to 1.5 per 100,000.[20]

TYPES OF CHILD MURDER BY PARENTS
Neonaticide

Neonaticide is the murder of an infant in the first day of its life. Neonaticide has consistently been described as being different than other filicides in motive and characteristics of the perpetrator.[21,22] In developing nations, there has been differential killing of female newborns for economic reasons.[23,24] Although this does not obviously match predictions according to Fisher's concept of maintaining a 1:1 sex ratio, it does reflect a type of coercion strategy as discussed by Daly and Wilson.

Neonaticide is almost always committed by the mother acting alone. The biologic father is frequently no longer a part of the mother's life. Neonaticidal mothers are often in their teens or 20s; unmarried; and of lower socioeconomic status (with limited resources).[21,22] The pregnancy is unwanted. These mothers rarely experience a mental illness before the homicide. Neonaticide is not associated with maternal suicide. The perpetrator often experiences denial or concealment of pregnancy.[22] Denial of pregnancy is defined as a woman's lack of awareness of her pregnancy, whereas concealment of pregnancy involves a woman who has knowledge that she is pregnant, but chooses to hide it from others.[25] The most common motive for neonaticide is simply that the infant is unwanted.[21,22]

It is very rare for fathers or couples to commit neonaticide. This may be because of the frequent concealment or denial of the pregnancy, coupled with the lack opportunity by the father of the baby. The unwanted birth creates a much more immediate crisis for the mother than the father. Just as the pregnancy had been hidden, infant bodies may be hidden. This may lead to underestimation of the frequency of neonaticide.

A Finnish study[26] involved forensic psychiatric interviews with women who had committed neonaticide. Just over a tenth (4 of 32) of the Finnish perpetrators was diagnosed with psychosis. These four women were older, married, with other children, and pursued prenatal care. These women likely killed for a different motive than the others. A larger percentage (10 of 32) was diagnosed with personality disorders. Similarly, a recent Federal Bureau of Investigation study[27] found that although most neonaticide offenders were single young women without criminal or psychiatric histories, about a quarter of the sample did not have these characteristics. Despite the frequent denial of pregnancy and concealment of pregnancy, the murdered infant is not always the first child of the mother. In the Finnish study, two-thirds of the time the index child was not the mother's first pregnancy,[26] and in an American study, 35% of the neonaticidal mothers had other children.[19]

In Japan[28] two types of neonaticide have been described, *mabiki* and *anomie*. *Anomie* has similar characteristics to other maternal neonaticides described in the current literature. However, *mabiki* translates to "thinning out" and usually involves married couples who are impoverished. They kill their neonate together because of their financial inability to care for the infant. This is consistent with Daly and Wilson's discussion of the adaptive evolutionary rationale of killing when there are scarce resources.

Overall, women who commit neonaticide are often younger and lack family support. Neonaticidal women usually do not have psychiatric disorders and are not suicidal. Rather, from an evolutionary perspective, young mothers with scarce resources are ridding themselves of an unwanted infant who may decrease their own reproductive capacity. The smaller group of older mothers was psychotic: they would be considered mentally abnormal killings. They were older and had relatively less opportunity for future reproductive capacity.

Infanticide

Infanticide is a generic term for child homicide by parents, but often refers to child homicide in the first year of life. It has even included murder sanctioned by the state in Biblical times. Currently, two dozen nations have laws defining infanticide as child homicide by the mother, usually within the first year of life.[29] Conviction of infanticide decreases the punishment for mothers but not fathers. This is because of notions from the early 1900s about "lactational insanity" and hormonal aspects of childbirth. Although the United States does not have an infanticide statute, Canada, the United Kingdom, and Australia do have such a statute.

In the United States, in the first week of life, the most likely perpetrator of child homicide is the mother.[30] Epidemiologic risk factors included a lack of prenatal care, lack of completion of formal high school education, and the victim was not the only child of a mother under 19 years old. These risk factors are unrelated to mental illness and are expected by evolutionary theory. They reflect reproductive pressures and include variables suggesting scarce resources available to raise the child.

Factors in the infant that may elevate the risk of being abused or killed include colic, developmental disability, and autism.[31] Infant behavior, such as persistent crying, was reported, as has been the belief that the child was "abnormal."[32] In a sample of mothers with colicky infants, 70% reported "explicit aggressive thoughts and fantasies" and 26% had infanticidal thoughts during colic episodes.[33] These factors, too, are consistent with evolutionary theory. The child is likely to require more parental investment, with perhaps less future potential for reproduction in those with developmental disability or autism.

Infanticide is, however, related to mental illness in a substantial number of cases. A study of infant homicide in England and Wales[34] found one-quarter of the maternal and paternal offenders were mentally ill at the time of the filicide. Mood disorders and substance use disorders were common. The time of a woman's life when she is at highest risk for mental illness is the postpartum. Untreated postpartum psychosis carries a 4% risk of infanticide and a 5% risk of suicide.[35] Jennings and colleagues[36] reported that 41% of depressed mothers of infants and toddlers had thoughts of harming their child. Among mothers in India hospitalized for postpartum mental illness, 43% had infanticidal ideas, 36% had infanticidal behavior, and 34% had both.[37] Fathers sometimes kill during postpartum exacerbations of mental illness.[38]

Filicide

A pattern of powerlessness, poverty, and emotional isolation is common among mothers who kill their children.[32] Other factors noted among mothers who kill vary with the type of population studied.[32] In general population studies, mothers who commit filicide are often poor, relatively isolated, and were victims of abuse themselves. They experience stressors, such as failed relationships, financial strain, or abuse. They sometimes experience substance abuse, depression, or psychosis. Mothers in correctional studies were often abuse victims themselves, had poor social support, were under educated, and had substance abuse.[32] In contrast, mothers in psychiatric studies often evidenced psychosis, with delusions about the child, depression, suicidality, and some had intellectual limitations. They often were "motherless mothers" (who had lost their own mothers because of death or desertion, or who had been abused at their mothers' hands themselves, and did not develop a concept of mothering).

A Denmark study found that the absolute risk of child homicide victimization was 0.009%; this was elevated to 0.051% if the parent had previously been admitted to a psychiatric hospital. At highest risk were children younger than 5, whose mothers were diagnosed with psychotic or mood disorders.[39] A quarter century of records from Statistics Finland[40] found that mothers killed younger children. Fathers were more likely to commit suicide at the time of their filicide than mothers. Parents often were under a great deal of stress and had little support.

Fathers who kill their children share much in common with filicidal mothers. A recent review of the literature by our group[38] revealed a mean age of fathers in their mid-30s and the mean age of the child victims was 5. Fathers often killed multiple children and their partner. Common themes included physical abuse, mental illness, and revenge. Fathers were often suffering financial stressors and frequently also committed suicide.

Stone and colleagues[41] hypothesized that mentally ill mothers would behave in a way that differed significantly from evolutionary expectations. Comparing a New York forensic psychiatric sample with a Canadian general population sample, they found that mentally ill mothers were generally older when they killed their children and naturally the child victims were older. Poverty, low education level (or low intellectual capacity), and lack of a partner were common in both samples.

Severely mentally ill women who were found not guilty by reason of insanity (NGRI) for filicide in Ohio and Michigan[42] were studied. These mothers were frequently in their late 20s, unmarried, unemployed, and had a high school education. Most had planned a filicide-suicide but had been unsuccessful in killing themselves after killing their child (56%). Most (69%) had auditory hallucinations and 74% were delusional. The mean age of child victims who were attacked was 4 years old; most (56%) attempted to kill all their children.

Stepparent Filicide

Daly and Wilson[1,43] noted that having a stepfather in the home increased the risk of child homicide many times over. In the United States, the rates of stepfather fatal child abuse were 100-fold higher. A Canadian child abuse registry found rates of stepparents 40 times higher than genetic parents. They also found that stepparents were 70 times as likely to kill a child younger than age 2 years, and they were 15 times more likely to kill teenage victims.[44] Daly and Wilson found, using Canadian and British databases, that stepfathers were more likely to kill by beating or bludgeoning, whereas genetic fathers shot or asphyxiated their offspring.[1] This suggests differential concerns about child suffering, and a different degree of anger. Weekes-Shackelford and Shackelford[45] replicated these findings in a US database. Whereas stepmothers less commonly kill than stepfathers, it should be recalled that it is relatively rare for a child to live with the father and stepmother, rather than the reverse.

Filicide-Suicide

Filicide-suicide occurs when a parent kills their child or children, and then kills themselves in the immediate aftermath, usually within 24 hours.[46] Fathers more commonly complete suicide after their filicides than mothers. Although 16% to 29% of mothers who commit filicide also kill themselves, 40% to 60% of fathers do so.[47] This is consistent with the fact that men more often complete suicide than women, and men tend to use more lethal means (ie, guns) rather than overdose.

In a study of filicide-suicide based on coroner files in Cleveland, Ohio, the motive in mothers and fathers was most often altruistic (70%).[46] Although mothers often killed all of their children, they did not kill their partner. However, fathers often killed their wives in addition to their children. Similar stressors (eg, financial and relationship issues) were noted in this study as in others.

An Australian study of coroner records of filicide-suicide found that the child victims had a mean age of 4 years; mothers had a mean age older than 30 years.[48] Maternal perpetrators often had a mental health history, life stressors, cultural conflict, and isolation. The authors noted that these cases had much in common with cases of "extreme psychiatric disturbance." Paternal perpetrators of filicide-suicide were sometimes involved in custody battles. The fathers were in their 30s, killed all their children, and sometimes their wife. A New Zealand study also found more fathers than mothers committed filicide-suicide. Mental illness and substance abuse histories were common.[49]

Dietz[50] described perpetrators of familicide, murder of the whole family. Fathers who killed often had a proprietary view of the family, and were depressed, paranoid, or intoxicated. They killed each member of the family, sometimes including their pets, and sometimes also killed themselves. Men commit 95% of familicides.

Filicide-suicide is not considered evolutionarily adaptive except in certain situations, such as serving to remove shame, which could limit future resource allocation for biologic relatives. In the absence of such incentive, filicide-suicide becomes a strong marker for a disturbance, such as mental illness. Similar to other cases of mentally abnormal filicide, victims of filicide-suicide are often older.

MOTIVES OF CHILD MURDER BY PARENTS AND THE ROLE OF MENTAL ILLNESS

Motives for filicide include fatal child maltreatment, unwanted child, partner revenge, altruistic, and acutely psychotic (**Table 2**).[51]

Fatal Maltreatment

Fatal maltreatment is the most common type of filicide.[35] In cases of fatal child maltreatment, the parent has often been either abusing or neglecting the child for a period of time. The child's death is not anticipated on a specific date, but occurs after the victim has been unable to withstand further trauma or lack of nutrition. Although parents who kill by fatal maltreatment may have severe mental illness,

Table 2 Contemporary motives for filicide	
Fatal child maltreatment	Death as result of chronic abuse, neglect, or Munchausen syndrome by proxy; most common type
Partner (spouse) revenge	Least common type; expression of rage at partner or ex-partner
Unwanted child	Most common motive in neonaticide
Altruistic	Murder "out of love," may be psychotic or nonpsychotic; common in filicide-suicide cases
Acutely psychotic	With psychosis, mania, or delirium; no comprehensible motive

they are more likely to have a personality disorder, anger problems, mental retardation, or substance abuse. Abusive behaviors are more consistent with anger and violence as generically adaptive control strategies that may suggest less likelihood of mental illness. Substance use or personality issues may override the control switch in otherwise adaptive nonlethal behavior. When Adler and Polk reviewed the Australian coronial cases of fatal assaults, they found maternal and paternal perpetrators had intent to punish, but not to kill their children.[48] These parents lashed out in response to perceived child misbehaviors. The children were young, usually younger than age 2 years, whereas the mean parental age was in the mid-20s.

Fatal child maltreatment cases also include the uncommon phenomenon of Munchausen syndrome by proxy. In Munchausen syndrome by proxy, most of the perpetrators are mothers. The mother's goal is to receive attention from others because of how she "heroically cares" for her ill child. She usually does not intend that child's death.[52] Munchausen syndrome by proxy has been noted to occur across cultures. The ultimate explanation may be the "dark side of parental investment theory."[52] The mother, who may have a personality disorder, seeks attention from higher-status medical professionals (often men) in a symbolic manner commensurate with otherwise legitimate female reproductive strategy.

Unwanted Child

The second motive, unwanted child filicide, occurs when unwanted children are killed because they are considered a hindrance to the parent. This may be for social reasons, such as limiting the opportunity for remarriage or financial reasons. These filicides usually occur in the absence of any severe mental illness. Women who commit neonaticide may believe they lack the resources to raise the unwanted child. In addition, historically neonaticide occurred in the presence of poor quality offspring.

Partner Revenge

Spouse (partner) revenge filicide, also known as the Medea syndrome, is the least common reason that parents kill their children. An angry vindictive parent kills one or more children to cause the other parent extreme psychological pain. If only one child is killed, it is often the favorite child of the parent against whom revenge is being sought. The perpetrator may have a severe personality disorder. These filicides typically occur after spousal infidelity or after a parent loses a bitter child custody battle.

Altruistic

Altruistic filicide is described as "murder out of love." A loving parent without mental illness may rarely kill a child who is suffering from a painful terminal disease, to prevent further suffering (euthanasia). A severely depressed parent, who is planning suicide, may kill their child as part of an extended suicide. The parent does not want their beloved child to have to fare for themselves in what the depressed parent sees as a miserable world. A psychotic parent may perceive the act of killing their child as the "lesser of evils" if they believe their child is experiencing a fate worse than death. These parents may delusionally believe that their child is being forced into white slavery or child pornography. Altruistic filicide most often occurs during psychosis or suicidal depression.

Acutely Psychotic

A parent suddenly may kill their child while in an acutely psychotic state. The filicide may be in the throes of delirium, mania, or psychosis, or in response to command hallucinations. There is no comprehensible motive. Acutely psychotic filicide is, by definition, related to mental illness (psychosis, mania, or rarely delirium).

Motives and Mental Illness

In the study of mothers who committed filicide and were found NGRI in Ohio and Michigan,[42] most had altruistic or acutely psychotic motives. The other motives for filicide (fatal maltreatment, unwanted child, and partner revenge) are not usually related to serious mental illness. However, this is not to say that these filicidal parents do not have some diagnosable condition, such as a personality disorder, substance abuse, or intellectual limitations.[51,53–55] Conversely, parents may have a serious mental illness, such as depression or schizophrenia, and still may kill for a motive that is self-serving. That is, the mental illness is coincidental rather than causally related to the filicide.

FORENSIC EVALUATION OF THE FILICIDE OFFENDER
Preparation for the Forensic Evaluation

For general recommendations regarding conducting forensic evaluations, refer to the American Academy of Psychiatry and the Law guidelines.[56] Specific recommendations are provided here for the evaluator in cases of filicide. When evaluating a parent charged with filicide, the forensic examiner should obtain the precise standard for NGRI in the relevant jurisdiction from the referring attorney. Reviewing a copy of jury instructions is also useful. The attorney can also be asked to research whether the "wrongfulness" in the NGRI standard has been defined by case law to refer to legal wrongfulness or moral wrongfulness. Most state supreme courts have not specified either.

Review of Collateral Records

Aside from the collateral records that would be sought in any forensic evaluation, in a case of filicide or neonaticide some additional records may assist in understanding the parent-child relationship. For example, the prenatal care records and delivery records may yield contemporaneous statements to physicians and social workers regarding the "wanted-ness" of the pregnancy. The victim's pediatric records may yield information about parenting, bonding, and abuse. Evidence of overprotectiveness or neglect may be gleaned from pediatric or social work records. Psychotic concerns and notes about the parent's appropriate or inappropriate behaviors during pediatric visits may be found. Furthermore, a lack of appropriate pediatric visits may be seen.[42]

Records from child protective services should be sought, and interviews conducted if indicated. Interviews with family members, friends, and neighbors may also provide information about the parent's mental state before the offense. Collateral records should be reviewed before the psychiatric evaluation, so that the evaluator can inquire about specific behavior and resolve any inconsistencies between the records and the parent's account.

Forensic Interview

The motive for the filicide should be explored in detail. The evaluator should consider potential motives, ranging from motives that reflect evolutionary adaptive reproductive strategies that are often considered culpable, to the mentally abnormal motives that may be more likely to qualify for the insanity defense. If there were any recent marital problems, the possibility of spouse revenge filicide should be investigated. The offender's relationship to the child victim and the question of child abuse should be explored.

Altruistic filicides are often performed in the delusional belief that the parent is doing what is best for the child. Such parents often believe they are doing what is morally right even though they know that killing a child is against the law. In assessing whether a parent believed their killing was morally wrong, the evaluator could ask perpetrators whether they believe they will meet their Maker with a pure heart.

Some altruistic filicides have an element of spouse revenge, even though that was not the primary motive. An altruistic murder that falls short of NGRI may still be seen by the court as mitigating, when contrasted with an unwanted child or child maltreatment filicide. In cases of attempted suicide along with filicide, the forensic examiner should ask the defendant whether the decision to commit suicide occurred before or after the decision to kill the child or children.

The evaluator should inquire about planning, and the offender's thinking, feelings, and behaviors around the time of their offense. Limited information is available about the length of time spent contemplating filicide by mentally ill parents before their filicide. In one small qualitative study, Stanton and colleagues reported that psychotic mothers developed no plans for killing their children in advance, whereas depressed mothers contemplated killing their children for days to weeks.[2]

Psychological Testing

No psychological test has been designed to ascertain the motive or culpability for filicide or neonaticide. One American study of 16 young women referred for NGRI evaluation, primarily by the defense, after commission of neonaticide, used the Dissociative Experiences Scale.[57] This study found high self-reported rates of depersonalization, dissociative hallucinations, and intermittent amnesia at the time of the delivery and homicide. However, this study has been criticized[58,59] because of the strong motive to exaggerate symptoms after neonaticide and the lack of a scale for malingering.

One study compared psychological testing results among women charged with child murder, partner murder, and homicide of a nonrelative.[60] Minnesota Multiphasic Personality Inventory-2 (MMPI-2) testing did not reveal significant differences across the groups on clinical or content scales. However, MMPI-2 profiles of the filicide group revealed a six to eight mean profile, in contrast with the two to six mean profile for matricidal women and four to eight mean profile for homicidal women. Psychological testing may be useful to ascertain information about personality traits, intellectual level, and the validity of psychotic symptoms. However, psychological testing is not mandatory in all filicide cases.

Formulating an Opinion on Sanity

The evaluator must initially determine whether mental illness was present at the time of the offense. Claims of mental illness are suspect if no symptoms were noted by professionals, friends, or family before the filicide. However, postpartum psychosis can begin quite quickly, with rapid worsening of symptoms. The reader is referred elsewhere[35] for a full discussion of postpartum psychosis. The fact that postpartum psychosis is not in the Diagnostic and Statistical Manual has led to some difficulties in testimony about this entity, which presents very dramatically and differently than schizophrenia, although it has been described since the time of Hippocrates.[61]

Diminished capacity to form the requisite intent for murder is a consideration in some jurisdictions. Fatal child maltreatment cases are more likely to be charged with manslaughter than murder, compared with altruistic filicides.

The evaluator should consider the parent's motive for the homicide. This sets the stage to examine the parent's knowledge of wrongfulness of the filicide. Mothers found insane in a Michigan and Ohio study overwhelmingly had motives that were altruistic or acutely psychotic.[42] Mothers with an altruistic motive may delusionally believe that murdering their child was right because a child would otherwise suffer a fate worse than death.

Mothers who killed in an acute psychosis sometimes believed that they were responding to the commanding voice of God. This is called a "deific decree" defense. This stems from Genesis 22 when God commanded Abraham to kill his son Isaac, as a test of his faith. Parents acting on a deific decree qualify for NGRI in some states that otherwise limit their NGRI test to legal wrongfulness.

Parents who kill as a result of fatal maltreatment have often engaged in a long pattern of child harm. They have no belief that they were doing what was right. Parents who kill a child simply because the child is unwanted are usually free of mental illness. Those who murder to emotionally upset the other parent are usually acting out of anger and revenge rather than because of a major mental illness.

In cases of filicide, knowledge of wrongfulness may be indicated by attempts to hide the child's death, claims of stranger kidnapping, and attempts to hide information about the child's death. In filicide cases with accomplices, it is rare to find lack of knowledge of wrongfulness.

Gender bias and "chivalry justice" are concerns specific to filicide.[62] Society tends to think of mothers who kill their children as "mad," whereas fathers who kill are often viewed as "bad." In reality, fathers who kill have many characteristics in common with mothers who commit filicide. Societies often try to explain away various forms of female aggression. The evaluator may need to explain to the court that not all female aggression is related to mental illness and that there are some rational motives for maternal filicide.

SUMMARY

Despite public perception, a large percentage of filicides are committed by parents who are not seriously mentally ill. In the evaluation of parents who have killed, the motive for the filicide must be elucidated. Motives include fatal child maltreatment, unwanted child, partner revenge, altruistic, and acutely psychotic. The likelihood of mental illness varies with the motive for the filicide. Evolutionary psychology helps explain differences between evolutionarily normal rationales for filicide and mentally abnormal filicides. Neonaticides are distinct from other cases of filicide. They usually occur because the child is unwanted in a context of scarce resources. Evolutionary psychology demonstrates that some filicides are rational acts, specifically by identifying contemporary parental motives that may have equivalence to the adaptive pressures of our evolutionary past. To the extent that these motives could be considered as adaptive, the clinician is presented with a useful reference point to consider divergence of maladaptive motives in filicide cases. This ultimately provides a theoretical framework to approach the consideration of the role of mental illness in such cases.

REFERENCES

1. Daly M, Wilson M. Killing children: parental homicide in the modern west. In: Homicide. New York: Aldine De Grutyer; 1988. p. 61–93.
2. Stanton J, Simpson A, Wouldes T. A qualitative study of filicide by mentally ill mothers. Child Abuse Negl 2000;24:1451–60.

3. Hrdy S. The Langurs of Abu: female and male strategies of reproduction. Cambridge (MA): Harvard University Press; 1977.
4. Hrdy S. Infanticide among animals: a review, classification, and examination of the implications for the reproductive strategies of females. Ethol Sociobiol 1979;1:13–40.
5. Wilson DS. Evolution for everyone: how Darwin's theory can change the way we think about our lives. New York: Delacorte Press; 2007.
6. Kuhn TS. The Structure of scientific revolutions. Chicago: University of Chicago Press; 1962.
7. Darwin C. On the origin of species by means of natural selection. London: John Murray; 1859.
8. Spencer H. Principles of biology. London: Williams and Norgate; 1864.
9. Trivers RL. Social evolution. Menlo Park (CA): Benjamin/Cummings; 1985.
10. Daly M, Wilson M. The truth about Cinderella: a Darwinian view of parental love. New Haven (CT): Yale University Press; 1999.
11. Fisher R. The genetical theory of natural selection. Oxford: Clarendon; 1930.
12. Maynard Smith J, Price GR. The logic of animal conflict. Nature 1973;246:15–8.
13. Hamilton WD. The genetical evolution of social behaviour. J Theor Biol 1964;7:1–16.
14. Hamilton WD. Extraordinary sex ratios: a sex-ratio theory for sex linkage and inbreeding has new implications in cytogenetics and entomology. Science 1967;156:477–88.
15. Cosmides L, Tooby J. From evolution to behavior: evolutionary psychology as the missing link. In: Dupre J, editor. The latest on the best: essays on evolution and optimality. Cambridge (MA): The MIT Press; 1987.
16. Nisbett RE. Evolutionary psychology, biology, and cultural evolution. Motivat Emot 1990;14:255–63.
17. Marks MN, Kumar R. Infanticide in Scotland. Med Sci Law 1996;36:299–305.
18. Marks MN, Kumar R. Infanticide in England and Wales. Med Sci Law 1993;33: 329–39.
19. Herman-Giddens ME, Smith JB, Mittal M, et al. Newborns killed or left to die by a parent: a population-based study. JAMA 2003;189:1425–9.
20. Finkelhor D. The homicides of children and youth: a developmental perspective. In: Kantor GK, Jasinski JL, editors. Out of the darkness: contemporary perspectives on family violence. Thousand Oaks (CA): Sage; 1997. p. 17–34.
21. Resnick PJ. Murder of the newborn: a psychiatric review of neonaticide. Am J Psychiatry 1970;26:1414–20.
22. Friedman SH, Resnick PJ. Neonaticide: phenomenology and considerations for prevention. Int J Law Psychiatry 2009;32:43–7.
23. Hesketh T, Xing ZW. Abnormal sex ratios in human populations: causes and consequences. Proc Natl Acad Sci U S A 2006;103:13271–5.
24. Wu Z, Viisainen K, Hemminki E. Determinants of high sex ratio among newborns: a cohort study from rural Anhui province, China. Reprod Health Matters 2006;14: 172–80.
25. Friedman SH, Heneghan A, Rosenthal M. Characteristics of women who deny or conceal pregnancy. Psychosomatics 2004;48:117–22.
26. Putkonen H, Weizmann-Henelius G, Collander J, et al. Neonaticides may be more preventable and heterogeneous than previously thought: neonaticides in Finland 1980–2000. Arch Womens Ment Health 2007;10:15–23.
27. Beyer K, Mack SM, Shelton JL. Investigative analysis of neonaticide: an exploratory study. Crim Justice Behav 2008;35:522–53.
28. Sakuta T, Saito S. A socio-medical study on 71 cases of infanticide in Japan. Keio J Med 1981;30:155–68.

29. Friedman SH, Resnick PJ. Child murder by mothers: patterns and prevention. World Psych 2007;6:137–41.
30. Overpeck MD, Brenner RA, Trumble AC, et al. Risk factors for infant homicide in the United States. N Engl J Med 1998;339:1211–6.
31. Friedman SH, Friedman JB. Parents who kill their children. Pediatr Rev 2010;31: e10–6.
32. Friedman SH, Horwitz SM, Resnick PJ. Child murder by mothers: a critical analysis of the current state of knowledge and a research agenda. Am J Psychiatry 2005;162:1578–87.
33. Levitzky S, Cooper R. Infant colic syndrome: maternal fantasies of aggression and infanticide. Clin Pediatr 2000;39:395–400.
34. Flynn SM, Shaw JJ, Abel KM. Homicide of infants: a cross-sectional study. J Clin Psychiatry 2007;68:1501–9.
35. Friedman SH, Resnick PJ, Rosenthal M. Postpartum psychosis: strategies to protect infant and mother from harm. Curr Psychol 2009;8:40–6.
36. Jennings KD, Ross S, Popper S, et al. Thoughts of harming infants in depressed and nondepressed mothers. J Affect Disord 1999;54:21–8.
37. Chandra PS, Venkatasubramanian G, Thomas T. Infanticidal ideas and infanticidal behavior in Indian women with severe postpartum psychiatric disorders. J Nerv Ment Dis 2002;190:457–61.
38. West SG, Friedman SH, Resnick PJ. Fathers who kill their children: an analysis of the literature. J Forensic Sci 2009;54:463–8.
39. Laursen TM, Munk-Olsen T, Mortensen PB, et al. Filicide in offspring of parents with severe psychiatric disorders. J Clin Psychiatry 2010;71:698–703.
40. Kauppi A, Kumpulainen K, Karkola K, et al. Maternal and paternal filicides: a retrospective review of filicides in Finland. J Am Acad Psychiatry Law 2010;38:229–38.
41. Stone MH, Steinmeyer E, Dreher J, et al. Infanticide in female forensic patients: the view from the evolutionary standpoint. J Psychiatr Pract 2005;11:35–45.
42. Friedman SH, Hrouda DR, Holden CE, et al. Child murder committed by mentally ill mothers: an examination of mothers found not guilty by reason of insanity. J Forensic Sci 2005;50:1466–71.
43. Daly M, Wilson M. Some differential attributes of lethal assaults on small children by stepfathers versus genetic fathers. Ethol Sociobiol 1994;15:207–17.
44. Daly M, Wilson M. Evolutionary social psychology and family homicide. Science 1988;242:519–24.
45. Weekes-Shackelford VA, Shackelford TK. Methods of filicide: stepparents and genetic parents kill differently. Violence Vict 2004;19:75–81.
46. Friedman SH, Hrouda DR, Holden CE, et al. Filicide- suicide: common characteristics of parents who kill their children and themselves. J Am Acad Psychiatry Law 2005;33:496–504.
47. Nock MK, Marzuk PM. Murder-suicide: phenomenology and clinical implications. In: Jacobs DG, editor. The Harvard Medical School guide to suicide assessment and intervention. San Francisco (CA): Jossey-Bass; 1999. p. 188–209.
48. Alder C, Polk K. Child victims of homicide. Cambridge (United Kingdom): Cambridge University Press; 2001.
49. Friedman SH, Cavney J, Simpson AIF, et al. Child murder by parents: epidemiology, assessment, treatment and recovery. Presented at the Royal Australia and New Zealand College of Psychiatry, forensic section, annual meeting. Prato, Italy, October 2010.
50. Dietz PE. Mass, serial and sensational homicides. Bull N Y Acad Med 1986;62: 477–91.

51. Resnick PJ. Child murder by parents: a psychiatric review of filicide. Am J Psychiatry 1969;126:325–34.
52. Saad G. Munchausen by proxy: the dark side of parental investment theory? Med Hypotheses 2010;75:479–81.
53. d'Orban PT. Women who kill their children. Br J Psychiatry 1979;134:560–71.
54. Farooque R, Ernst FA. Filicide: a review of eight years of clinical experience. J Natl Med Assoc 2003;95:90–4.
55. Oberman M. Mothers who kill: coming to terms with modern American infanticide. Am Crim Law Rev 1996;34:2–109.
56. Glancy G, Norko M, Pinals D, et al. Forensic psychiatric evaluation guidelines. J Am Acad Psychiatry Law 2012; in press.
57. Spinelli MG. A systematic investigation of 16 cases of neonaticide. Am J Psychiatry 2001;158:811–3.
58. Mendlowicz MV, Rapaport MH, Fontenelle L, et al. Amnesia and neonaticide. Am J Psychiatry 2002;159:498.
59. Resnick PJ, Friedman SH. Book review: infanticide: psychosocial and legal perspectives on mothers who kill. Psych Serv 2003;54:1172.
60. McKee GR, Shea SJ, Mogy RB, et al. MMPI-2 profiles of filicidal, mariticidal, and homicidal women. J Clin Psychol 2001;57:367–74.
61. Friedman SH, Sorrentino RM, Stankowski JE. Postpartum psychosis, forensic psychiatry and the DSM. Newslett Amer Acad Psych Law 2011;36:24–30.
62. Stangle HL. Murderous Madonna: femininity, violence, and the myth of postpartum mental disorder in cases of maternal infanticide and filicide. Wm Mary L Rev 2008;699.

Evaluating Amnesia for Criminal Behavior: A Guide to Remember

Charles L. Scott, MD

KEYWORDS

- Amnesia • Malingering • Memory • Intoxication • Dissociative • Criminal
- Defendant

KEY POINTS

- Memory stages include acquisition, storage, and retrieval of information.
- Anterograde amnesia involves difficulty in recalling new facts or life events after the onset of a particular condition or incident.
- Retrograde amnesia occurs when people have impaired retrieval of information that they had learned before the onset of a condition or situation.
- Alcohol blackouts are most commonly caused by rapid alcohol consumption on an empty stomach.
- Presentations suggestive of malingered amnesia include a focal retrograde amnesia for the crime period alone combined with preoffense planning and atypical presentation of amnesic symptoms.
- Malingering assessments specific to amnesia claims are available and are important to conduct in forensic evaluations.

INTRODUCTION

Amnesia involves a loss of memory. Of defendants who have committed a violent offense, 20% to 30% claim amnesia for their crime.[1,2] Despite this high frequency, structured evidenced-based assessment of criminal offenders' amnesia claims is shockingly absent in most evaluations. In their review of psychiatric reports from 2001 to 2007 on 102 Norwegian defendants charged with homicide, Grondahl and colleagues[3] determined that of the 40% defendants claiming amnesia, none were evaluated with a memory test. The authors noted that despite the seriousness of the crimes and claims, the forensic experts did not apply psychological testing of memory function or appropriate tests of malingering. The need for a structured approach is essential when evaluating an offender's claim of memory loss. This article

Division of Psychiatry and the Law, Department of Psychiatry and Behavioral Sciences, UC Davis School of Medicine, University of California, Davis Medical Center, 2230 Stockton Boulevard, Sacramento, CA 95817, USA
E-mail address: charles.scott@ucdmc.ucdavis.edu

Psychiatr Clin N Am 35 (2012) 797–819
http://dx.doi.org/10.1016/j.psc.2012.08.003
0193-953X/12/$ – see front matter Published by Elsevier Inc.

reviews important concepts to understand regarding memory formation and memory systems, proposed causes of amnesia, reasons why amnesia claims may be true or false, and important strategies to implement as part of the evaluation process.

MEMORY OVERVIEW

Memory has 3 sequential stages, commonly described as encoding, storage, and retrieval.

Encoding represents the initial registration and interpretation of stimuli. The encoding process is also referred to as *registration* or *sensory memory*.

The subsequent storage stage signifies the consolidation and maintenance of encoded stimuli over time.

Retrieval, the third stage, involves the search and recovery of stored stimuli, a process commonly referred to as *remembering*.

Two conscious approaches to memory retrieval have been described: free recall and recognition recall.

Free recall of a memory involves an active complex search process to open-ended questions. For example, when asked, "Who is the first President of the United States?" the person's unassisted answer is a result of the ability or inability to freely recall the information.

In contrast, *recognition recall* references those memories that come to the person's awareness as a result of a cue or other reminder. Recognition memory can be tested by asking people to choose whether or not they have previously seen an item presented to them or to select an item they have presently known from 2 or more presented alternatives. In a recognition memory testing scenario, rather than being asked to recall the name of the first U.S. President, the individual might be asked, "Who was the first President of the U.S.? A. George Washington; or B. Grover Cleveland?"[4]

In addition to memory formation stages, numerous complex memory systems have been described. One fairly straightforward system categorizes memory into the following 2 primary subcategories[4]:

1. Explicit memory, also known as *declarative memory*
2. Implicit memory, also known as *implicit memory*

Explicit memory involves personally experienced events and facts that are available to consciousness and can be internally recalled. In other words, people actively remember specific information that they previously learned or experienced. Explicit memory is subject to various influences, and therefore recall is not always highly accurate.[4] Tulving[5] divides explicit memory into semantic or episodic memory. Semantic memory (also known as *fact memory*) includes memories for specific information previously learned, although the exact place and time at which the information was learned may not be recalled. Examples of semantic memory include knowing the meaning of the word "milk," the capital of France, how many states comprise the United States of America, or recognizing the face of a famous person.[4,5]

In contrast, episodic memory (sometimes referenced as *autobiographical memory*) includes a person's recall of past incidents and events that occurred at a particular time and location. Examples of episodic memory include the recall of details of a person's wedding or graduation from high school, both of which are highly associated with a location and specific date. The distinction between episodic and semantic memory may have particular relevance in assessing retrograde memory difficulties, because various neurologic impairments may differentially impact these abilities.[4]

For clinical purposes, understanding how explicit memories are initially experienced and subsequently stored can be conceptualized as consisting of the following 3 memory stages[4,6]:

1. Registration memory: Registration memory is responsible for holding large amounts of incoming information in a sensory store for a very brief period. The experienced information either quickly fades or becomes further processed in short-term memory.
2. Short-term memory: Short-term memory has been described as consisting of 3 main components. First, immediate memory represents that information retained from the initial registration process. Immediate memory lasts between 30 seconds to several minutes and allows a person to respond to the situation actively before them.[6] Asking a person to repeat a series of digits is a common component of the mental status examination, which assesses a person's immediate memory. The concept of "working memory" has been described as one aspect of immediate memory that involves the cognitive processing of language and visuospatial data to help guide behavior. "Rehearsal" represents the second component of short-term memory and involves the mental process of repeating information. Through rehearsal, the information is more likely to be stored in the short term. An example of rehearsal might include a person repeating over and over a newly acquired telephone number. Although rehearsal may help this person remember the number for a few hours, there is no guarantee that the number will become part of the long-term memory. The third component of short-term memory involves information that may be retained from an hour up to 1 or 2 days but is not yet consolidated as part of long-term memory.
3. Long-term memory: Long-term memory represents the consolidation of information that may occur quickly or occur over longer lengths of time. No precise dividing line exists between what is considered a recent versus a remote memory.[6]

In contrast to explicit memory, implicit memory does not require conscious efforts to retrieve stored information. Implicit memory involves knowledge that the person can use and actions that the person can perform without conscious awareness. Two clinically relevant types of implicit memory include procedural memory and priming. Procedural memory is sometimes referred to as *skill memory*. Procedural memory involves motor and cognitive activities that do not require conscious awareness. Examples include retaining the ability to dress, walk, or speak despite explicit memory impairments (eg, an inability to recall important past autobiographic information or facts). Other examples of procedural memory include activities such as typing, playing, tennis, or playing the piano. People claiming that they cannot remember important facts of their life should nevertheless remember how to ride a bike if they had previously learned this skill.

Priming represents a second type of implicit memory. Priming involves a cued recall situation in which prior exposure to information enhances a person's subsequent performance without awareness. Evaluating procedural memory and priming are relevant to assessing claimed amnesia because both are usually preserved in amnesic patients.[6] **Fig. 1** provides a simplified overview a more complex long-term memory system proposed by Squire.[7] **Fig. 1** summarizes the memory systems described earlier and is not inclusive of all types of memory described in the literature.

AMNESIA OVERVIEW

For the purposes of this review, amnesia represents memory impairment while other basic cognitive functioning remains intact. Disorders that involve marked impairment in multiple cognitive domains, such as dementia or other progressive neurologic

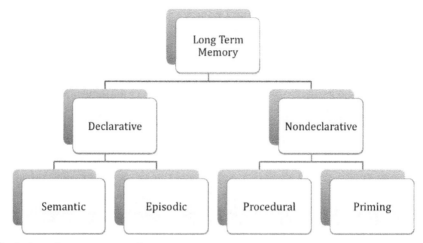

Fig. 1. Long-term memory systems.

disorders, are not typified by isolated memory impairments. Amnesia can be divided into 2 main types based on how the memory loss is referenced to a particular point in time. Anterograde amnesia involves difficulty in recalling new facts or life events after the onset of a particular condition or incident. Anterograde amnesia is typically global in that memory for all newly presented information (both verbal and nonverbal) is impaired regardless of how the information is presented. Most patients with antero-grade amnesia have some degree of retrograde amnesia.[8] However, this pattern is not absolute. In fact, cases have been reported of people with particular brain injuries or diseases who experience anterograde amnesia with minimal or no associated retro-grade amnesia.[9]

The term *transient global amnesia* (TGA) was coined by Fisher and Adams.[10] TGA is characterized by complete anterograde amnesia, which may result in the person experiencing disorientation to time and place. Because affected persons are able to use their long-term memory, they retain knowledge about who they are and are often able to make logical interpretations of their circumstances. Common characteristics of TGA include repetitive questioning and answering, repetitive behaviors, apathy or agitation, and a transient memory loss usually lasting between 1 to 24 hours. The exact cause of TGA is unclear, although many cases seem to be triggered by precipitating events, such as physical exertion, sexual intercourse, emotional stress related to arguing, or certain medical procedures. TGA is distinguished from other forms of anterograde amnesia by its short duration and memory recovery.[11]

Retrograde amnesia occurs when a person has impaired retrieval of information that they had learned before the onset of a condition or situation.[12] Focal retrograde amnesia is defined as a memory loss for an isolated circumscribed period of a person's life. Offenders who claim amnesia only for the period of their criminal behavior without other memory deficits are reporting a focal (ie, circumscribed) retrograde amnesia.

PROPOSED CAUSES OF AMNESIA

For the purposes of this paper, normal forgetting for events of nonsignificance is not considered amnesia. Three proposed causes of amnesia that are commonly described are organic, psychological, and malingering. Each of these is considered in the following sections.

Organic Causes

A variety of circumstances may impact brain structures that relate to the encoding and consolidation of memories. For example, medical conditions (eg, diabetic hypoglycemia, traumatic head injury) may interfere with the brain's ability to input and store the memory.[9] The list of possible medical conditions affecting memory is extensive, and careful consideration of an organic cause is important when evaluating amnesia claims. **Box 1** lists some known organic causes of amnesia.

Psychological Causes

Numerous potential emotional triggers for situation-specific amnesia have been described in the literature. Suggested psychological causes center on the theory that an altered emotional state or level of consciousness results in memories being stored in some type of exceptional or alternate context.[13] When the person attempts to retrieve the memory in a calmer state, the memories are theoretically not accessible because of this state-dependent memory. Emotional states that have been suggested to cause or contribute to amnesia include extreme rage, anger, psychosis, or dissociation resulting from severe trauma. In line with this theory, researchers have found that defendants with more emotionally driven and reactive murders are more likely to claim amnesia (56%) than defendants whose homicides involved planning (30%).[14]

Memory loss caused by a rageful state usually related to a crime of passion has been referred to as a *red out*. Swihart and colleagues[15] present 2 cases to support this proposed this red-out phenomena, which they report involves a sudden rush of anger toward a known victim resulting in homicidal violence. In this red-out scenario, the perpetrator describes a loss of memory that begins at the peak of the violent act, with memory returning after the completion of the violence. These authors propose 4 key elements of a red-out:

1. An intact memory for events before and after the violent attack
2. An unusual level of anger associated with the attack

Box 1
Potential medical causes of amnesia

- Alcohol and/or substance use
- Aneurysm rupture of the anterior communicating artery
- Anoxia
- Brain disease, impairment, or injury
- Cerebrovascular accident
- Delirium
- Dementia
- Electroconvulsive therapy
- Encephalitis
- Hypoglycemia
- Somnambulism
- Transient epileptic forms of amnesia
- Wernicke-Korsakoff syndrome

3. Amnesia for the most violent part of the event
4. The absence of any alcohol, drugs, or organic basis for the amnesia

Although the investigators suggested malingering was unlikely in their 2 case reports, no structured assessments of malingering were described in their review. A self-report of a person's "emotionality" before the claimed amnesia may need to be viewed with some skepticism. For example, one study found that murderers nearly always provided an exaggerated account of their emotionality at the time of the crime, as determined through comparing their statements to official crime reports.[16]

The *Diagnostic and Statistical Manual of Mental Disorders* (Fourth Edition, Text Revision) (*DSM-IV-TR*) uses the term *dissociative amnesia* when describing psychological states associated with memory loss. According to the *DSM-IV-TR*, the diagnosis of dissociative amnesia is "an inability to recall important personal information, usually of a traumatic or stressful nature, that is too extensive to be explained by normal forgetfulness."[17(p.520)] The *DSM-IV-TR* provides several definitions of specific memory disturbances that may appear in individuals with dissociative amnesia, including

1. Localized amnesia: the person is unable to describe events that occurred during a localized timeframe, usually the first few hours after an upsetting event.
2. Selective amnesia: The person can recall some, but not all, events that occurred during a circumscribed period of time.
3. Generalized amnesia: The person is unable to remember events after a specific time, and the amnesia continues to the present.
4. Systematized amnesia: The person reports a memory loss for certain categories of information, such as an inability to remember a particular person or family members.

The *DSM IV-TR* distinguishes the diagnosis of dissociative amnesia from other diagnoses that may include an amnesic or dissociative state as one of the diagnostic criteria. The alternate diagnoses that should be considered in the differential diagnosis of amnesia are summarized in **Table 1**, and the specific words or phrases referencing memory loss are italicized. In each of these diagnoses, the memory loss cannot result from substances used (such as alcohol, drugs, or medications) or from any type of neurologic condition or head trauma.[17(p.463–533)]

Psychogenic amnesia and *dissociative amnesia* have both been used to describe situations in which psychological factors affect memory. However, Kopelman[12] suggests that *psychogenic amnesia* is the preferable term because it does not assume any particular cause for the underlying memory loss, as is suggested by term *dissociative amnesia*.

Malingering

The *DSM-IV-TR* defines malingering as the "intentional production of false or grossly exaggerated physical or psychological symptoms motivated by external incentives."[17(p.739)] Avoidance or mitigation of criminal responsibility represents a significant external incentive for defendants charged with a criminal offense.

The precise prevalence rate of malingered amnesia in criminal cases is difficult to establish. However, when research subjects are asked to think of a way to defend against a hypothetical murder charge, amnesia combined with blaming the act on an internal force (eg, an alternate personality) is the most commonly chosen strategy.[18,19] Surveys of forensic psychologists indicate the base rate of malingering in referred cases is in the range of 11% to 20%.[20] Likewise, in one of the first studies examining offenders who claim amnesia, Hopwood and Snell[21] found that nearly 20%

Table 1 Nonmedical *DSM-IV-TR* disorders that include amnesia as symptom	
DSM-IV Diagnosis	**Amnesia Diagnostic Component**
Dissociative amnesia	• One or more episodes *involving an inability to remember personal information* • *Lost memories* are usually related to stressful or traumatic event
Dissociative fugue	• Sudden unexpected travel from one's home or workplace • *Inability to recall one's past* • Confusion about one's personal identity or assumption of new identity
Dissociative identify disorder	• Two or more distinct personality states or identities • At least 2 states currently take control of person's behavior • *Inability to recall important personal information* that is too extensive to be explained by ordinary forgetfulness
Posttraumatic stress disorder and acute stress disorder	• Person has been exposed to a traumatic event that involved actual or threatened death or serious injury, or threat to physical integrity of others • Person's response involved intense fear, helplessness, or horror • *An inability to recall an important aspect of the trauma*
Somatization disorder	• A history of many physical complaints beginning before 30 years of age that occur over a period of several years • Results in treatment being sought or significant impairment in social, occupational, or other areas of functioning • One pseudoneurologic symptom including *dissociative symptoms, such as amnesia*

of offenders reporting no recollections of their criminal acts were feigning their memory loss. Kopelman[12] notes that there are at least 4 reasons to suggest that some amnesia claims are genuine and should not automatically be discounted.

1. Different offenders' descriptions of their memory gaps are similar to each other, with the reported memory loss for the offense period typically lasting an hour or less.
2. Some victims or witnesses of violent crime who experience emotional arousal and/ or alcohol intoxication have also claimed amnesia. Despite these associated factors (which are often present in offenders), victim and witness claims are rarely questioned.
3. Offenders' amnesia claims may not help in their defense or may prevent important information they know from coming forward, yet they persist in reporting a loss of memory for their actions.
4. Many offenders claiming amnesia have actually turned themselves into the police or failed to take steps to prevent their apprehension, indicating that they are not malingering amnesia to avoid punishment.[12]

Even though some offenders turn themselves in to police, they may still have multiple reasons to feign memory loss. First, falsely claiming amnesia allows the defendant to potentially testify while remaining silent about the crime. A defendant who reports no memory for the crime can significantly evade cross-examination for his criminal actions.[14] Along these same lines, a defendant may find it easier to claim amnesia as opposed to taking the riskier approach of lying or creating a fake alibi.[13]

Second, Oorsouw and Cima[22] showed that pretrial inmates were significantly more likely to claim amnesia for their crime compared with convicted inmates. Defendants who claim amnesia are likely to have an extensive psychiatric evaluation.[14] Because experts may not be adequately trained in assessing amnesia and/or may not conduct structured memory assessment, defendants may be inappropriately diagnosed as genuinely amnesic when they are faking. For example, one study indicated that trained forensic experts failed to identify 50% of malingerers when they relied solely on the defendant's self-report or failed to conduct or review appropriate psychological tests.[23,24] Finally, claiming amnesia provides the defendant a reason not to discuss the crime and thereby avoid potentially painful memories.[14]

Suspecting that a defendant may feign memory loss is justified for several reasons, as summarized by Jelicic and Merckelbach.[2] First, complete amnesia is rare, even in situations in which a person may be in a different emotional state when the crime occurs from when later questioned about the crime.[2] Second, significant research notes that actions performed by a person are remembered better than other types of information[25] or other events witnessed.[26] Third, individuals who witness a violent crime do not typically report memory loss of the traumatic event, suggesting that emotional trauma is an unlikely explanation for complete memory loss. In particular, concentration camp survivors maintain memories of the brutal violence they experienced when examined 40 years later.[27] Likewise, children between the ages of 5 and 10 who witness their parents being murdered maintain vivid recollections of the trauma.[28] Fourth, polled sexual and homicide offenders overwhelmingly report that feigning memory loss is common when charged with these offenses. Finally, studies of convicted offenders who claimed crime-related amnesia show that these individuals are more likely to score in the malingering range on a self-reported instrument to assess feigned rare and bizarre cognitive and psychiatric symptoms compared with prison inmates who have not claimed amnesia.[2]

The presence of psychopathy has been suggested as a factor that might increase the likelihood that an offender will malinger amnesia. Psychopathy represents a personality construct characterized by severe personality defects (eg, lack of empathy, callousness, lack of remorse, pathologic lying, conning others) and disruptive behaviors (eg, juvenile delinquency, early childhood behavioral problems, adult arrests).[29] One study sometimes cited to suggest that psychopaths facing legal charges are more likely to feign amnesia for their crime involves research conducted by Lynch and Bradford.[30] In this study, 22 pretrial defendants, all of whom reported some type of alcohol and/or drug amnesia regarding their offense, were referred for a forensic psychiatric evaluation. A polygraph was given to the defendants to evaluate the truthfulness of their amnesia claims. The authors noted that 63% of offenders with psychopathic features were deceptive in their amnesia claims compared with 50% of those without personality disorders. The study, however, did not incorporate any measure of psychopathy. Instead, all personality disorders were grouped together into one personality group. The study results also did not show how any subject met diagnostic criteria for antisocial personality disorder or psychopathy.

Subsequent research indicates that, contrary to what might be expected, psychopathic criminal defendants are not more likely to feign a psychiatric disorder[31] or be particularly adept at malingering.[32] Currently, psychopathy alone cannot be cited as a reliable indicator that the person is malingering amnesia. Finally, no precise feigned-amnesia profile exists. Research studies are mixed regarding the demographics of those who falsely claim amnesia,[3] although some evidence indicates that older offenders more commonly claim amnesia.[33]

EVALUATING AMNESIA CLAIMS IN CRIMINAL OFFENDERS

In addition to conducting a thorough biopsychosocial psychiatric evaluation, evaluators assigned the challenging task of evaluating an offender's claim of amnesia should approach the case with an organized methodology. Important components of the assessment process described by Merckelbach and Christianson[14] are summarized, with some additional components recommended.

Conduct a Relevant Medical and Psychiatric Examination

The evaluator should first clarify that the reported problem is one of amnesia rather than memory problems associated with dementia, delirium, or a developmental disability, such as mental retardation. A memory evaluation should be comprehensive and in many circumstances will be aided by neuropsychological testing. Basic components of a memory evaluation include the following[34]:

1. Orientation to time and place
2. Ability to recall prose
3. Rote learning
4. Visuospatial memory and retention
5. Remote memory and fund of information
6. Autobiographic memory

Potential medical contributions to memory loss must be investigated with appropriate laboratory testing, physical and neurologic examinations, and imaging when indicated. In cases involving retrograde amnesia resulting from severe head trauma, older memories more commonly return than more recent ones. Over time, the amnesia substantially resolves, with the amnesic period limited to the traumatic event and the few seconds before the event. Offenders claiming amnesia as a result of brain trauma whose memory recovery does not follow this pattern should be carefully screened for malingering.[14]

In addition to the disorders highlighted in **Table 1**, mood disorders[35] and psychotic disorders[36] may also be associated with memory deficits, although complete amnesia is not the usual presenting symptom.

Semistructured diagnostic assessment tools may assist in better understanding memory loss complaints. Numerous instruments are available to guide the evaluator in asking questions specific to amnesia associated with a wide variety of conditions. Semistructured interviews that have been used to assess amnesia associated with posttraumatic stress disorder (PTSD) include the Clinician-Administered PTSD Scale,[37] the Peritraumatic Dissociation Experiences-Rater version,[38] and the PTSD Symptom Scale Interview.[39]

Similarly, a variety of semistructured interview instruments to assess dissociation (with related amnesic components) have also been published. One commonly used screening instrument for dissociation is the Dissociative Experience Scale (DES).[40] The DES consists of 28 statements that relate to a range of dissociative symptoms, and the person evaluated is asked to note how often they have these experiences when they are not under the influence of alcohol or drugs. Scores of 30 or higher have been noted to suggest severe dissociation. Two other structured interviews to evaluate potential dissociative disorders include the Dissociative Disorders Interview Schedule[41] and the Structured Interview for DSM-IV Dissociative Disorders.[42]

Although semistructured interview instruments may help the evaluator ask specific symptom-related questions, most of these instruments rely on self-reports alone to code and score the responses. Therefore, in individuals feigning memory loss, a "finding" of amnesia or dissociation does not prove that the claimed memory impairment is genuine or related to the crime. For example, McLeod and colleagues[43] noted that male prisoners' high levels of dissociative symptoms were unrelated to their violent crimes. Furthermore, in their study of Canadian homicide offenders, Woodworth and colleagues[44] found that although dissociative tendencies measured with the DES were associated with a self-reported memory loss, objective measures of memory quality did not reflect this perceived impairment.

Clarify the Characteristics of Claimed Amnesia

When an alleged offender claims amnesia, the evaluator should carefully determine the type (eg, anterograde, retrograde, or both) and extent of memory deficit reported. The following symptoms of extreme specificity regarding amnesia reports have been described as consistent with malingering[13,45,46]:

1. A circumscribed memory loss for the crime with recall of events before and after the crime. In one study of murderers who claimed amnesia, most (60%) reported that their memory loss was limited to the crime itself.[47] This isolated pattern of memory loss contrasts with studies of memory and emotional events, which generally find that people remember the event very well but have some memory loss for information before and after the emotionally arousing incident.[45]
2. A sharp and sudden onset and ending of the circumscribed amnesic period. Genuine amnesia more characteristically has a blurred beginning and ending.[45,48]
3. A complete loss of memory for a circumscribed period. In a study of 21 convicted male offenders claiming amnesia, 20 claimed partial amnesia and only 1 claimed complete amnesia. These findings indicate that complete amnesia for a criminal act is rare[1] and amnesia for the complete act of killing is unlikely.[45]
4. An attitude by the offender that nothing can possibly help their memory recovery. Schacter[46] assessed offenders' "feeling-of-knowing" regarding their beliefs that their memory return could be assisted by cues, reminders, reenactments, or a return to the crime scene. Offenders with low "feeling-of-knowing" ratings were dogmatic that their memory could not be helped by any assistance, and this pattern was described as characteristic of malingerers.
5. An overly dramatic presentation with reports that the symptoms experienced were extremely severe.[45]
6. A report of extremely specific symptoms (ie, "I can't remember anything from precisely 8:00 AM until 12:00 PM").[45]
7. A report that the amnesia was caused by intoxication contrary to available evidence.[45]

Most of these factors suggested to be consistent with malingering did not derive from studies that included specific tests to evaluate malingering. Therefore, evaluations of genuine versus malingered amnesia will need to consider multiple factors unique to the case, with an understanding of how the defendant's presentation compares with genuine cases. A review of the literature suggests that important areas to review should include the following:

1. What type of amnesia is being reported? In particular, is the amnesia anterograde, retrograde, or some combination of both?
2. What is the last memory before the onset of amnesia?
3. What does the defendant think caused the amnesia?
4. What is the length of the claimed amnesic period?

5. How did the amnesia begin and end? Was there a sudden onset and ending or was there a blurring between the beginning and end of the amnesic episode?
6. Does the amnesia represent a patchy loss of memory with some preserved memories or is there a complete loss of all memory for a defined period?
7. What emotions was the defendant experiencing before the onset of the amnesia?
8. Does the defendant have any particular close or emotional relationship to the victim?
9. Was there any use of alcohol or other substances around the time of the amnesia? (See section below on evaluating alcohol and substance use in amnesia claims.)
10. Was there any head trauma related to the period of claimed amnesia?
11. Have any lost memories returned? If so, which ones and when?
12. Is there anything the defendant thinks could possibly help with memory recovery?
13. Has the defendant experienced other memory problems, such as forgetting how to ride a bike, type, or get dressed?
14. Have there been any prior amnesic episodes?
15. Has the defendant read any literature about memory loss?
16. Has the defendant had any exposure to others who have experienced amnesia, either in person or through the media? If so, describe.

Evaluate the Relationship of Alcohol and/or Substance Use to Claimed Amnesia

Alcohol use is common in violent offenders who claim amnesia. In their study of criminal offenders, Taylor and Kopelman[49] noted that more than half of those claiming amnesia were under the influence of alcohol in the hours before their offense. Persons who consumed the most alcohol were more likely to report amnesia. Other studies have indicated that more than 85% of offenders claiming amnesia were under the influence of alcohol and/or drugs when they committed their crime.[50] Evaluators, however, should not assume that an offender's reported alcohol or drug use has resulted in genuine amnesia. For example, Cima and colleagues[33] found that although substance-abuse-disordered forensic patients were more likely than controls to claim amnesia, only a minority of them had a sufficiently high alcohol or drug level to actually produce amnesia. This finding indicates that an offender may falsely claim that their substance use caused memory loss for their crime to minimize their personal responsibility.[51]

Although alcohol likely impacts most stages of memory processing, it primarily interferes with the transfer of information from short-term to long-term storage. People are usually able to recall long-term memories they had prior to becoming intoxicated.[52] Ryback[53] described memory impairments that occur after a person has consumed a smaller amount of alcohol, such as the number of drinks that would result in a blood alcohol level (BAL) less than 0.15 g/dL. These characteristic memory impairments (sometimes referred to as "cocktail-party" memory deficits) are manifested after a person has had a few drinks and include difficulty remembering what was said or parts of a conversation. Other studies have shown that even at a low BAL, persons can experience difficulty forming memories for items on word lists or recognizing new faces.[54,55]

No clear evidence exists of "state-dependent" learning with alcohol or other drugs. State-dependent learning references the theory that information learned in an intoxicated or drugged state is best recalled when the person is placed back in that state. Current evidence does not support the notion that information learned while intoxicated can be retrieved through resuming intoxication.[56] In a study by Wolf,[57] criminals who claimed amnesia under the influence of alcohol did not recover their memory when placed back in a state of alcohol intoxication.

Alcohol impairs a person's ability to store information across delays longer than a few seconds, particularly if the person is distracted between the time they are given the new information and the time they are tested.[52] Perhaps the most extreme memory impairment resulting from alcohol intoxication is an alcohol "blackout." Goodwin[58] estimated that a person would need to consume approximately 5 glasses of whiskey or 20 glasses of beer within a 5-hour period to achieve a blackout. High BALs have been associated with a higher risk of experiencing a blackout. For example, in a study of 65 adults arrested with a corresponding BAL of 310 g/dL or higher had a 0.50 or greater probability of having an alcoholic blackout.[59] One suggested threshold BAC necessary for producing an alcoholic blackout is 0.25 g/dL.[60] However, Ryback's[53] study of alcohol on memory in 7 hospitalized alcoholics estimated that blackouts often began at levels around 0.20 g/dL and as low as 0.14 g/dL. Heavy drinking alone is insufficient to result in a blackout. More important is the rate of alcohol consumption (ie, "gulping" drinks) combined with drinking on an empty stomach. A rapid rise in the blood alcohol level is a particularly significant risk factor for inducing a blackout.[53,61]

The National Longitudinal Survey of Youth characterized blackout drinkers compared with nonblackout drinkers.[62] This information may assist in evaluating the likelihood that alcohol caused a blackout. In this study, blackout drinkers were more likely to have a significantly greater number of days they drank alcohol, had a greater frequency of drinking 6 or more drinks during one drinking episode, and had a greater number of drinks on an average day.

Although individuals with a history of frequent and heavy alcohol consumption are at risk for developing blackouts, social drinkers are also vulnerable to having an alcohol blackout. In their survey of 772 undergraduates, White and colleagues[63] asked the following question: "Have you ever awoken after a night of drinking not able to remember things that you did or places that you went?" Fifty-one percent of students answered that they had experienced a blackout during the course of their lifetime. On average, students estimated that they consumed approximately 11.5 drinks before the onset of a blackout. Female undergraduate students in this survey were noted to have a higher risk of experiencing a blackout compared with males at any level of alcohol consumption.

An alcohol blackout is not the same as passing out and falling asleep. Blackouts occur when a person is unable to recall critical elements of events, or even entire events, that occurred while he or she was intoxicated and awake. People experiencing a blackout can participate in salient, emotionally charged events and even more routine actions that they cannot later remember.[58] Persons who experience a blackout have anterograde memory impairments while intoxicated but retain memories that occurred before they became intoxicated. Two types of blackouts have been described: en bloc blackouts and fragmentary blackouts.[61] En bloc blackouts are characterized by a person's inability to recall any details from events that occurred while intoxicated. The use of other substances, including marijuana and benzodiazepines, increases the likelihood that the person will experience an en bloc blackout. Persons who have experienced an en bloc blackout do not recover memories of what happened during the blackout when told about what they did.[64] Common features of en bloc blackouts include the following[61]:

- A distinct onset
- The ability to keep information active in short-term memory for a few seconds up to 2 minutes but not much longer
- The ability to have conversations with others or drive a car
- Falling asleep and later waking up from the blackout

In contrast to en bloc blackouts, fragmentary blackouts involve memory loss that can later be recalled when the person is provided cues about what happened while they were intoxicated. Fragmentary blackouts are more common than en bloc blackouts. When substances (such as marijuana or benzodiazepines) are combined with alcohol, en bloc blackouts are more commonly experienced than fragmentary blackouts.[64]

Various substances, including benzodiazepines and barbiturates, have also been described to independently impair memory when not combined with alcohol. When determining a possible relationship between any substance and amnesia, the evaluator should be familiar with the literature specific to that medication. Evaluating a possible relationship of alcohol to claimed amnesia requires detailed questioning. Important questions and areas to review when making this determination are summarized in **Box 2**. Many of these questions will be relevant when investigating the possible relationship of a particular substance to an amnesia claim.

Evaluate Degree of Offense Planning

Criminal behavior is often described as either instrumental or impulsive. Instrumental crimes are those that involve a degree of planning compared with more impulsive crimes, which are typically sudden, emotionally driven, with little or no preparation. In reality, both instrumental and reactive components may be involved in a crime. Nevertheless, this distinction is important in evaluating authenticity of memory claims. Because elaborative processing and rehearsal actually improves memory,[65] planning and premeditation should enhance an offender's memory for the crime. As a result, genuine amnesia for instrumental criminal behavior would not be expected.[2]

To evaluate an offender's memory regarding the alleged criminal act, the examiner might find it helpful to systematically follow Calhoun and Weston's[66] proposed pathway model to homicidal violence. **Table 2** summarizes the first 6 steps to violent homicides in this model pathway, with 2 additional subsequent steps (steps 7 and 8) suggested by Christianson and colleagues.[45]

Obtain Relevant Collateral Information

Relying on the defendant's self-report alone is inadequate when evaluating amnesia claims for a criminal act. A thorough review of available collateral records is essential. Important records to consider include the following:

- Police reports
- Defendant's statements (at time of and after arrest)
- Witness statements
- Investigation reports
- Alcohol and drug levels for period of claimed amnesia
- Jail records
- Laboratory data associated with alcohol use (eg, liver function tests)
- Medical records (including neurologic workup)
- Relevant neuroimaging studies
- Psychiatric records
- Alcohol and drug treatment records
- Education records
- Observations by others regarding prior memory functioning
- Observations by others regarding current memory functioning
- Prior exposure to media regarding amnesia cases or presentation
- General psychological testing
- Specific malingering testing
- Neuropsychological testing

Box 2
Alcohol and amnesia interview questions

1. When was the last time you ate before drinking?
2. Were you drinking on an empty stomach?
3. Did you eat during your drinking period?
4. What time did you start drinking alcohol?
5. What were you drinking?
6. How many drinks were consumed over what period of time?
7. How soon after drinking did you lose your memory?
8. What is your last memory before you experienced a memory loss?
9. What is the time period of your memory loss?
10. What is your first memory after this period of memory loss?
11. Do you have a partial or complete loss of memory for that time period?
12. Was the onset of your memory loss sudden or gradual?
13. Was the return of your memory sudden or gradual?
14. Are your memory problems only for events that happened while you were drinking alcohol or do you have problems remembering things before you began drinking alcohol?
15. Have you noticed any problems now remembering things when you are not drinking alcohol?
16. Have cues or reminders from others about what happened while you were drinking helped restore your memory?
17. Have you remembered anything that you did not initially? If yes, what do you think helped you remember?
18. Do you know your blood alcohol level related to this episode? If yes, what was it?
19. Did you use any other drugs (such a marijuana or benzodiazepines) in combination with alcohol for the drinking episode in question?
20. How many days a week do you drink alcohol?
21. How often do you consume 6 or more drinks when you drink alcohol?
22. What is the average number of drinks you consume on an average day?
23. Have you ever awoken after a night of drinking not able to remember things that you did or places that you went (ie, blackouts)? If yes, how often?
24. What type of blackouts have you experienced in the past (ie, en bloc, fragmentary, or both)?
25. Do you have any history of drinking alcohol more than planned?
26. Did you have any head injury during the drinking episode in question?
27. Have you had any history of head injury outside of this drinking episode in question?

Conduct Appropriate Psychological Testing

Psychological testing is often a useful adjunct when evaluating malingered amnesia, and represents a valuable component in the multimethod assessment process. The specific tests selected for the evaluation vary depending on the individual case specifics and symptoms reported. The article by McDermott elsewhere in this issue provides an excellent overview of malingering assessment strategies, many of which are relevant for

Table 2
Proposed pathway to violence

Violent Crime Stages	Associated Feeling and Action Memories
Step 1: Grievance	Feelings include anger, revenge, and being wronged
Step 2: Ideation	Accepting use of violence to correct wrong or fulfill violent/sexual fantasies May identify with other assailants and discuss fantasies with others
Step 3: Research and planning	May include gathering information to enact plan, inquiring about target, and conducting surveillance
Step 4: Preparations	May involve assembling equipment, practicing firing gun, choosing clothing, writing messages to others, making will
Step 5: Breach	Positioning oneself close to the potential victim
Step 6: Attack	Enacting a plan, which requires commitment and resolve
Step 7: Realization	Actions on the victim's body, including additional violence or sexual acts
Step 7: Postcrime behavior	Behaviors aimed at avoiding discovery or staging the crime scene

Data from Christianson SA, Freij I, Vogelsang E. Searching for offenders' memories of violent crimes. In: Christianson SA, editor. Offenders' memories of violent crimes. Chichester (England): John Wiley & Sons; 2007. p. 3–35; and *From* Brown SC, Craik FI. Encoding and retrieval of information. In: Tulvig E, Craik FI, editors. The Oxford handbook of memory. New York: Oxford University Press; 2000. p. 93–107.

assessing malingered memory loss. Instruments often used to detect possible malingering of psychiatric symptoms include the Structured Interview of Reported Symptoms[67] and Minnesota Multiphasic Personality Inventory, Second Edition.[68] Assessment tools that specifically address potential malingered amnesia include the Test of Memory Malingering,[69] Word Memory Test,[70] Structured Inventory of Malingered Symptomatology,[71] Rey's 15-Item Memory Test,[72] and Coin in the Hand Test.[72]

Neuropsychological testing is often essential to substantiate specific cognitive deficits that are consistent with genuine forms of organic amnesia. Professionals skilled in the administration and interpretation of neuropsychology testing can play an invaluable role in evaluating memory loss claims. Many of these assessment tools evaluate the person's performance on both free-recall tests and recognition tests. Because recognition memory is generally easier than free-recall memory, individuals who perform worse on recognition memory tests than free-recall tests should be suspected of foigning.[73] Furthermore, simulators portraying amnesia often perform worse than brain-damaged memory-disordered patients on tests of recognition memory.[74] Evaluating the person's immediate recall may also provide clues to possible amnesia feigning. In general, individuals with anterograde or retrograde amnesia do not typically exhibit deficits in immediate memory recall.[75]

Symptom validity testing (SVT) is often used to assess complaints of impaired memory. SVT involves asking the patient to choose 1 of 2 items relevant to the complaint. For example, if a person reports having impaired memory, a series of words, pictures, or even numbers can be shown. The person is then presented 2 items, only 1 of which was presented previously. The person is then asked to make a forced choice, or identify which item had been previously shown. Individuals with genuine memory loss are expected to correctly identify at least 50% of the items by chance alone. Through the use of statistics, the evaluator can determine the probability that a person with genuine amnesia would score below chance levels.[76] Numerous symptom validity tests are available to assess whether subjects are putting forth their best effort when their memory is tested. Because the use of multiple tests is more likely to detect below-chance results than a single test, the examiner should consider using multiple tests in forensic neuropsychological evaluations.[77] Many commonly used tests to assess memory loss use this SVT approach.

For individuals claiming a retrograde memory loss, tests evaluating a person's remote memory may be particularly relevant. There are 2 general categories of remote memory testing. The first assesses a person's recall of public events and famous persons. Examples of these tests include the Public Events Tests,[78] News Events Test,[79] Dead-or-Alive Memory Test,[80] Famous Faces Test,[81] and the President Test.[82] The underlying test strategy involves presenting famous faces or well-known events that have occurred over various decades to determine the degree of memory prominence (if any) associated with any particular period. Limitations of this testing include the possibility that the person could have relearned information about famous past people or events and answer items correctly despite impairment, events or individuals selected as "famous" may not be as familiar to all persons in all cultures, and the information designated as historically significant becomes less well-known with the passage of time. Because of these concerns, the evaluator should carefully select tests that have been updated and are likely to include items relevant to the tested individual's culture.[34]

The second category of remote memory tests evaluates subjects' capacity to recall their own history (ie, their autobiographical memory). Assessing remote memory for both famous persons/events and autobiographical memory is particularly relevant in evaluating amnesia for 2 reasons. First, genuine retrograde amnesia rarely involves a loss of autobiographical memory. Second, it is extremely rare for a person to have a greater loss of their autobiographical memory than impaired memory for public events and people.[83] Two tests frequently used to evaluate autobiographical memory include The Crovitz Test[84] and the Autobiographical Memory Interview.[85]

In addition to these specific tests of retrograde memory, the principles of SVT can be used to evaluate an individual who claims a focused retrograde memory loss for their alleged crime. For example, if a person reports having no memory of the crime, the person can be instructed to answer a series of questions based on what is remembered about the circumstances of the crime, if anything. Each question has 2 possible answers: one is a correct fact about the crime and the other is not. To illustrate, consider the case of a man charged with shooting and killing 3 people in a crowded mall at 11:00 AM on March 22, 5 minutes after handing a note reading "beware" to a female store clerk.

Potential forced-choice questions that could be developed from this scenario include the following:

1. What date did the crime occur?
   a. March 22
   b. March 24
2. What time did the crime occur?
   a. 11:00 AM
   b. 3:00 PM
3. What weapon was used?
   a. Knife
   b. Gun
4. What was the store clerk's gender?
   a. Male
   b. Female

5. What did the note say?
   a. Beware
   b. Peace

The questions are worded in a way to prevent the person from having a direct admission of guilt. Sample introductions to the presented questions include, "Police reports allege…" or "The investigation reports claim…" Based on the number of incorrect answers, the probability that the person's responses are from chance alone or worse than chance can then be calculated. Obviously, the worse the person performs below chance the greater the likelihood they are feigning.

Denney[86] applied this SVT approach in evaluating 3 defendants claiming amnesia who were referred for an assessment of their trial competency. Recommended procedures for organizing an SVT to assess crime-related amnesia are summarized in **Box 3**. If the defendant has acquired significant information about the crime, the SVT procedure may not be useful. In particular, the defendant could select the right answer based on what was learned about the crime and still claim to not have any independent memory of it.

Potential Psychophysiological Tools to Evaluate Amnesia

A variety of assessments that evaluate the body and/or brain's reaction to presented stimuli are potentially promising in evaluating feigned amnesia. These techniques are generally not admissible in court in regard to determining malingered amnesia, although they may meet the admissibility standard for expert testimony in the future.

Box 3
Suggested SVT procedure to evaluate crime-related amnesia claim

1. Acquire specific investigative information regarding details of the crime events during the claimed amnesic period to create a list of items specific to the crime.

2. Create questions that include crime specific items that one could reasonably expect a person without a memory loss to correctly answer.

3. Have the questions with item content reviewed by a colleague to help validate the question detail.

4. Word questions in a manner to avoid direct admissions of guilt (ie, "Investigative records allege…" or "The indictment claims…").

5. Develop answers for each question that represent reasonably plausible alternatives.

6. Avoid creating an alternative answer that seems more likely than the correct answer

7. Present each question to the individual to identify whether or not they report a memory for the item in the question.

8. Discard questions for which the person reports adequate memory for items in the question and for which the person could reasonably deduce the correct answer. Attempt to acquire 25 effective questions.

9. Ask the person to choose the correct answer to each remaining question or to guess if they cannot remember. Inform the person after the select an answer if the response was correct or incorrect.

10. Total the correct responses and use the appropriate statistical measures to calculate the probability of correct discrimination with genuine amnesia.

Data from Denney RL. Symptom validity testing of remote memory in a criminal forensic setting. Arch Clin Neuropsychol 1996;7:589–603.

These emerging evaluation approaches include the Guilty Knowledge Test (GKT), event-related brain potentials (ERPs), pupil changes to recognition tests, and brain imaging techniques.

The GKT measures a person's electrodermal response to questions about the crime. Electrodermal responses are recorded through measuring the person's palmar sweat reactions. In general, a person exhibits a sweat response when they are presented with familiar stimuli, particularly those with an emotional content. Genuinely amnesic persons would not be expected to have a palmar sweat reaction when crime-related information is introduced because this information should be unfamiliar to them.[87,88] Some concerns have been raised that the GKT approach may not work with psychopathic individuals because they are known to have decreased autonomic responses, such as those measured by electrodermal reactions.[89]

A second psychophysiologic approach uses the electroencephalogram (EEG), which records ERPs. Because ERPs are associated with recognition memory tasks, using an EEG to monitor these events may help detect the malingering of amnesia.[87,90] In this proposed technique, the GKT uses an EEG to monitor ERPs instead of electrodermal responses measured through palm sweating. In one study to examine ERPs as a measure of detecting feigned amnesia, Rosenfeld and colleagues[90] asked subjects to feign amnesia for autobiographical facts, such as their birth date. When the correct birth date was presented to them along with incorrect dates, the authors were able to measure the ERP response to each item. In this study, the investigators were able to identify 77% of the instances in which the subjects had falsely claimed amnesia for the target fact based on the ERP magnitudes.

A third psychophysiologic approach measures a person's change in pupil size when old versus new items are presented during recognition memory tests. When a person sees information that is known, the pupils generally dilate. This phenomenon has been coined the "pupil old/new effect".[91] For individuals feigning memory loss, an increase in pupil size might be expected when they are shown old information that they claim to not know. In line with this hypothesis, Heaver and Hutton[92] compared changes in pupil size during recognition memory tests under 3 conditions: when participants were given standard recognition memory instructions, instructed to feign amnesia, and instructed to report that all items (both old and new) were new to them. Participants' pupils dilated more to old items under all 3 instruction conditions. The authors note that because these changes in pupil size are not under conscious control, pupil measurements may help determine whether a person is feigning memory loss. Finally, an increasing number of brain imaging studies (eg, functional magnetic resonance imaging and positron emission tomography scans) are exploring potential relationships among abnormal brain findings, aggression, and amnesia.[93] Although abnormalities may be found on imaging studies, they may not be causally related to amnesia. Therefore, experts should use caution when interpreting their results and disclose the limitations of current research in this area.

Assessments Not Recommended

Although hypnosis has been used in the past to assist individuals in memory recovery, this technique is generally not recommended in the assessment of a defendant's amnesia. Memories recovered under hypnosis are vulnerable to suggestion. Although witnesses may recover more correct information while hypnotized, they also provide more incorrect information. Neither examiners nor examinees have shown an ability to distinguish true versus false recovered memories. For these reasons, hypnosis is not generally recommended for the purposes of memory recall in criminal cases, and evidence emerging from hypnosis is rarely admissible in court.[94] Likewise, proposed "truth-serums," such as Amytal or sodium pentothal, should be avoided, because these drugs have shown a memory-distorting effect, including confabulations and reporting fantasies as actual memory.[95]

SUMMARY

A structured approach to evaluating amnesia claims by defendants is critical. The evaluator should be familiar with key memory systems, types of memory impairment, and the proposed causes of amnesia. Particular skill in evaluating the relationship between alcohol and memory impairment is crucial in a large percentage of claimed amnesia cases. The evaluator also must carefully consider the relationship, if any, of a medical or psychiatric disorder to the reported memory loss. The presence of any disorder or stressor does not automatically equate with the presence of a genuine crime-related amnesia. The evaluator must review collateral records and include relevant neuropsychological testing and structured malingering assessments to adequately assess amnesia claims. This article provides a general guide to assist experts in remembering how to evaluate those persons who claim they cannot.

REFERENCES

1. Evans C, Mezey G, Ehlers A. Amnesia for violent crime among young offenders. J Forens Psychiatry Psychol 2009;20(1):85–106.
2. Jelicic M, Merckelbach H. Evaluating the authenticity of crime-related amnesia. In: Christianson SA, editor. Offenders' memories of violent crimes. Chichester (England): John Wiley & Sons; 2007. p. 215–33.
3. Grondahl P, Vaeroy H, Dahl A. A study of amnesia in homicide cases and forensic psychiatric experts' examination of such claims. Int J Law Psychiatry 2009;32: 281–7.
4. Baddeley AD. The psychology of memory. In: Baddeley AD, Kopelman MD, Wilson BA, editors. The handbook of memory disorders. 2nd edition. Chichester (England): John Wiley & Sons; 2002. p. 3–15.
5. Tulving E. Episodic and semantic memory. In: Tulving E, Donaldson W, editors. Organization of memory. New York: Academic Press; 1972. p. 381–403.
6. Lezak MD, Howieson DB, Loring DW. Basic concepts. In: Lezak MD, Howieson DB, Loring DW, editors. Neuropsychological assessment. 4th edition. New York: Oxford University Press; 2004. p. 15–38.
7. Squire LR. Declarative and non-declarative memory: multiple brain systems supporting learning and memory. J Cogn Neurosci 1992;4:232–43.
8. O'Connor M, Verfaellie M. The amnesic syndrome: overview and subtypes. In: Baddeley AD, Kopelman MD, Wilson BA, editors. The handbook of memory disorders. 2nd edition. Chichester (England): John Wiley & Sons; 2002. p. 145–66.
9. Kopelman MD. Retrograde amnesia. In: Baddeley AD, Kopelman MD, Wilson BA, editors. The handbook of memory disorders. 2nd edition. Chichester (England): John Wiley & Sons; 2002. p. 189–207.
10. Fisher CM, Adams RD. Transient global amnesia. Acta Neurol Scand 1964; 24(Suppl 9):1–83.
11. Goldenberg G. Transient global amnesia. In: Baddeley AD, Kopelman MD, Wilson BA, editors. The handbook of memory disorders. 2nd edition. Chichester (England): John Wiley & Sons; 2002. p. 209–31.
12. Kopelman MD. Psychogenic amnesia. In: Baddeley AD, Kopelman MD, Wilson BA, editors. The handbook of memory disorders. 2nd edition. Chichester (England): John Wiley & Sons; 2002. p. 451–71.

13. Porter S, Birt AR, Yuille JC, et al. Memory for murder: a psychological perspective on dissociative amnesia in legal contexts. Int J Law Psychiatry 2001;24:23–42.
14. Merckelbach H, Christianson SA. Amnesia for homicide as a form of malingering. In: Christianson SA, editor. Offenders' memories of violent crimes. Chichester (England): John Wiley & Sons; 2007. p. 165–90.
15. Swihart G, Yuille Y, Porter S. The role of state-dependent memory in "red-outs". Int J Law Psychiatry 1999;22:199–212.
16. Porter S, Woodworth M, Doucette NL. Memory for murder: the qualities and credibility of homicide narrative by perpetrators. In: Christianson SA, editor. Offenders' memories of violent crimes. Chichester (England): John Wiley & Sons; 2007. p. 115–34.
17. American Psychiatric Association. Diagnostic and statistical manual of mental disorders. 4th edition, text revision. Washington, (DC): American Psychiatric Association; 2000.
18. Rabinowitz FE. Creating the multiple personality: an experimental demonstration for an undergraduate abnormal psychology class. Teach Psychol 1989;16:69–71.
19. Spanos NP, Weekes JR, Bertrand LD. Multiple personality: a social psychological perspective. J Abnorm Psychol 1986;94:362–76.
20. Mittenberg W, Patton C, Canyock EM, et al. Base rates of malingering and symptom exaggeration. J Clin Exp Neuropsychol 2002;24:1094–102.
21. Hopwood JS, Snell HK. Amnesia in relation to crime. J Ment Sci 1933;79:27–41.
22. Oorsouw KV, Cima M. The role of malingering and expectations in claims of crime-related amnesia. In: Christianson SA, editor. Offenders' memories of violent crimes. Chichester (England): John Wiley & Sons; 2007. p. 191–213.
23. Rosen GM, Phillips WR. A cautionary lesson from simulated patients. J Am Acad Psychiatry Law 2004;32:132–3.
24. Rubenzer S. Malingering, incompetence to stand trial, insanity, and mental retardation. The Texas Prosecutor 2004;6:17–23.
25. Engelkamp J, Zimmer HD. Human memory. Seattle (WA): Hogrefe; 1994.
26. Symons CS, Johnson BT. The self-reference effect in memory: a meta-analysis. Psychol Bull 1997;121:371–94.
27. Wagenaar WA, Grownewed J. The memory of concentration camp survivors. Appl Cognit Psychol 1990;4:77–87.
28. Malmquist CP. Children who witness pretrial parental murder: posttraumatic aspects. J Am Acad Child Psychiatry 1986;25:320–5.
29. Hare RD. Without conscience: the disturbing world of psychopaths among us. New York: Pocket Books; 1993.
30. Lynch BE, Bradford JM. Amnesia. Detection by psychophysiological measures. J Am Acad Psychiatry Law 1998;8:288–97.
31. Kucharski LT, Duncon S, Egan SS, et al. Psychopathy and malingering of psychiatric disorder in criminal defendants. Behav Sci Law 2006;24:633–44.
32. Poythress NG, Edens JF, Watkins MM. The relationship between psychopathic personality features and malingering symptoms of major mental illness. Law Hum Behav 2001;25:567–82.
33. Cima M, Jijman H, Merckelbach H, et al. Claims of crime-related amnesia in forensic patients. Int J Law Psychiatry 2004;27:215–21.
34. Lezak MD, Howieson DB, Loring DW. Memory I: tests. In: Lezak MD, Howieson DB, Loring DW, editors. Neuropsychological assessment. 4th edition. New York: Oxford University Press; 2004. p. 414–79.
35. Dalgleish T, Cox SG. Memory and emotional disorder. In: Baddeley AD, Kopelman MD, Wilson BA, editors. The handbook of memory disorders. 2nd edition. Chichester (England): John Wiley & Sons; 2002. p. 437–49.

36. McKenna P, Ornstein T, Baddeley AD. Schizophrenia. In: Baddeley AD, Kopelman MD, Wilson BA, editors. The handbook of memory disorders. 2nd edition. Chichester (England): John Wiley & Sons; 2002. p. 413–35.

37. Blake DD, Weathers FW, Nagy LM, et al. The development of a clinician-administered PTSD scale. J Trauma Stress 1995;8:75–90.

38. Marmar CR, Weiss DS, Meltzer TJ. The peritraumatic dissociative experiences questionnaire. In: Wilson JP, Keane TM, editors. Assessing psychological trauma and PTSD. New York: Guilford Press; 1997. p. 412–28.

39. Foa EB, Tolin DF. Comparison of the PTSD symptom scale-interview version and the clinician-administered PTSD scale. J Trauma Stress 2000;13:181–91.

40. Carlson EB, Putnam FW. An update on the dissociative experiences scale. Dissociation 1993;6:16–27.

41. Ross CA, Heber S, Norton CA, et al. The dissociative disorders interview schedule: a structured interview. Dissociation 1989;2:169–89.

42. Steinberg M. Structured clinical interview for DSM-IV dissociative disorders (SCID-D), revised. Washington, (DC): American Psychiatric Press; 1994.

43. McLeod HJ, Byrne MK, Aitken R. Automatism and dissociation: disturbances of consciousness and volition from a psychological perspective. Int J Law Psychiatry 2004;27:471–87.

44. Woodworth M, Porter S, Brinke LT, et al. A comparison of memory for homicide, non-homicidal violence, and positive life experiences. Int J Law Psychiatry 2009;32:329–34.

45. Christianson SA, Freij I, Vogelsang E. Searching for offenders' memories of violent crimes. In: Christianson SA, editor. Offenders' memories of violent crimes. Chichester (England): John Wiley & Sons; 2007. p. 3–35.

46. Schacter DL. Amnesia and crime. How much do we really know? Am Psychol 1986;41:286–95.

47. Bradford JW, Smith SM. Amnesia and homicide: the Padola case and a study of thirty cases. Bulletin of the J Am Acad Psychiatry Law 1979;7:219–31.

48. Power DJ. Memory, identification and crime. Med Sci Law 1977;17:132–9.

49. Taylor PJ, Kopelman MD. Amnesia for criminal offenses. Psychol Med 1984;14:581–8.

50. Parwatikar SD, Holcomb WR, Menninger KA. The detection of malingered amnesia in accused murderers. Bull Am Acad Psychiatry Law 1985;13:97–103.

51. Cima M, Merckelbach H, Nijman H, et al. I can't remember your honour: offenders who claim amnesia. Ger J Psychiatr 2002;5:24–34.

52. White AM. What happened? Alcohol, memory blackouts, and the brain. Alcohol Res Health 2003;27:186–96.

53. Ryback RS. The continuum and specificity of the effects of alcohol on memory. Q J Stud Alcohol 1971;32:995–1016.

54. Mintzer MA, Griffiths RR. Alcohol and triazolam: differential effects on memory, psychomotor performance and subjective ratings of effects. Behav Pharmacol 2002;13:653–8.

55. Westrick ER, Shapiro AP, Nathan PE, et al. Dietary tryptophan reverses alcohol-induced memory impairment of facial recognition but not verbal recall. Alcohol Clin Exp Res 1988;12:531–3.

56. Weissenborn R, Duka T. State-dependent effects of alcohol on explicit memory: the role of semantic associations. Psychopharmacology 2000;149:98–106.

57. Wolf AS. Homicide and blackout in Alaskan natives. J Stud Alcohol 1980;41:456–62.

58. Goodwin DW. Alcohol amnesia. Addiction 1995;90:315–7.

59. Perry PJ, Argo T, Barnett MJ, et al. The association of alcohol-induced blackouts and grayouts to blood alcohol concentrations. J Forensic Sci 2006;51:896–9.
60. Sweeney DF. Alcoholic blackouts. Legal implications. J Subst Abuse Treat 1990; 7:155–9.
61. Goodwin DW, Crane JB, Guze SB. Alcoholic "blackouts": a review and clinical study of 100 alcoholics. Am J Psychiatry 1969;126:191–8.
62. Jennison KM, Johnson KA. Drinking-induced blackouts among young adults: results from a national longitudinal study. Int J Addict 1994;29:23–51.
63. White AM, Jamieson-Drake DW, Swartzwelder HS. Prevalence and correlates of alcohol-induced blackouts among college students: results of an e-mail survey. J Am Coll Health 2002;51:117–31.
64. Hartzler B, Fromme K. Fragmentary and en bloc blackouts: similarity and distinction among episodes of alcohol-induced memory loss. J Stud Alcohol 2003;64: 547–50.
65. Brown SC, Craik FI. Encoding and retrieval of information. In: Tulvig E, Craik FI, editors. The oxford handbook of memory. New York: Oxford University Press; 2000. p. 93–107.
66. Calhoun FS, Weston SW. Contemporary threat management: a practical guide for identifying, assessing and managing individuals of violent intent. San Diego (CA): Specialized Training Services; 2003.
67. Rogers R, Bagby RM, Dickens SE. Structured interview of reported symptoms: professional manual. Odessa (FL): Psychological Assessment Resources; 1992.
68. Butcher JN, Dahlstrom WG, Graham JIR, et al. MMPI-2: manual for administration and scoring. Minneapolis (MN): University of Minnesota Press; 1989.
69. Tombaugh TN. Test of memory malingering. North Tonawanda (NY): Multi Health Systems; 1996.
70. Green P, Lees-Haley PR, Allen LM. The word memory test and the validity of neuropsychological test scores. J Forensic Neuropsychol 2002;2:97–124.
71. Widows MR, Smith GP. Structured inventory of malingered symptomatology professional manual. Odessa (FL): Psychological Assessment Resources; 2005.
72. Kelly PJ, Baker GA, van den Broek MD, et al. The detection of malingering in memory performance: the sensitive and specificity of four measures in a UK population. Br J Clin Psychol 2005;44:333–41.
73. Denney RL, Wynkoop TF. Clinical neuropsychology in the criminal forensic setting. J Head Trauma Rehabil 2000;15:804–28.
74. Wiggins EC, Brandt J. The detection of simulated amnesia. Law Hum Behav 1988;12:57–77.
75. Cave C, Squire L. Intact and long-lasting repetition priming in amnesia. J Exp Psychol Learn Mem Cogn 1992;18:509–20.
76. Binder LM, Pankratz L. Neuropsychological evidence of a factitious memory complaint. J Clin Exp Neuropsychol 1987;9:167–71.
77. Greve KW, Binder LM, Bianchini J. Rates of below-chance performance in forced-choice symptom validity tests. Clin Neuropsychol 2009;23:533–44.
78. Reed JM, Squire LR. Retrograde amnesia for facts and events: findings from four new cases. J Neurosci 1998;18:3943–54.
79. Kopelman MD, Stahhope M, Kingsley D. Retrograde amnesia in patients with diencephalic, temporal lobe or frontal lobe lesions. Neuropsychologia 1999;37: 939–58.
80. Kapur N, Young A, Bateman D, et al. Focal retrograde amnesia: a long term clinical and neuropsychological follow-up. Cortex 1989;25:387–402.

81. Albert MS, Butters N, Brandt J. Memory for remote events in alcoholics. J Stud Alcohol 1980;41:1071–81.
82. Hamsher K, Roberts RJ. Memory for recent U.S. presidents in patients with cerebral disease. J Clin Exp Neuropsychol 1985;7:1–13.
83. Evans JJ, Breen EK, Antoun N, et al. Focal retrograde amnesia for autobiographical events following cerebral vasculitis: a connectionist account. Neurocase 1998;2:1–11.
84. Crovitz HF, Schiffman H. Frequency of episodic memories as a function of their age. Bull Psychon Soc 1974;4:517–8.
85. Kopelman MD. The autobiographical memory interview (AMI) in organic and psychogenic amnesia. Memory 1994;2:211–35.
86. Denney RL. Symptom validity testing of remote memory in a criminal forensic setting. Arch Clin Neuropsychol 1996;7:589–603.
87. Allen JJ, Iacono WG. Assessing the validity of amnesia in dissociative identity disorder: a dilemma for the DSM and the courts. Psychol Publ Pol 2001;7:311–44.
88. Lykken DT. A tremor in the blood. Reading (England): Perseus Publishing; 1998.
89. Lorber MF. Psychophysiology of aggression, psychopathy, and conduct problems: a meta-analysis. Psychol Bull 2004;130:531–2.
90. Rosenfeld JP, Willwanger J, Sweet J. Detecting simulated amnesia with event-related brain potentials. Int J Psychophysiol 1995;19:1–11.
91. Vo ML, Jacobs AM, Kuchinke L, et al. The coupling of emotion and cognition in the eye: introducing the pupil old/new effect. Psychophysiology 2008;45:130–40.
92. Heaver B, Hutton SB. Keeping an eye on the truth? Pupil size changes associated with recognition memory. Memory 2011;19:398–405.
93. Markowitsch HJ, Kalbe E. Neuroimaging and crime. In: Christianson SA, editor. Offenders' memories of violent crimes. Chichester (England): John Wiley & Sons; 2007. p. 137–64.
94. Spiegel D. Forensic uses of hypnosis. In: Rosner R, editor. Principles and practice of forensic psychiatry. New York: Chapman & Hall; 1994. p. 485–9.
95. Piper A. Truth serum and recovered memories of sexual abuse: a review of the evidence. J Psychiatry Law 1993;21:447–71.

Child Pornography and the Internet

Humberto Temporini, MD

KEYWORDS

• Child pornography • Internet • Sex offender • Risk assessment

KEY POINTS

- Possession of child pornography is a felony crime in the United States.
- The incidence of child pornography offenses has increased as a result of the availability, affordability, and anonymity provided by the Internet.
- Several types of offenders have been proposed based on behavior and motivation.
- Child pornography offenses are indicators of pedophilia.
- Child pornography offenses increase the risk of contact offenses in individuals with a prior history of contact offenses.

INTRODUCTION

There are few crimes that carry almost universal condemnation and are viewed as despicable by society as a whole. Sexual contact with children is one of them. Pedophiles do not elicit sympathy or compassion, unlike other criminals may. Adults engaging in sexual activity with children inspire an innate disgust in most people.[1] In addition, the public tends to perceive sex offenders who victimize children as more dangerous and in need of more supervision in comparison with those charged with other sexual offenses, like nonconsensual spousal intercourse or statutory rape.[2]

While the actual number of reported instances of sexual abuse in the United States has decreased steadily over the past 2 decades,[3,4] the number of cases involving the possession and production of child pornography are on the rise.[5] Over the past 15 years, as the Internet has become an almost essential part of our lives, pornography has increasingly shifted from videotapes and DVDs, magazines, and photos to a variety of electronic formats. Today, movies and pictures of all kinds can be streamed to desktop and laptop computers, personal tablet devices (iPad), and mobile phones. It is no surprise that child pornography has undergone a similar transformation. Once a difficult to find and rather costly possession for individuals with

Department of Psychiatry, Kaiser Permanente South Sacramento Medical Center, 7300 Wyndham Drive, Sacramento, CA 95823, USA
E-mail address: Humberto.D.Temporini@kp.org

Psychiatr Clin N Am 35 (2012) 821–835
http://dx.doi.org/10.1016/j.psc.2012.08.004
0193-953X/12/$ – see front matter © 2012 Elsevier Inc. All rights reserved.

sexual interest in children, child pornography is now available free of charge from any mobile phone with data access.

CHILD PORNOGRAPHY OVERVIEW

The definition of what constitutes child pornography varies depending on jurisdiction. Federal law in the United States defines child pornography as any visual depiction of sexually explicit conduct involving a minor (someone under 18 years of age).[6] The US Code further establishes that "visual depictions" include photographs, videos, digital or computer-generated images indistinguishable from an actual minor, and images created, adapted, or modified, but appearing to depict an identifiable, actual minor. United States law does not require that a minor be involved in sexual activity to meet the definition of child pornography. In fact, a photograph of a naked child may constitute child pornography if it is suggestive enough. Furthermore, the definition also includes virtual child pornography: computer-generated images of children that meet the criteria described.

In the United States the production, distribution, and possession of these images are considered criminal behaviors. Images of child pornography are not protected under First Amendment rights and are illegal contraband under federal law.[6] Most cases of possession and production are prosecuted in US Federal court, as they usually involve the Internet or other means of interstate commerce (ie, postal service or couriers). Penalties for these crimes are severe: the production of child pornography in an individual with no prior record carries a minimum sentence of 15 years. The distribution of child pornography via the Internet or interstate commerce carries a 5-year mandatory minimum sentence. The penalties may increase if aggravating factors are present. Examples of these include the presence of sadistic, masochistic, or violent images, sexual abuse of the child at the hands of the convicted individual, and prior convictions for child sexual exploitation.

Images and movies depicting sexual abuse of children are easily obtained online. The actual amount available is exceedingly difficult to ascertain, given the decentralized nature of the Internet and the disparate types of network where these images and movies can be found. Most users are familiar with email, the Web, and using browsers to access the Web. Internet relay chat (IRC), Usenet newsgroups, and peer-to-peer (P2P) networks are also part of the Internet, and have come to constitute common sources of child pornography.

CHILD PORNOGRAPHY AND INTERNET COMMUNICATION METHODS
Internet Relay Chat

IRC is a system that allows users to talk to each other in real time. IRC is organized into "channels" where users share a common interest. A good analogy to these channels is a CB radio: a user tunes into a channel by logging in and is then able to see the real-time messages posted by other users.[7] In addition, IRC allows for private communication between users, as well as transfer of files. Common chat programs, such as MSN or Yahoo messenger, are similar to IRC as they allow group chats, private chats, and file transfers.

An early survey of IRC networks found that there were 55 channels with titles related to child pornography.[7,8] The names of these channels can be very descriptive at times (eg, #babysex, #kinky_preteensex) but they may also use monikers that are not indicative of child pornography. In addition, the number channels that are publicly viewable is dwarfed by the number of so-called private channels: unlisted forums that can be accessed via invitation only.

The importance of IRC as a source of abusive material became clear in a sample of individuals arrested for possession of child pornography between 1996 and 2001: 78% had obtained at least some of their content from an IRC network.[9]

Newsgroups

Newsgroups are public discussion forums that cover a very large number of topics. Individuals can post, read, and reply to "articles" posted by others. Internet service providers (ISPs) subscribe to particular newsgroups, which are then available for the users. Most email programs include a newsgroup feature that allows for easy access to the material. There are several thousands of newsgroups, in different languages, and stored on separate computers called news servers. Individuals can post a variety of different materials to these groups, such as movies and pictures, which can then be accessed by others. The names of the newsgroups may quickly identify the material in the articles (ie, alt.fan.barry-manilow or alt.sex.bestiality).

In the 1990s, as newsgroups emerged as the first social networks, several studies attempted to quantify the amount of pornography and child pornography accessible from these sources. Of 9800 pornographic images retrieved from 32 newsgroups between July 1995 and July 1996, approximately 20% included children and adolescents. Nearly half of these (5.1% of the total sample) were identified as "nudity only," while another 40% (4.4% of the total number of images) were identified as pedophilic.[10] Another survey of newsgroups from one week in January 1998 suggested that there were approximately 40,000 newsgroups, and that 0.07% of them contained major elements of child pornography. The survey identified approximately 6058 pictures, a third of which could be considered pornographic.[7] Most of the images identified in that survey appeared to be 20 to 30 years old.

While Internet traffic in the newsgroups has continued to grow over the past 15 years and reached 9.29 terabytes per day in January 2012, the amount of traffic in P2P networks and the Web has grown much more. It is likely that the bulk of traffic in child pornography material online has switched from newsgroups and IRC to the Web and P2P networks.

World Wide Web

According to statistics from the Internet Watch Foundation (IWF), a United Kingdom–based watchdog organization, at the end of 2011 there were 12,966 URLs (Web addresses) containing child pornography.[11] These addresses were hosted in 1595 domains located in 39 countries. As high as these figures may appear, they are approximately 50% lower than they were in 2006. Some of this material was hosted in sites that provided movies and pictures on a commercial basis. Such Web sites can be accessed only after paying a fee, and thus profit financially from the sale of images of child sexual abuse. Since 2009, the IWF has identified 998 unique sources of commercial child pornography. Of these, 440 were active in 2011.

While the World Wide Web (WWW) continues to be the most accessible way to find child pornography, there is evidence that searches for terms associated with this kind of material have decreased. Between January 2004 and November 2008, Google queries for key terms associated with child pornography (eg, Lolita, underage porn, preteen sex) declined by approximately 60%.[12] This change does not appear secondary to users switching to a different search engine; in fact, searches for the comparison term "xxx" have actually increased in the same period. The most likely explanation is that highly publicized operations against child pornography[13,14] have resulted in a shift in searches toward other media that increase the user's perception of anonymity, such as P2P networks.

Peer-to-Peer Networks

P2P file-sharing networks allow for the search and transfer of files directly from one computer to another without the use of an intermediate storing site. This scenario is clearly different from newsgroups and the WWW, where content is hosted on a server. To participate in P2P networking, individuals download software that connects them to a network of users. These programs can index the content of a specific folder or folders in a computer and make that content available to other users. P2P networks have received a fair amount of attention, as they are a source of all kinds of pirated material, from major movies and music to full software programs.

P2P networks have become the most common sources of child pornography material at present.[15] A report from 2003 by the US Government accountability office indicates that a simple search of key words on the KaZaA network yielded a large number of different files. Approximately 42% to 44% of these were images of child pornography.[16] In addition, a review of all the queries on the P2P network Gnutella over a period of several weeks showed that the unique term most commonly searched for was PTHC, an acronym for preteen hard core. This term is unmistakably associated with child pornography, as it is improbable that individuals without knowledge of the matter would randomly search for it. Searches for popular movies were second. In addition, the study showed that approximately 1% of all queries were related to child pornography, and that 7% of the hosts (individuals in the network) were sharing child pornography material. A review of the queries also showed that the predominant age searched for was 13 to 14 years old, with 76% of searches looking for material involving children ages 11 to 16. Approximately 30% of the searches originated in computers based in the United States, whereas 90% of the responses (ie, the computers where the material was located) were located in Brazil.[17]

A review of the arrests for possession of child pornography in the United States between 2000 and 2009 shows that the use of P2P to obtain this type of material has grown from 4% in 2000 to 28% in 2006 and 61% in 2009 (**Fig. 1**).[18]

When P2P users are compared with those who use other means to access child pornography, they tend to have the following characteristics:

- More likely to be younger (under 25 years old)
- More likely to have images of children younger than 3 years
- More likely to have images depicting sexual penetration and violence
- More likely to have videos
- More likely to have more than 1000 images
- More likely to distribute images

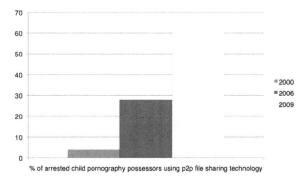

Fig. 1. Percentage of arrested child pornography possessors using peer-to-peer file-sharing technology.

OFFENDER CHARACTERISTICS
Why Individuals Access Child Pornography

The most common question that arises in the context of child pornography is the issue of motivation. Media reports tend to describe cases where the offenders are educated and employed men, often with no prior criminal record, who are arrested and found in possession of vast amounts of illicit material.[19] These cases are often perplexing to others as they search to understand the reasons behind this behavior. From a clinical standpoint, the rationale behind the possession of this material is very relevant. For example, an offender who collects child pornography as part of an interest in bizarre or taboo sexual practices is different from an offender who uses child pornography to entice minors to meet him for sex. Similarly, someone who distributes child pornography for financial profit has a clearly different motivation from someone who collects this material for his own sexual gratification.[20]

One of the first analyses of the reasons behind accessing child pornography identified 6 categories of explanations provided by 13 men arrested for downloading child pornography. These 6 reasons include the following[21]:

1. For sexual arousal, whether as a substitute or a stimulus for contact sexual offending
2. As part of an interest in collecting a complete set or series of images
3. As part of online networking with like-minded individuals
4. To fulfill a lack of satisfying relationships
5. To assist in self discovery and exploration of one's own problems
6. Part of a larger pattern of behavior including Internet addiction

Recent studies have highlighted a relationship between pedophilia and possession of child pornography. Although clearly not the only explanation for the collection of this material, sexual interest in children is a powerful motivator in these cases. For example, an examination of the sexual interest and behavior of 685 male patients showed that child pornography offenders were more likely to be sexually aroused by children (as measured by phallometric testing) than actual contact sexual offenders who had either child or adult victims.[22] Given this information, the possession of child pornography strongly suggests that the individual has an underlying diagnosis of pedophilia. Another indication of the relationship between pedophilia and child pornography comes from an online survey of the responses of 290 individuals who characterized themselves as boy-attracted pedophiles.[23] The respondents were recruited from among those visiting www.boylinks.net, a Web site frequented by men interested in boys. Approximately 95% of this sample reported using child pornography for sexual purposes at some point in their lives.

A more recent study explored reasons given by 2 groups of child pornography offenders when asked about the motivation for their crimes.[24] One group comprised offenders interviewed by police in the context of investigating their crime while the other group consisted of convicted individuals who were evaluated in a forensic setting. Notably, less than 50% of each sample admitted to sexual interest in child pornography or children. Approximately 40% of the sample interviewed by police indicated that they had accessed the material accidentally or out of curiosity, whereas almost 30% of the sample assessed in a forensic setting claimed an addiction to pornography in general as the principal motivator for having obtained child pornography. Although this study may seem to contradict the previously described association between possession of child pornography and pedophilia, the role that social desirability plays in these individual's deceptive responses must be emphasized.

This minimization regarding the relationship of child pornography to deviant sexual fantasies and masturbation was illustrated in a Dutch study where researchers polygraphed 38 offenders convicted of child pornography offenses. During an initial interview, 55% of the sample denied ever masturbating to child pornography. Those who admitted to masturbating to child pornography reported that they had done so using only material depicting a single child in an erotic pose or naked. All offenders denied sexual interest in material depicting sexual contact between a child and an adult, sadistic sexual conduct, or sexual contact between children and animals. In addition, when asked about preferred material, the sample indicated that they were most interested in images of single naked children. After the polygraph evaluation, all 21 individuals who had originally denied masturbating to child pornography admitted masturbating to pornographic images of children. Furthermore, 32 of the 38 individuals in the sample admitted to masturbating to material depicting sexual contact between a child and an adult, with 10 individuals reporting masturbation to images of bestiality. The reported preferred type of images also changed after the polygraph evaluation, with most of the sample describing interest in images depicting children having sex with other children or with adults.[25]

As outlined below, to accurately assess the risk that these offenders may pose to the community it is essential to consider collateral sources of information. Mental health professionals evaluating or treating child pornography offenders frequently hear that the access to the material was "one time only" or accidental, only to find out that a forensic analysis of the computer used revealed a pattern of frequent and deliberate attempts to find child pornography.

Types of Child Pornography Offenders

Even before the Internet appeared, researchers attempted to develop typologies for child pornography offenders. An early classification scheme[26] based on men involved in 55 child pornography rings identified 4 different types of child pornography possessors: closet collectors; pedophile collectors; cottage collectors; and commercial collectors. Closet collectors are secretive about their interest in child pornography; they lack communication with other individuals with similar sexual interest and they do not have contact with children. Pedophile collectors have pornographic material and have sexual contact with children. Their collections may include material obtained from their own sexual abuse of children. Cottage collectors are those who abuse children and share their material with other individuals with similar interests. Finally, commercial collectors are those who financially profit from the distribution of child pornography.

A more recent classification scheme takes into account the behavior of the offender and suggests the presence of 3 different types of offenders: traders, travelers, and trader-travelers.[19] Traders are offenders who amass and share collections of child pornography. Travelers are those who use the Internet to arrange in person meetings with children for the purpose of sexual contact. Trader-travelers collect and share child pornography while using the Internet to set up in-person encounters. This particular typology derives from the analysis of 225 cases publicized in news media articles. This sample may not be representative of all child pornography offenders, as it represents the more sensational cases that make the news and lacks more detailed clinical information that would typically be obtained from direct interviews. Though imperfect, both classifications suggest that child pornography offenders are a heterogeneous group of individuals with different levels of risk for contact offenses.

Other typologies classify child pornography offenders based on their behavior and motivation, and suggest a continuum of increased seriousness of offending. The Australian Institute of Criminology classification,[27] developed in 2004, uses 3 factors to rate the seriousness of the offense:

1. The nature of the abuse, from indirect to direct victimization of the child
2. The level of networking by the offender
3. The level of security used to avoid detection

According to this scheme, offense severity increases depending on the number and intensity of these factors. **Table 1** describes the different types of offenders based on this classification.

The different levels of offending highlighted in this typology clearly describe the behavior of the individual engaged in Internet child pornography. However, this scheme does not provide a clear assessment of the risk for crossover into contact offenses. For example, can a browser become a trawler and then a groomer?

A 2010 behavioral analysis of child pornography offenders attempts to improve the attribution of risk for crossing over from simple possession to contact offender by evaluating the offender's motivation.[20] This typology classifies offenders into the following 3 categories:

1. Situational offenders
2. Preferential offenders
3. Miscellaneous offenders.

Situational offenders
Situational offenders are individuals who possess child pornography but who may not have actual pedophilic interests. Examples of situational offenders include the following:

a. Normal adolescent/adult: persons who are searching online for pornography and sex and stumble onto child pornography. This category includes adolescents sharing sexually explicit photos/videos of themselves or peers.
b. Morally indiscriminate: individuals with antisocial traits and a history of criminal offenses. Parents who make their children available for sex online fit this definition.
c. Profiteers: criminals who traffic in child pornography for financial or sexual gain. For example, those who blackmail victims, demanding more material after getting them to engage in sexual conduct.

Preferential offenders
Preferential offenders are Individuals who have sexual interest in children, ranging from a mild interest to a primary interest. Examples include:

a. Pedophiles: individuals who have a sexual preference for minors.
b. Diverse: individuals with a wide variety of sexual interests but no strong sexual preference for children. Such offenders are also described as sexually indiscriminate.
c. Latent: individuals with potentially illegal, but previously latent sexual preferences. It is not uncommon for these individuals to experience a decrease in their sexual inhibitions following contact with like-minded peers online.

Miscellaneous offenders
Miscellaneous offenders are individuals who break the law without sexual interest or intent. Examples include media reporters researching child pornography or naively

Table 1
Krone's typology of Internet offenders

Type of Involvement	Features	Level of Networking by Offender	Security Used	Nature of Abuse
Browser	Response to spam, accidental hit on suspect site—material knowingly saved	Nil	Nil	Indirect
Private fantasy	Conscious creation of online text or digital images for private use	Nil	Nil	Indirect
Trawler	Actively seeking child pornography using openly available browsers	Low	Nil	Indirect
Nonsecure collector	Actively seeking material often through peer-to-peer networks	High	Nil	Indirect
Secure collector	Actively seeking material but only through secure networks. Collector syndrome and exchange as an entry barrier	High	Secure	Indirect
Groomer	Cultivating an online relationship with one or more children. The offender may or may not seek material in any of the above ways. Pornography may be used to facilitate abuse	Varies—online contact with individual children	Security depends on child	Direct
Physical abuser	Abusing a child who may have been introduced to the offender online. The offender may or may not seek material in any of the above ways. Pornography may be used to facilitate abuse	Varies—physical contact with individual children	Security depends on child	Direct
Producer	Records own abuse or that of others (or induces children to submit images of themselves)	Varies—may depend on whether becomes a distributor	Security depends on child	Direct
Distributor	May distribute at any of the above levels	Varies	Tends to be secure	Indirect

attempting to arrange meetings with sex offenders, as well as pranksters and over-zealous civilians attempting sting operations.

Taken together, these different typologies suggest the presence of 4 groups of offenders[8]:

1. Individuals who access child pornography sporadically, impulsively, or out of curiosity

2. Individuals who access and trade child pornography images to fuel their sexual interest in children
3. Individuals who use the Internet as a pattern of offline contact offending
4. Individuals who access child pornography for nonsexual reasons, such as financial profit.

INTERNET OFFENDERS AND CONTACT OFFENDERS: ARE THEY SIMILAR OR NOT?

Evidence exists supporting both answers to this question. Many studies have found that a subgroup of Internet offenders have had prior sexual contact with a child.[20,28,29] Sexual attraction to children has been described as a significant risk factor in the commission of sexual offenses against minors.[30] As already described, the majority of online offenders display a pedophilic pattern of sexual arousal that becomes evident when assessed with penile plethysmography.[22]

By contrast, a meta-analysis of 9 studies that compared samples of child pornography offenders with contact sexual offenders identified several differences between the 2 groups[31]:

- Online offenders tend to have higher IQs and are better educated than sex offenders who have no history of accessing child pornography.[32]
- Online offenders tend to be younger and are less likely to be of a racial minority.
- Online offenders report lower rates of physical abuse than contact sex offenders.
- Online offenders have greater levels of sexual deviancy, more victim empathy, and less manipulation of others to view them in a positive light.
- Online offenders are more likely to have had mental health contact in adulthood.

Characteristics of those who committed actual contact offenses include the following:

- Contact offenders tended to have higher levels of psychopathy and antisocial attitudes than online offenders.
- Contact offenders had more instances of substance misuse during the commission of the offense.
- Contact offenders tended to have greater emotional identification with children, as well as more cognitive distortions regarding their deviant sexual activity.

Child pornography offenders who have not had actual sexual contact with children are generally aware of the damaging consequences that may result from sexual contact between children and adults. Still, they often fail to acknowledge that they have committed a crime or that they have any responsibility for the harm caused by the sexual activities depicted in child pornography.[33] In addition, although child pornography offenders demonstrate a lower frequency of cognitive distortions than contact sexual offenders, cognitive distortions are by no means absent. As frequently seen with other types of sex offenders, cognitive distortions are used to downplay the seriousness of the crime and minimize accountability.[34] Child pornography offenders may indicate that they have not created victims, that they are not sex offenders, and that their activities are almost inoffensive when compared with those of contact offenders.[35] To justify their minimizing of the potential harm of child pornography to children involved, child pornography collectors may indicate that the children in the pictures or videos were smiling and therefore were enjoying the activity.

RELATIONSHIP OF POSSESSION OF CHILD PORNOGRAPHY WITH CONTACT SEXUAL OFFENDING

The main concern for both lawmakers and evaluators in the area of Internet offenders is whether there is a relationship between viewing or collecting child pornography and contact sexual offenses. Questions usually arise in 2 areas:

1. The offender's background and the possibility of prior undisclosed or unknown sexual offenses
2. The possibility that someone who downloads child pornography will progress to committing a contact sexual offense

The answer to these questions continues to be somewhat equivocal, although there is evidence that these individuals are a rather heterogeneous group, with different levels of risk depending on motivation, personality traits, and history.

Assessing Risk of Contact

A large number of individuals express their sexual interest in children by collecting child pornography, and never engage in contact offenses.[28] These offenders most commonly use illicit material for sexual stimulation (ie, masturbation), although other purported motivations include networking with like-minded peers, addiction to pornography, or even an attempt at decreasing the likelihood of engaging in a contact sexual offense. In others, this conduct is not the result of a sexual interest in children, but rather an indicator of a general pattern of impulsive and rather indiscriminate sexual behavior. Finally, another group of individuals go on to commit sexual offenses against children after viewing this material. The identification of factors that distinguish these groups is of utmost importance, as it could guide policy, treatment decisions, and allocation of resources toward offenders posing the highest levels of risk.

Although the use of actuarial risk-assessment instruments (eg, Static-99, Sex Offender Risk Appraisal Guide [SORAG]) is commonplace in the evaluation of sex offenders, there is little evidence of their utility in a group of individuals without a history of contact offenses. These instruments were developed to identify individuals who are more likely to engage in contact sexual reoffending and not those who may sexually offend for the first time. In the case of child pornography offenders without a history of contact offenses, the goal is to identify factors that would predict the onset of contact sexual offending, as opposed to the persistence of sexual offending after a first incident.[36] There is evidence that these instruments may overpredict the risk of future reoffending.[37,38] The use of a modified version of the Risk Matrix 2000 (RM2000) has yielded positive preliminary results in the prediction of recidivism in this group.[37,39]

Assessing Prior Sexual Offenders

The importance of obtaining accurate information about an individual's history of sexual offenses in the context of a risk assessment cannot be overemphasized. For example, if the evaluator is aware of a prior contact offense, actuarial instruments may be used to provide a preliminary idea of the individual's likelihood to reoffend. Common instruments, such as the Static-99 or the SORAG, do not include child pornography offenses as variables considered in the assessment of risk. Instead, they focus on static factors that are unlikely to change (ie, age at offense, criminal history, type of victims). There is significant evidence, however, that the use of child pornography in individuals with a prior history of contact offenses increases the risk for contact reoffending.

For example, a study of criminal recidivism in a sample of 341 child molesters found that those individuals who viewed child pornography were 233% more likely to commit a new sexual offense than those who did not use such material.[40] In a sample of 541 online offenders followed for an average of 4.1 years after the index offense, 4.1% of the total sample went on to commit a new contact sex offense and 7% were charged with a new child pornography offense. Only 3 of 228 individuals with no record of prior contact offenses and a current child pornography offense went on to commit a contact sexual offense. By contrast, 16% of child pornography offenders with a prior history of contact sexual offenses went on to commit a new contact sexual offense.[41]

The rates of prior contact sexual offending among child pornography offenders have been reviewed in a recent meta-analysis.[28] Of a total sample of 4697 online offenders, 17.3% were known to have committed a contact sexual offense, mostly against a child. There was significant variability in the rates of contact sexual offenses reported in the study depending on the sample type: arrested (ie, pretrial) suspects tend to have lower reported rates of prior sexual offenses than samples of incarcerated offenders. In addition, clinical samples (ie, offenders referred for treatment) have the highest rates of reported prior contact sexual offending of any kind.

There is considerable debate about the accuracy of the reported rates of prior contact sexual offending by online offenders. In particular, these rates are significantly different depending on the source of information. It is expected that rates of prior contact sexual offending derived from self report will be higher than those provided by official records because not all crimes are reported, investigated, or prosecuted. Still, some studies have described very high rates of prior offending that appear to be clear outliers when compared with the rest of the data available. For example, a well-publicized report from the US Federal Bureau of Prisons[29] indicated that approximately 85% of a sample of incarcerated child pornography offenders in a treatment program described that they had committed a previous hands-on sex offense. This study has been criticized for the possibility that the participants had an incentive to disclose prior sexual contacts, even if they had not occurred, as a sign of progress in their treatment.[28]

The polygraph has also been used in an effort to identify those Internet child pornography offenders with prior histories of contact sexual offenses. In a Dutch sample of 25 child pornography offenders, the number of individuals who acknowledged having sought sex with children increased from 1 individual to 15 after a polygraph interview.[42] Despite this promising finding, the use of the polygraph continues to be controversial, and its use in the evaluation of child pornography offenders demands caution.[43]

If the accurate assessment of a prior history of contact sexual offenses seems difficult, the question of future offending in this group is even more controversial. The role that possession of child pornography by itself plays in the genesis of contact sexual offenses appears to be minimal. To date, there is no evidence of a direct causal link between Internet offending and the commission of a contact offense.[37] In fact, pornography seems to play a role in sexual offenses only in individuals who are "predisposed" to do so. If the predisposition is present, then pornography use may increase the risk. Otherwise, pornography possession alone does not appear to be sufficient to originate sexual offending.[25]

Assessing Internet Offenders in Comparison with Contact Offenders

A recent study sought to identify factors that would differentiate between Internet-only offenders, those that had both Internet offenses and contact offenses, and a group of child molesters with no Internet offenses. Using two scales, one measuring antisocial behavior and another assessing Internet preoccupation, the investigators were able to predict membership in each group (Internet offenders only, Internet offenders with contact offenses, and child molesters) with reasonable accuracy.[44] The Internet-only offenders were low on the antisocial behavior scale and high on Internet preoccupation. The child molesters with no Internet offenses were, as expected, low on Internet preoccupation and high on antisocial behavior. Finally, the child pornography offenders with a history of contact offenses were high on both scales. This finding adds to the existing evidence linking the commission of hands-on sexual offense with the presence of antisocial behavior. For example, child pornography offenders with a prior history of criminal behavior were significantly more likely to reoffend, either sexually or generally.[45] Other factors associated with increased risk of sexual contact reoffending include offender age at first offense (the younger the age, the higher the risk), the presence of a juvenile record, substance-abuse problems, prior violent offenses, and admitted hebephilic interests.[46] These risk factors are consistent with the evidence available regarding risk to reoffend in other types of sex offenders, such as rapists and child molesters. In these groups, the likelihood to recidivate increases with the presence of antisocial behavior and deviant sexual interests.[30]

SUMMARY

The Internet is a ubiquitous part of our lives. Its role has affected many aspects of our daily activities, communications, and entertainment. The increase in cybercrime has been a by-product of this popularity. Fueled by the feeling of anonymity that the Internet provides, many individuals have engaged in behaviors that would have been unlikely before its advent. Using the Internet to obtain or trade child pornography is one of them. Child pornography offenses have increased dramatically over the past 10 years, even as the rates of child sexual abuse have decreased significantly in the same period. The significance of this surge in interest in material considered abhorrent by the majority of society continues to be unclear. Is this a crime brought on by the anonymity of the Internet and availability of the material, or is it a blueprint for the commission of a contact sexual offense?

The vast majority of individuals found in possession of this material are likely to meet the diagnostic criteria for pedophilia. Although pedophilic interest is a risk factor for sexual reoffending, it is unlikely that its presence alone would result in sexual contact with a child in an individual without a prior history of such offenses. Research suggests that the risk to commit a hands-on sexual crime results from the interplay between deviant sexual interests, antisocial tendencies, and difficulties in the ability to control one's behavior.

REFERENCES

1. Finkelhor D. What's wrong with sex between adults and children? Ethics and the problem of sexual abuse. Am J Orthop 1979;49(4):692–7.
2. Kernsmith P, Craun S, Foster J. Public attitudes toward sexual offenders and sex offender registration. J Child Sex Abus 2009;18(3):290–301.
3. US Department of Health and Human Services, Administration for Children and Families. Bureau of children research statistics [internet]. Available at: http://www.acf.hhs.gov/programs/cb/stats_research/. Accessed June 30, 2012.
4. Finkelhor D, Turner H, Ormrod R, et al. Trends in childhood violence and abuse exposure: evidence from 2 national surveys. Arch Pediatr Adolesc Med 2010; 164(3):238–42.

5. Motivans M, Kyckelhahn T. Federal prosecution of child sex exploitation offenders, 2006 [internet] Bureau of Justice Statistics. 2007. Available at: http://bjs.ojp.usdoj.gov/index.cfm?ty=pbdetail&iid=886. Accessed July1, 2012.
6. Citizens guide to US federal law in child pornography [internet]. USDOJ: CRM: Child Exploitation and Obscenity Section. Available at: http://www.justice.gov/criminal/ceos/citizensguide/citizensguide_porn.html. Accessed June 30, 2012.
7. The Department of Justice and Equality. Illegal and harmful use of the internet—first report of the working group [internet]. Available at: http://www.inis.gov.ie/en/JELR/Pages/Illegal_use_of_the_Internet_report. Accessed June 30, 2012.
8. Beech A, Elliott IA, Birgden A, et al. The internet and child sexual offending: a criminological review. Aggression Violent Behaviour 2008;13(3):216–28.
9. Carr A. Internet traders of child pornography and other censorship offenders in New Zealand [internet]. Available at: http://www.dia.govt.nz/Pubforms.nsf/URL/entirereport.pdf/$file/entirereport.pdf. Accessed June 30, 2012.
10. Mehta MD. Pornography in Usenet: a study of 9,800 randomly selected images. Cyberpsychol Behav 2001;4(6):695–703.
11. 2011 annual report | internet watch foundation (IWF) [internet]. Available at: http://www.iwf.org.uk/accountability/annual-reports/2011-annual-report. Accessed June 30, 2012.
12. Steel C. Web-based child pornography: quantification and qualification of demand. International Journal Digital Crime Forensics 2009;1(4):58.
13. FBI—overview and history: innocent images national initiative [internet]. Available at: http://www.fbi.gov/stats-services/publications/innocent-images-1. Accessed June 30, 2012.
14. Krone T. International police operations against online child pornography. Crime Justice Int 2005;21(89):11–20.
15. Wolak J, Finkelhor D, Mitchell K. Child pornography possessors: trends in offender and case characteristics. Sex Abuse 2011;23(1):22–4.
16. U.S. GAO-file-sharing programs: peer-to-peer networks provide ready access to child pornography [internet]. Available at: http://www.gao.gov/products/gao-03-351. Accessed June 30, 2012.
17. Steel CM. Child pornography in peer-to-peer networks. Child Abuse Negl 2009;33(8):560–8.
18. Wolak J, Finkelhor D, Mitchell K. Trends in arrests for child pornography possession: the third national juvenile online victimization study (NJOV-3) [internet]. Crimes Against Children Research Center 2012. Available at: http://www.unh.edu/ccrc/internet-crimes/paper.html. Accessed June 30, 2012.
19. Alexy E, Burgess A, Baker T. Internet offenders: traders, travelers, and combination trader-travelers. J Interpers Violence 2005;20(7):804–12.
20. Lanning K. Child molesters: a behavioral analysis [internet]. National Center for Missing and Exploited Children 2010. Available at: http://www.missingkids.com/en_US/publications/NC70.pdf. Accessed June 30, 2012.
21. Quayle E, Taylor M. Child pornography and the internet: perpetuating a cycle of abuse. Deviant Behav 2002;23(4):331–6.
22. Seto M, Cantor J, Blanchard R. Child pornography offenses are a valid diagnostic indicator of pedophilia. J Abnorm Psychol 2006;115(3):610–5.
23. Riegel D. Effects on boy-attracted pedosexual males of viewing boy erotica. Arch Sex Behav 2004;33(4):321–3.
24. Seto M, Reeves L, Jung S. Explanations given by child pornography offenders for their crimes. Journal of Sexual Aggression 2010;16(2):169–80.

25. Seto MC, Maric A, Barbaree HE. The role of pornography in the etiology of sexual aggression. Aggression Violent Behaviour 2001;6(1):35–53.

26. Hartmann C, Burgess A, Lanning K. Typology of collectors. In: Burgess A, editor. Child pornography and sex rings. Toronto: Lexington Books; 1984. p. 93.

27. Krone T. A typology of online child pornography offending [internet]. Australian Institute of Criminology. 2004. Available at: http://www.aic.gov.au/publications/current series/cfi/81-100/cfi084.aspx. Accessed June 30, 2012.

28. Seto M, Hanson RK, Babchishin K. Contact sexual offending by men with online sexual offenses. Sex Abuse 2011;23(1):124–45.

29. Bourke ML, Hernandez AE. The 'Butner study' redux: a report of the incidence of hands-on child victimization by child pornography offenders. J Fam Violence 2009;24(3):183–91.

30. Hanson RK, Morton Bourgon K. The characteristics of persistent sexual offenders: a meta-analysis of recidivism studies. J Consult Clin Psychol 2005; 73(6):1154–63.

31. Babchishin K, Hanson RK, Hermann C. The characteristics of online sex offenders: a meta-analysis. Sex Abuse 2011;23(1):92–123.

32. Blanchard R, Kolla N, Cantor J, et al. IQ, handedness, and pedophilia in adult male patients stratified by referral source. Sex Abuse 2007;19(3):285–309.

33. Winder B, Gough B. "I never touched anybody—that's my defence": a qualitative analysis of internet sex offender accounts. Journal of Sexual Aggression 2010; 16(2):125–41.

34. Abel GG, Becker JV, Cunningham Rathner J. Complications, consent, and cognitions in sex between children and adults. Int J Law Psychiatry 1984;7(1):89–103.

35. Howitt D, Sheldon K. The role of cognitive distortions in paedophilic offending: internet and contact offenders compared. Psychol Crime Law 2007;13(5):469–86.

36. Seto M. In: Assessing the risk posed by child pornography offenders. Global symposium for examining the relationship between online and offline offenses and preventing the sexual exploitation of children; 2009; University of North Carolina, Durham, April 5–7, 2009.

37. Webb L, Craissati J, Keen S. Characteristics of internet child pornography offenders: a comparison with child molesters. Sex Abuse 2007;19(4):449–65.

38. Osborn J, Elliott I, Middleton D, et al. The use of actuarial risk assessment measures with UK internet child pornography offenders. Journal of Aggression, Conflict and Peace Research 2010;2(3):16–24.

39. Wakeling H, Howard P, Barnett G. Comparing the validity of the RM2000 scales and OGRS3 for predicting recidivism by internet sexual offenders. Sex Abuse 2011;23(1):146–68.

40. Kingston D, Fedoroff P, Firestone P, et al. Pornography use and sexual aggression: the impact of frequency and type of pornography use on recidivism among sexual offenders. Aggress Behav 2008;34(4):341–5.

41. Eke A, Seto M, Williams J. Examining the criminal history and future offending of child pornography offenders: an extended prospective follow-up study. Law Hum Behav 2011;35(6):466–78.

42. Buschman J, Bogaerts S, Foulger S, et al. Sexual history disclosure polygraph examinations with cybercrime offences: a first Dutch explorative study. Int J Offender Ther Comp Criminol 2010;54(3):395–411.

43. Robilotta SA, Mercado CC, DeGue S. Application of the polygraph examination in the assessment and treatment of internet sex offenders. J Forensic Psychol Pract 2008;8(4):383–9.

44. Lee A, Li N, Lamade R, et al. Predicting hands-on child sexual offenses among possessors of internet child pornography. Psychol Publ Pol Law 2012. Advance online publication.
45. Seto M, Eke A. The criminal histories and later offending of child pornography offenders. Sex Abuse 2005;17(2):201–10.
46. Seto M. In: A picture is worth a thousand words: what do we know about child pornography offenders? Association for the Treatment of Sex Offenders annual conference. Montreal, October 1, 2009.

Juvenile Offenders
Competence to Stand Trial

Matthew Soulier, MD

KEYWORDS

- Juvenile justice • Competency • Immaturity

KEY POINTS

- All states, except Oklahoma, have recognized the right of juveniles to be competent to stand trial.
- The standard for juvenile competency to stand trial has not been determined by the US Supreme Court.
- Incompetency of a juvenile may by caused by "developmental immaturity."
- The assessment of juvenile adjudicative competency should include a structured instrument to aid the evaluator in making a forensic opinion within reasonable medical certainty.

INTRODUCTION

A juvenile required to stand before an early twentieth-century judge would hardly recognize the same juvenile justice system he or she would face today. Such a juvenile might wonder why an attorney was present and what to say to their newly appointed counsel. A more formal juvenile justice system developed in the late 1800s as a byproduct of social reformers concerned about the abused, neglected, and delinquent youths who were being treated and punished as adults. These reformers believed that such wayward children deserved a chance at rehabilitation consistent with the *parens patriae* doctrine,[1] a philosophy that emphasized the role of the state functioning in a parental, rather than a punitive role. Early juvenile courts were not intended to be adversarial or resemble adult court in form or function.

The first juvenile court was established in 1899 in Chicago, Illinois.[2] This court's mission was to help youths become productive and law-abiding adults. The early juvenile court was civil in nature and various legal rights provided to defendants in adult court were not applied to juvenile proceedings. In contrast to adult defendants, juveniles were not necessarily ensured adjudicative competence, or competence to stand trial. Competency to stand trial is a legal principle that defendants should have the

No disclosures.
Division of the Psychiatry and Law, University of California, Davis Medical Center, 2230 Stockton Boulevard, Sacramento, CA 95817, USA
E-mail address: matthew.soulier@ucdmc.ucdavis.edu

Psychiatr Clin N Am 35 (2012) 837–854
http://dx.doi.org/10.1016/j.psc.2012.08.005
0193-953X/12/$ – see front matter

ability to participate in their own trial proceedings. Although adult trials sought to maintain procedural protections of defendants (due process), the early American juvenile court system authorized the judge to determine how to best protect the youth before the court. The judge had ample latitude and authority in efforts to rehabilitate these deviant and often neglected youths. The juvenile court system grew throughout the country while operating under these ideals. Within 25 years, most states had created juvenile court systems.

This newly created system's attempt to rehabilitate delinquent juveniles without offering due process went virtually unchecked until the US Supreme Court heard the landmark juvenile justice case, *Kent V United States* (1966).[3] *Kent* concerned the constitutionality of a juvenile court judge having the authority to send a juvenile case to the adult criminal justice system instead of remaining before the juvenile court, a process known as "judicial waiver." Morris Kent was a 16-year-old boy alleged to have committed robbery, housebreaking, and rape. He was not informed of his right to remain silent while he was interrogated without a lawyer present. Kent admitted to the crimes. Kent's attorney arranged for a psychiatric evaluation. The evaluation concluded that Kent suffered from "severe psychopathology" and recommended psychiatric hospitalization. The juvenile court judge had the authority to waive Kent to an adult court. Kent's lawyer opposed the waiver and motioned to prove that Kent was suitable for rehabilitation if offered psychiatric hospitalization. This motion was ignored by the juvenile court judge and Kent was waived to the criminal court without a hearing. Kent was then found guilty and sentenced to 30–90 years in prison. Kent appealed his conviction to the US Supreme Court on the basis that his due process rights had been violated when he was not allowed a waiver hearing. The *Kent* Court held that a juvenile should receive a waiver hearing with appointed defense counsel, access to all records, and a written statement by the judge explaining the circumstances for the waiver. The *Kent* holding was the first of multiple decisions[4,5] by the Supreme Court in the ensuing decade, which forever altered the landscape of juvenile justice.

The year following *Kent*, the US Supreme Court continued its analysis of the inadequacies of the juvenile justice system in the case of *In Re Gault* (1967).[6] Gerald Gault was a fifteen-year-old-boy who was taken into custody without notice to his parents after he made a lewd telephone call to a neighbor. A deputy Sherriff filed a petition in a juvenile court, stating only that Gerald was a juvenile delinquent. During the hearing, Gerald was not offered counsel and the only witness was an unsworn deputy who said that Gerald admitted to the offense during questioning. On appeal, the US Supreme Court held that the Due Process Clause of the Fourteenth Amendment applied to juveniles. The Court famously reasoned, "Under our Constitution, the condition of being a boy does not justify a kangaroo court.[7]" As a result of this decision, new significant due process rights outlined in **Box 1** were extended to juveniles in the juvenile court system.

Box 1
Due process protections extended to juveniles as a result of *Gault*

- Notice of charges
- A hearing with represented counsel
- Protection against self-incrimination
- The right to confront and cross-examine witnesses

As a product of these 2 cases, the US Supreme Court extended many of the constitutional protections afforded to adults in the criminal justice system to youths involved in the juvenile justice system. Prominent exceptions included *McKeiver v Pennsylvania* (1976),[8] in which the US Supreme Court ruled that a jury trial was not required for juvenile court and the US Supreme Court in *Schall v Martin* (1984),[9] which upheld the constitutionality of pretrial preventive detention for juveniles. Despite these differences, the overall outcome of the US Supreme Court decisions following *Kent* has been a modern adversarial juvenile court with due process afforded to minors who potentially face severe penalties for offenses found true. Despite juveniles equipped with counsel, new rights, and safeguards, the issue of juvenile competency to stand trial was rarely raised until the 1990s.

LEGAL STANDARD FOR COMPETENCY TO STAND TRIAL

The legal foundation for the right of a defendant to be competent to stand trial begins in mid-17th century English common law.[10] English Courts recognized that mentally ill or cognitively impaired individuals were not able to understand the proceedings or assist counsel in their defense. Without a defendant's full participation in assisting counsel, testifying, and effectively cross-examining witnesses, a trial was considered unfair and undignified. As a result, common law recognized that such disadvantaged individuals would not face trials until they had understanding or ability to assist counsel.[11]

English common law additionally sought fairness for juveniles, but through a unique finding of culpability. The moral responsibility for a juvenile was determined by age: minors older than 14 were treated as adults; the ability to form criminal intent was disputable for minors between ages 7 and 14; children younger than age 7 were not sufficiently culpable to hold responsible for their offenses.[12] The mitigating effect of age on culpability continued its influence in the initial creation of juvenile courts in the United States.

For adult criminal defendants, the common law traditions regarding competency were continued in 1960 when the US Supreme Court articulated in *Dusky v United States*[13] the minimum standard for competency to stand trial. In *Dusky*, the Court held that a defendant is competent to stand trial if he or she "has sufficient present ability to consult with his lawyer with a reasonable degree of rational understanding and… a rational as well as factual understanding of the proceedings against him."

Whenever a defendant's competency is questioned, this issue must be raised before the court.[14] Proceedings are then stayed until an evaluation can be conducted and the factfinder (ie, judge or jury) determines a defendant's competence to proceed. A diagnosis of mental illness or intellectual disability does not define competency, but instead it is the impaired understanding or ability to assist counsel that can lead to a finding of incompetency. The *Dusky* Court did not state which conditions may render a defendant incompetent to stand trial and left open the possibility that circumstances such as immaturity could influence competency. Most jurisdictions' criminal statutes necessitate the presence of some mental defect or condition for a finding of incompetence. Evaluators of a defendant's competence should consult their jurisdictional statutes to ascertain the range of conditions for which a defendant may be found incompetent to stand trial.

The US Supreme Court has not specified whether *Dusky* applies equally to a juvenile court or whether the *Dusky* standard should change for juvenile defendants transferred to an adult criminal court. Transferred juvenile defendants are typically afforded all of the due process protections given to adult criminal defendants, but their competence standard has not been specifically stated by the US Supreme Court.

All state appellate courts, with the exception of Oklahoma, have held that youths have to be competent to stand trial in a juvenile court. (The Oklahoma Court of Criminal Appeals held that competency is not required because of the original rehabilitative nature of juvenile proceedings).[15] However, most states lack statutory guidance regarding competency to stand trial in juvenile proceedings. Evaluators of juvenile competence to stand trial must consult their individual state statutes and case law to precisely know their competency standards.

Twenty states lack a defined competency standard for juveniles to stand trial. In jurisdictions that have proscribed standards, juvenile justice has relied on case law, juvenile court statutes, or the application of adult court statutes to determine competency to stand trial in a juvenile court. Thirteen states have applied the *Dusky* standard to stand trial to the juvenile court.[16] Of these 13 states, 4 have specifications such as Arkansas law, which only requires *Dusky* abilities if the defendant is younger than age 13 and charged with capital or first degree murder.[17] Additionally, Ohio appellate courts apply the adult statute on competency to juvenile courts, but suggest using "juvenile norms.[18]"

Although the concept of "juvenile norms" is poorly defined, an Ohio forensic examiner in the case of *In re Bailey*[19] concluded that the juvenile was not competent to stand trial in an adult court but was competent to enter a guilty plea or admit to aggravated robbery in juvenile court. In oral testimony, the examiner testified that Bailey did not understand everything in court and he could not effectively assist counsel in his defense, but he was competent to enter a guilty plea in a juvenile court. At the conclusion of the hearing, Bailey entered a plea agreement with the state and he was committed to the Department of Youth Services for 4 years. The juvenile court never made a determination regarding Bailey's competence to stand trial. On appeal, Bailey argued that the juvenile court erred by accepting his guilty plea when the competency evaluation showed that he was not competent to stand trial yet contended that he was competent to admit to the offense. The prosecutor agreed with Bailey and argued on appeal that the competency standard to stand trial was equivalent to competency to enter a guilty plea. The Ohio Court of Appeals disagreed with the prosecutor's claim, but reversed the judgment because the trial court failed to make *any* formal finding regarding Bailey's competency. The Ohio Court of Appeals stated, "There is authority to support a juvenile court's finding that although a child may be incompetent to stand trial in adult court, he or she may nevertheless be competent to enter an admission and stand for adjudication in juvenile court, because of the differences in the complexities in adult criminal proceedings versus juvenile proceedings…A juvenile court can properly consider those differences in determining whether a child is competent to enter an admission…"[20] Such language from the Ohio appellate court hints at a potential lower bar than *Dusky* for juvenile competency-related matters, but this nuance is yet to reach broader legal acceptance.

Eighteen jurisdictions have determined their standard for competency to stand trial in a juvenile court includes the ability to assist counsel and understand the proceedings.[16] Such standards slightly differ from *Dusky* in that they do not specify the need for factual and rational understanding of the proceedings. Factual understanding includes a basic knowledge or understanding of definitions of participants and concepts in a trial proceeding, but rational understanding is a higher level of appreciation and includes an ability to apply factual knowledge. For instance, a minor may factually know that the prosecutor is seeking his conviction in a trial, but the same minor may not appreciate the difference between the prosecutor and defense counsel when asked to compare their roles. Without a rational understanding of the difference, a minor may hold back from telling counsel everything if the minor fails to appreciate their distinct roles despite their apparent friendliness between proceedings.

DEVELOPMENTAL IMMATURITY

CASE VIGNETTE 1

Erik is a 12-year-old charged with vandalism after he spray-painted the classroom windows of his prior seventh grade while he was bored during the summer vacation. Erik was caught by the school janitor and he immediately confessed before the janitor called the police to the scene. Erik is an average student without any history of special education or psychiatric services. He has never been charged with a crime. His parents were shocked by his behavior and pledged to provide better supervision of him during the summer months. When Erik met with his court appointed attorney, Erik was unable to let go of his mother. He made no eye contact except to briefly ask his attorney if he was going to suspend him from school. Erik promised never to lie even "to that guy who wears a black dress on TV" Erik then looked at the ground and refused to answer any questions, even with his mother's support. Erik began crying and his mother said, "I don't think he has any idea what we are doing with you." Erik's attorney later questioned his competency to stand trial in juvenile court and asked for a court appointed evaluation.

Erik's case illustrates how developmental immaturity may impact a juvenile's ability to assist their counsel in any meaningful way. Such considerations are even more important when a juvenile is transferred to adult court or faces serious consequences in juvenile court. Both situations are increasingly likely considering juvenile violence trends during the last several decades. In particular, during the late 1980's and mid 1990s, juvenile violence reached an all time high in the United States. In response, state legislators crafted laws, which increased penalties in juvenile courts. In addition, many states passed laws that provided additional mechanisms to transfer youths to adult courts, where they were subject to criminal processes.[21] As the pendulum moved from the rehabilitative ideal of the early juvenile justice system to a more punitive model, attorneys representing juveniles sought additional legal safeguards for their young defendants by raising inquiries into the youth's mental status and competence to stand trial.[22] In the absence of US Supreme Court or initial statutory guidance regarding juvenile competency, juvenile courts did not have a clear directive as to how to best handle these inquiries.

Confusion arose because juvenile competency raised additional distinct questions. For example, *Dusky* did not ponder or address the effect of development on the decision-making process of a juvenile. Appellate courts were confronted with juveniles contesting their competence to stand trial who were not mentally ill or mentally retarded, but were young and significantly developmentally immature.

In California, *Timothy J. v Superior Court*[23] was typical of related cases heard by appellate courts around the United States. In *Timothy J.*, a 12-year-old based his claim of incompetence on developmental immaturity. Timothy, age 12, entered his elementary school after being suspended and stole personal property from the premises. The court placed Timothy on informal probation, during which time he was caught with a knife on school grounds. Timothy's counsel declared doubt regarding the minor's competency to stand trial. Counsel informed the court that when Timothy was asked what trial was or its purpose, Timothy responded "[w]hen you do something bad. I don't know." Counsel also advised the court that Timothy did not understand the gravity of his situation, the potential consequences of his acts, or what constitutes probation. The trial court subsequently denied the request regarding competency on the grounds Timothy did not have a mental disorder.

Timothy appealed his denial for a competency hearing to the California Court of Appeals. The Court of Appeals agreed with Timothy, asking the trial court to reconsider

Timothy's adjudicative competency. The California Court of Appeals stated "for purposes of determining competency to stand trial, we see no significant difference between an incompetent adult who functions mentally at the level of a 10- or 11-year-old because of a developmental disability and that of a normal 11-year-old whose mental development and capacity is likewise not equal to that of a normal adult."[23] The California Court of Appeals clarified that juvenile incompetence may be based on immaturity, mental disorder, or developmental disability.

In California, the basis of developmental maturity was codified into formal juvenile court statutes in 2011. California Welfare and Institutions Code § 709 (b) states: "Upon suspension of proceedings, the court shall order that the question of the minor's competence be determined at a hearing. The court shall appoint an expert to evaluate whether the minor suffers from a mental disorder, developmental disability, developmental immaturity, or other condition and, if so, whether the condition or conditions impair the minor's competency." An increasing number of states have recognized "developmental immaturity" by statute or case law as a specific cause for incompetence in juvenile court. The most significant difference between juvenile and adult competency is that juveniles can be found incompetent if they are unable to understand the nature of the proceedings or assist counsel in their defense because of "developmental immaturity."

Developmentally immature youths exhibit incomplete development in regards to perceived autonomy, risk perception, time perspective, or abstract thinking.[24] Chronologic age is not equal to maturational age, but research has shown age is a significant factor related to adjudicative competence. Grisso and colleagues[25] (2003) compared abilities associated with adjudicative competence among 927 adolescents (ages 12–17) in juvenile justice facilities and community settings with 466 young adults (ages 18–24) in jails or the community. Key findings from this study were as follows:

1. Juveniles younger than the age of 15 performed worse than young adults in trial-related abilities. 35% of 11- to 13-year-olds were significantly impaired.
2. Minors older than 16 years old with intelligence scores less than 75 were the most impaired in the study.
3. The 16- to 17-year-olds and young adults ages 18 to 24 performed similarly.
4. When presented with hypothetical decision-making vignettes, younger adolescents compared with young adults were more likely: to confess to police; not consult with a lawyer; and not evaluate the pros and cons of a plea agreement.
5. Younger children, ages 11 to 13, tended more often than young adults to make legal choices that reflected compliance with authority.

This direct relationship between age and competency related abilities has been replicated in several studies.[26,27] Grisso observed that particularly young children were more likely to function as incompetent mentally ill adults, but many of these incompetent youths were not mentally ill or mentally retarded—instead, they were solely too developmentally immature to participate and adequately understand the nature of delinquency proceedings. Grisso[25] observed that these younger children's psychosocial immaturity resulted in faulty decision making with less attention to long-term consequences of their decisions compared with older adolescents and adults. For such immature youths lacking appreciation of legal concepts, prior legal exposure has not been shown to predict or improve competence-related abilities.[28]

FUTURE POTENTIAL LEGAL DIRECTIONS IN JUVENILE ADJUDICATIVE COMPETENCY

For juvenile defendants who are tried in an adult criminal court, there is significantly less, if any, statutory guidance regarding competency to stand trial. The inquiry into a juvenile's competence to stand trial during the last decade has been partly driven by concern for the increased transfer of youths to adult criminal courts and yet transferred minors' standard for competency is not clarified. Some appellate courts have applied *Dusky* to such minors,[16] but further development in this legal area is still lacking. "Juvenile norms" such as those described *In re Bailey*[19] for competency to stand trial in a juvenile court could be found legal and different from what a juvenile would be expected to understand and participate in a criminal court. Similarly, a transferred youth's abilities to competently stand trial could also one day be adjudged differently than an adult in criminal court. Such a model of varying thresholds based on development and the stakes of the proceedings could preserve the worthy intentions of the early juvenile court with its emphasis on rehabilitation instead of punishment. Juvenile hearings could thus maintain some level of informality, flexibility, and low stigma. For now, the competency of a juvenile is presumed with the burden of proof lying with the defense to prove incompetence in all juvenile or transferred youths' legal proceedings.[29]

Though the US Supreme Court has not defined the standard for juvenile competence to stand trial, the Court has foreshadowed how it might consider a youth incompetent to stand trial because of developmental immaturity in an unrelated juvenile death penalty case. In the US Supreme Court case of *Roper v Simmons* (2005),[30] the Court was asked to evaluate the constitutionality of the death penalty for individuals 17 years or younger. In 1993, Christopher Simmons murdered a woman and a jury later recommended the death penalty. Mr Simmons' attorney disputed the constitutionality of the death penalty, citing the Eighth Amendment's prohibition against cruel and unusual punishment. The American Psychiatric Association and American Academy of Child and Adolescent Psychiatry submitted amicus briefs to the US Supreme Court, in support of abolishing capital punishment for juveniles.[31] These psychiatric groups argued that scientific evidence suggested youths were immature because of limited neurocognitive development. In a 5–4 ruling, the Court held that it was cruel and unusual punishment for a person who committed a crime less than 18 years to receive the death penalty. In its decision, the Court cited the submitted scientific evidence regarding developmental immaturity and diminished culpability. The Court additionally considered that states already had laws prohibiting juveniles from voting, marrying, or serving on juries because of concerns about their immaturity. The Supreme Court continued this trend in *Miller v Alabama* (2012),[32] ruling a mandatory life without parole sentence for juveniles was unconstitutional. As a result of *Roper v Simmons, Miller v Alabama,* and other cases,[33,34] juveniles who commit crimes will be exposed to diminished compulsory sentences. The Court's support of immaturity as a factor for diminished culpability suggests that the Court could be open to developmental immaturity as a predicate for trial incompetence. Without a US Supreme Court decision on this matter, states have continued to vary in their application of a juvenile's right to competence to stand trial.

CURRENT PRACTICE IN JUVENILE COMPETENCY TO STAND TRIAL

There is no national database that collects information on current juvenile court practice regarding evaluation of a juvenile's competence to stand trial. The California Youth Law Center attempted to investigate the prevalence of juvenile incompetency to stand trial by surveying California counties from October 2006 to June 2007 by telephone and email.[35] Their data had multiple acknowledged limitations such as the discovery that some counties actively and purposefully diverted potentially incompetent juveniles out of juvenile court before a determination of incompetence. According to this survey, nearly half of the 34 counties that responded had used a judicial hearing to find a juvenile incompetent. Thirteen counties reported no juvenile competency evaluations or judicial findings of trial incompetency. In 8 counties, officials reported that they did not recall if any juveniles in their jurisdiction had been found incompetent. There was wide discrepancy in the frequency that proceedings were used to investigate a juvenile's competency and the outcome of such proceedings. For instance, Sacramento County had 64 evaluations ordered during the surveyed year to determine competency, and approximately 10 juveniles were found incompetent. In Los Angeles County, carrying the largest caseload in the state, probation staff estimated that approximately 50 juveniles were found incompetent during the surveyed year. Although these numbers lack scientific rigor, they suggest that the evaluations and findings of juvenile competency to stand trial vary among California counties.

Extrapolating further, if this informal survey found this much variance among counties in the same state, uniformity among states regarding juvenile competence to stand trial is unlikely. For example, some states dismiss charges, others divert the youth before a finding of competency, and other jurisdictions attempt to remediate competency during a designated period of time.[36] Virginia is one of the few states that has statutory direction for an "unrestorably incompetent" juvenile. Charges are to be dismissed in 1 year for a misdemeanor offense and in 3 years from the date the juvenile is arrested for a felony case.[37] Most jurisdictions lack such statutory clarity. The lack of legal uniformity has the potential to create wide inconsistency in the quality and basis of evaluators' forensic opinions on this matter.

In *Jackson v Indiana*,[38] the US Supreme Court held that indefinite commitment of a pretrial defendant because of his incompetency to stand trial violated the defendant's due process. The *Jackson* Court further determined that if treatment could not restore a defendant to competence, the state must either begin civil commitment proceedings or release the defendant. The applicability of *Jackson* to incompetent to stand trial juveniles is not determined especially when considered that juveniles are not afforded the right to bail and they can be held for pretrial preventive detention (see *Schall v Martin* (1984)[9] described earlier).

FORENSIC EVALUATION OF JUVENILE COMPETENCY TO STAND TRIAL

CASE VIGNETTE 2

Roger is a 12-year-old charged with robbery. He is being held at Juvenile Hall after he violated probation for the third time in 2 weeks. His public defender is receiving daily phone calls from juvenile probation complaining of his inability or unwillingness to follow any directions. Probation has requested his first psychiatric evaluation because he seems to be talking to himself. Roger was doing very well in school until 6 months ago, when his grades began to rapidly decline. The school initially told the parents to not worry, but the parents later insisted that he receive a special education evaluation. The school had started the process of gathering information about his unexplained academic decline when he was arrested for robbery. Roger's attorney visited him and found him to be disheveled and bizarre. Roger's attorney expressed doubt to the juvenile court judge about his client's competency to stand trial.

The preceding scenario highlights obvious mental health concerns in this young juvenile that raises questions regarding his trial competency. Based on his research findings, Grisso (1987)[28] recommends that the question of juveniles' trial competence should be raised in cases involving any one of the conditions outlined in **Box 2**.

> **Box 2**
> **Conditions that should prompt an inquiry into a juvenile's adjudicative competence**
>
> • Age 12 or younger
> • Prior diagnosis/treatment for a mental illness or mental retardation
> • Borderline level of intellectual functioning or record of learning disability
> • Pretrial observations by others that suggest deficits in memory, attention, or appreciation of reality
>
> *Data from* Grisso T, Miller M, Sales B. Competency to stand trial in juvenile court. Int J Law Psychiatry 1987;10:1–20.

Organizing the Evaluation

Evaluators assigned to assess a juvenile's adjudicative competency should understand the specific forensic question and jurisdictional legal standard. The evaluator should avoid dual roles as much as possible (ie, the forensic evaluator should not be the juvenile's treatment provider). Such role confusion can disadvantage a youth who may feel a sense of trust with a prior treatment provider and raises issues of medicolegal confidentiality. If dual roles are unavoidable given circumstances (eg, being the treating psychiatrist in a forensic hospital), the roles should be clarified to the juvenile before beginning the examination.

Before the initiation of an interview with a juvenile, the forensic evaluator should inform the youth about the scope and nature of the evaluation. The minor should be told to whom the information of the interview will be shared. Evaluators should error cautiously, including probation, parents, and trial participants as potential receivers of the information from the interview. The examination should be voluntary, though the minor should be explicitly told that they are not required to answer every question, but their nonresponsiveness will be reported. Consent from minors is generally not required for court-ordered evaluations, but their assent is necessary. Developmentally appropriate language should be used by the evaluator during the assent process, and the minor's understanding should be documented.

Collateral Sources of Information

An evaluator of juvenile adjudicative competence should seek and review collateral sources of information before the interview. The forensic evaluator's report on juvenile adjudicative competency should include a description of all of the sources of information on which the opinion was based. Potential collateral sources of information should include contact with the defense counsel and parents or guardian when feasible. Parents can provide information regarding the youth's birth and early development and a perspective on the juvenile's behavior at home and school. Their information may contradict or be consistent with that which the juvenile reports. Inconsistencies are important to note as they may represent clues that a juvenile is malingering or minimizing symptoms. Defense counsel should also share their perspective of working with the youth. For instance, if defense counsel reports the primary concern with the juvenile involves a lack of appreciation regarding the ramifications of a plea bargain, the terms and implications of a plea bargain could be carefully explored with the juvenile during the evaluation. Comparing the youth's performance during the evaluation with the defense attorney's observations should be considered when evaluating a juvenile's ability to rationally assist counsel. An evaluator should be aware of the nature of the specific charges and the potential penalties so that a youth can be accurately assessed.

In addition to collateral contacts, a review of the following records is important: school records including special education evaluations and individualized education plans; medical records; court records; police reports; psychiatric and psychological evaluations. All of these sources of information may be helpful to clarify mental diagnoses and/or intellectual deficiencies. The records may also direct further remediation plans to restore competency. Restoration may be as simple as restarting a psychiatric medication from which the youth benefited in the past. Given the time constraints and difficulty in obtaining all of these records, forensic evaluators should work with local juvenile courts and probation departments to make the collection of the records standard practice for any accompanying request for an evaluation of a juvenile's competency to stand trial. With records, the report will be more reliable and the evaluator can possibly save time through the elimination of redundancy. For example, extensive intellectual testing would not be needed if it was documented that a juvenile had been a client of statewide services for the developmentally disabled because of mental retardation.

Psychiatric Evaluation of Juvenile Adjudicative Competency

Box 3 highlights the most essential components of a forensic evaluation of a juvenile's competency to stand trial. Each of these is discussed in more detail.
- Assessment of mental disorder and intellectual disability
- Assessment of developmental status
- Assessment of functional abilities for adjudicative competence

Assessment of mental disorder and intellectual disability
A forensic assessment of juvenile adjudicative competence includes the determination of the presence or absence of a mental illness or intellectual disability. Although no single deficit renders a juvenile incompetent, any deficit has the potential to negatively impact a youth's trial abilities. Because mental illness is more prevalent in the juvenile justice population, assessment of any potential mental disorder or disability is essential. Research indicates that more than 50% of juvenile delinquents and nearly 20% of nondelinquent minors have a mental disorder.[39] Many juveniles have a host of diagnoses, coupled with disadvantaged socioeconomic backgrounds, limited educational opportunities, and intellectual deficits. This combination of problems can create a complex puzzle for the evaluator to sort and evaluate how each piece contributes to a juvenile's competence abilities.

Many mental disorders could potentially impact juveniles' understanding of delinquency proceedings or their ability to assist defense counsel. For instance, even

---

Box 3
Essential components of a competency evaluation

a. Assessment of mental disorder and intellectual disability

b. Assessment of developmental status

c. Assessment of functional abilities for adjudicative competence

d. Linkage of deficits to functional abilities for adjudicative competence

e. Potential for remediation/restoration

a depressed youth may lack the energy, hope, concentration, or motivation to rationally assist counsel. Depressed juveniles may be irritable or hostile toward counsel. Traumatized children with posttraumatic symptoms may have a foreshortened sense of the future, behave in a guarded manner with their counsel, or be more reactive to perceived danger. Mental illnesses that are most likely to negatively impact juvenile competency include psychosis and attention-deficit/hyperactivity disorder (ADHD). Psychosis is the most typical mental illness of incompetent adult defendants,[40] but psychosis is rarer in children. ADHD, particularly untreated ADHD, can impair decision making, risk taking, and impulse control. Hyperactivity can lead to poor behavior in a courtroom and an inability to effectively communicate with counsel.

Juveniles' intellectual deficits are more likely than mental disorders to impair a youth's ability to understand proceedings and assist counsel. McGaha and colleagues[41] found that 58% of juveniles determined incompetent were a result of an underlying cognitive impairment, compared with 6% of incompetent adults. Juveniles can be mentally retarded, and/or they can also have multiple impaired cognitive domains in the setting of more normal intellectual potential. Deficits in attention, executive function, memory, or discreet learning disorders such as a nonverbal or auditory processing disorder could dramatically impact how a youth processes information, reacts, and behaves with a lawyer.

A competency to stand trial evaluator should conduct a thorough assessment and collect as much data as feasible regarding the juvenile's life course. The competency report should include a description of any psychiatric symptoms shown during the juvenile's life. A current assessment of the mental status of a juvenile should be conducted and clearly documented:

- Past psychiatric history including treatment, hospitalizations, suicide attempts, medications, substance abuse, and a family history of psychiatric illness should also be recorded.
- A medical history, including a history of head trauma or seizure activity can illuminate underlying causes for mental illness or intellectual difficulties.
- Side effects from medications can also impair competency, whereas some medications may be needed to maintain competency.

Intellectual testing should consist of at least the Mini-Mental State Examination and may require more refined assessment methods to objectively measure intelligence and learning achievement. Intelligence is made up of multiple cognitive components. Different cognitive domains are resourced according to the competency-related task. For instance, communicating to an attorney relies on strong verbal skills; however memory, attention, and reasoning are more important to a youth considering a plea. Challenging cases include intelligent youths with discrete learning challenges such as nonverbal or auditory processing disorders. Further neuropsychological testing may be needed to better define a youth's cognitive potential and achievement in all spheres.

There is no score, no bright line, or cut off that defines competency, but all deficits will ultimately need to directly affect trial-related functions to impact a competency finding. The results of any administered tests should be documented. School records, prior special education evaluations, and individualized education plans often sufficiently outline a history and current status of any intellectual disabilities. All diagnoses should be supported by data described in the body of the report.

Assessment of developmental status

Although the definition of what legally constitutes developmental immaturity remains poorly defined, forensic evaluators of juvenile competency have relied on developmental research conducted during the last 2 decades.[42–48] The evaluator of juvenile compe-tence should have training and experience specific to children and adolescents. The evaluator must be able to assess the juvenile's history and current development status. Larson and Grisso (2011) suggested considerations in the developmental assessment of juveniles, which are included in **Box 4**.[49]

Developmental maturity A birth and medical history should be documented and the timing of key developmental milestones. A juvenile's development must be compared with similar-aged peers. It is important to identify a 16-year-old who functioning on a maturational level as a 10-year-old, and conversely a 10-year-old who is functioning on a maturational level as a 16 year-old. The developmental level of a juvenile is more important to establish instead of relying on a specific age to speculate about a juve-nile's competence to stand trial. Developmental challenges can also complicate the impact of comorbid mental illness or intellectual deficits on a juvenile's trial abilities.

Psychosocial maturity Important aspects of psychosocial maturity and childhood development should also be considered. Psychosocial development concerns the social and emotional development of youth. The process of making legal decisions is different for youths compared with adults. On a functional level, social and emotional forces on a juvenile's decision making process can uniquely affect competence to stand trial. Youth's decisions are affected by their perception of autonomy from adults or persons of authority, risk, time, and ability to abstract.[42–48]

Identity Immature juveniles may make decisions based on imperfect presumptions. For example, adolescents' major developmental achievement includes the formation of identity and they may experiment with identities that are not commonly accepted by conventional adults. With greater maturity and frontal lobe development, adolescents are better able to control impulses, consider longer term consequences, and think

---

Box 4
Recommended considerations to assess the developmental status of the juvenile

Age and maturity level, including:

1. Responsibility (autonomy, self-reliance, clarity of identity)

2. Temperance (the ability to delay action and think through issues, seeking advice when needed)

3. Perspective (ability to acknowledge the complexity of a situation and frame a decision within the larger context)

4. Developmental stage

5. Judgment, reasoning, and decision-making ability

6. Future orientation

7. Risk perception

8. Peer influences

9. Influence of parental relationship

10. Suggestibility and compliance with others

Data from Larson K, Grisso T. Developing statutes for competence to stand trial in Juvenile delin-quency proceedings: a guide for lawmakers. National youth screening and assessment project. 2011. p. 1–104. Available at: http://www.umassmed.edu/uploadedFiles/cmhsr/Products_and_Publications/reports_papers_manuals/developing_statutes.pdf. Accessed April 21, 2012.

abstractly.[42] Younger adolescents value short-term benefits over long-term consequences and minimize the probability of a negative outcome. As youths develop, their own sense of autonomy increases.[50] Younger children are more reliant on adults to make decisions on their behalf and they are more susceptible to suggestion and influence from peers and parents. Youths ages 13 to 15 begin to seek their own ideas and desire to make their own decisions, eventually transforming into independent decision makers. Younger children may fail to conceptualize that they can make decisions outside of parents or a lawyer's guise and may instead seek to appease authority figures. The adolescent appreciation of risk similarly changes as the frequency of risky behaviors maximizes between ages 16 and 19. If juveniles fail to appreciate the inherent risk and long-term implications of a plea bargain, their decision making process would be undermined by their own immaturity.

Assessment of functional abilities for adjudicative competence

To be competent to stand trial, a juvenile must have 2 abilities:

1. Rationally assist counsel in the conduct of the defense
2. A rational and factual understanding of the legal proceedings

A psychological tool (see psychological testing later), such as the Juvenile Adjudicative Competency Interview (JACI),[24] is useful to guide an evaluator in the exploration of both competency-related abilities with a juvenile. With or without such a structured instrument, an evaluator should determine a juvenile's understanding of the proceedings in an open-ended and documented manner. Topics to address with a youth should include the:

- Alleged criminal offense including its relative seriousness and the potential penalties
- Roles of all of the participants in a trial including the prosecutor, defense attorney, judge, and witnesses
- Basic purpose of a trial and the adversarial nature of court procedures
- Implications, drawbacks, and benefits of a plea bargain
- Trial-related rights including the right to deny an offense and the avoidance of self-incrimination
- Reasoning a juvenile would use if faced with common legal choices and options such as a plea bargain

It is most helpful if an evaluator can document the juvenile's actual understanding instead of simply certifying "yes or no" regarding a juvenile's knowledge about a particular legal concept.

A forensic evaluator must also assess the juvenile's ability to assist counsel in the defense. Areas to address with the juvenile include the following:

- The name, purpose, and relationship of a defense attorney
- The level of motivation to help and trust a defense attorney
- An ability to communicate, understand, and retain information
- Process and respond rationally to new information
- An ability to articulate facts pertaining to the alleged offense
- The ability to maintain proper courtroom behavior
- The strengths and weaknesses of a potential trial

Psychological Testing

The assessment of impairments must be complete, thorough, and incorporate psychological testing as necessary to generate a specific DSM-IV TR diagnosis. Psychiatrists and psychologists will vary in their use of psychological instruments for diagnostic purposes, but they should all have at minimum enough familiarity to read and interpret school records and prior special education and psychological evaluations. In addition to knowledge about psychological testing for the purpose of diagnosis, evaluators should be familiar with and use a structured format to explore a juvenile's trial competency-related abilities in a developmentally appropriate fashion. Two psychological tools, among the many tools available, which would aid in forensic opinion regarding juvenile competence to stand trial include the MacArthur Competence Assessment Tool–Criminal Adjudication (MacCAT-CA)[51] and JACI.[24]

MacCAT-CA

The MacCAT-CA is a 22-item structured interview that uses a vignette format and scored questions to measure 3 competence-related abilities: understanding (factual understanding of the legal proceedings); reasoning (ability to determine the relevant information to reason about 2 legal options); appreciation (ability to understand personal legal circumstances). The vignette involves a hypothetical case in which 2 men argue and fight at a bar, resulting in an aggravated assault charge. The advantages of the MacCAT-CA include its prior use with more than 900 juveniles in Grisso's landmark study[25] that compared the adjudicative abilities of adolescents to young adults. The MacCAT-CA also generates an objective score that could be compared with an adult score, and may be particularly helpful for a transferred youth to adult criminal court. However, the MacCAT-CA has not been sufficiently validated or normed for a juvenile population. The MacCAT-CA inflexibly uses a hypothetical case with words more applicable to an adult legal proceeding, and it is not specifically designed to assess malingering.

JACI

The JACI is an instrument used to gauge the degree of competence and consists of questions, grouped into 12 different areas. The JACI is designed to assess a youth's decision-making abilities relevant in juvenile court. The strength of the JACI is that it tests the factual and rational understanding of a juvenile's particular offense, its implications, and the adjudicative procedures in a developmentally appropriate manner. For example, instead of relying on a juvenile to explain the purpose of a trial, the JACI asks a juvenile to compare a trial to going to a principal's office when the youth is also in trouble. A juvenile is usually quite aware of the conduct of a principal in a discipline matter and they can use this comparison to apply their factual knowledge to express their appreciation of the similarities and differences with a trial. The JACI also requires the evaluator to attempt to remediate deficiencies in a juvenile's knowledge, with a re-assessment to ensure retention. Dr Grisso is clear that the JACI has not been validated and it does not generate a score, or cutoff point for which a juvenile's competence can be determined. The JACI has also been criticized because it sometimes uses terms not found in a typical juvenile court such as "pleading guilty" when "admitting" would be a more appropriate term, and it is not able to detect malingering.[24]

Cross-validation of data

Currently, there is not a validated method or single psychological instrument that is able to detect juvenile adjudicative competency malingering. Therefore, the evaluator should instead rely on cross-validating data with multiple sources of information, always looking for inconsistencies, which could indicate the presence of feigned or inadequate effort from the juvenile. A juvenile forensic evaluator should be looking for and have an opinion regarding malingering during any forensic evaluation despite the lack of validated psychological instruments to aid in this assessment.

Reaching the Forensic Opinion

The first steps of reaching a forensic opinion about a juvenile's competency to stand trial have already been outlined:

1. Description of the presence or absence of a mental disorder, intellectual disability, or developmental immaturity
2. Identification of the specific deficits in a juvenile's ability to understand trial proceedings or assist counsel in the conduct of the defense

After these steps have been articulated in the report, an evaluator must identify the relationship between the functional competency deficits and the juvenile's predicate causes. The facts and reasoning defining this causal relationship should be described. If a forensic evaluator is able to link a deficit to a functional competency impairment, then the evaluator should opine that the juvenile is incompetent to stand trial.

An example opinion statement might read as follows: "In my opinion, within reasonable medical certainty, due to John's severe ADHD, which has been medication resistant since age 4, he would have an inability to adequately sit still, comport with courtroom procedures, attend to the proceedings, follow directions, or assist counsel in his defense."

A forensic opinion is given "with reasonable medical certainty" if a physician and "with reasonable scientific certainty" if a psychologist. Both phrases translate to rendering an opinion that is "more likely than not" as supported by the evidence. If the evaluator finds, with reasonable medical or scientific certainty, that there is an absence of a causal deficit or functional impairment in competency, then he or she should opine that the juvenile is competent to stand trial. The purpose of the evaluator is to provide information and expert opinion, which will aid the factfinder in making a finding about competency. Evaluators should be as descriptive as possible in their opinions. Limitations of the report and used psychological instruments should be discussed. If an opinion cannot be rendered within reasonable medical or scientific certainty, the evaluator should outline the particular ambiguity of the case, how the ambiguity could be potentially resolved (for example though more in depth psychological testing or collateral contact), and evidence for and against an opinion regarding the juvenile's competence. The fact-finder will find such a report more helpful than a haphazard opinion, which leads to contested hearings and the need for additional evaluations.

If an evaluator determines that a juvenile is incompetent to stand trial, the potential for restoration of competency should be discussed. An evaluator should consider the time needed to remediate competency, the appropriate methods most likely to restore competency, and the local community resources to accomplish such restoration. An evaluator may also have simple recommendations for accommodations that would maximize a juvenile's participation in the legal process such as more frequent breaks or an interpreter for a juvenile who speaks English, but whose fluency may reflect it being a secondary language. Each deficit will require its own discussion and plan for remediation. Some remediation plans will be as simple as restarting a stimulant medication for diagnosed ADHD. However, this plan presumes a child would assent and a guardian would consent to such medication. There is no legal precedent for forcing any kind of competency restoration plan on a child such as medications, creating further potential barriers or gaps that the adult competency legal landscape has already crossed. Statutes governing the time and method of remediation will differ among states, and the extent of resources will vary among counties. Further unresolved questions related to juvenile adjudicative competency are summarized in **Box 5**.

Box 5
Unresolved issues related to juvenile adjudicative competence

1. The remediation of youths found incompetent based on developmental immaturity. The time limits, place of restoration, and mode of restoration for immature defendants are yet to be universally determined.

2. Can an incompetent youth be committed, detained, or ordered to competency restoration?

3. How to assess the adjudicative competency of a youth who claims amnesia related to his charges as dealt with in *Wilson v United States*?[52]

4. Should there be different standards for juvenile competency based on the quality of the crime and whether the youth is transferred to a criminal court?

SUMMARY

The inquiry into a juvenile's competency to stand trial became prominent in the 1990s with increasingly severe dispositions in juvenile court and increased transfer rates to adult court. Courts and researchers have responded to the special developmental issues concerning a youth's competence and discovered that a strict application of adult competency standards has not entirely correlated with a youth's competency capacity. The concept of developmental immaturity has led to case law and court statutes that have recognized the psychosocial immaturity of a youth as a basis for finding incompetency. The current conduct of forensic evaluators in this area must be developmentally-minded and attune to unique issues a juvenile faces in legal proceedings. Juveniles can be incompetent to stand trial, using the *Dusky* standard as at least a yardstick at this point. Their deficits may be remediable, but the course of correction will vary among states. Although the legal system and forensic evaluators have moved juvenile competency forward, the US Supreme Court has yet to determine a standard for juvenile adjudicative competency. Evaluators will need to stay current on both the local and national decisions regarding juvenile competency as society, legislators, and courts continue to confront juvenile offenders, seeking their justice while ensuring a fair process. Likely legal holdings in the future may include more clarity on the thresholds for adjudicative competency in juvenile court and youths transferred to an adult court.

REFERENCES

1. Juvenile justice philosophy and the demise of Parens Patriae. In: Hancock BW, Sharp PM, editors. Criminal justice in America: theory, practice, and policy. Upper Saddle River (NJ): Prentice Hall; 1996. p. 321–32.
2. Tanenhaus D. The evolution of transfer out of the juvenile court. In: Jeffrey Fagan J, Zimring FE, editors. The changing borders of juvenile justice: transfer of adolescents to the criminal court. Chicago (IL): University of Chicago Press; 2000. p. 13. 17.
3. *Kent v United States*, 383 US 541 (1966).
4. In *Re Winship*, 397 US 359 (1970).
5. *Breed v Jones*, 421 US 519 (1975).
6. In *Re Gault*, 387 US 1 (1967).
7. In *Re Gault*, 1967, p. 387.
8. *McKeiver v Pennsylvania*, 403 US 528 (1971).
9. *Schall v Martin* 104 S Ct 2403 (1984).
10. Winick BJ, DeMeo TL. Competency to stand trial in Florida. Univ Miami Law Rev 1980;35:31.

11. Blackstone W. Commentaries on the Laws of England. Oxford (UK): Clarendon Press; 1884. p. 1765–9.
12. Malmquist C, Schetky D, Benedek E, editors. Overview of juvenile law. Principles and practice of child and adolescent forensic psychiatry. Washington DC: American Psychiatric Publishing; 2002. p. 259–66.
13. *Dusky v United States* 362 US 402 (1960).
14. *Drope v Missouri*, 420 US 162, 180–81 (1975).
15. *G.J.I. v State*, 778 P.2d 485, 487 (Okla. Crim. App. 1989).
16. Sanborn J. Juveniles' competency to stand trial wading through the rhetoric and the evidence. J Crim Law Criminol 2009;99:135–214.
17. 22 ARK. CODE ANN. § 9-27-502(b)(7)(C)(ix)(b)(1).
18. In *Re Bailey,* 782 N.E.2d 1177, 1179 (Ohio Ct App 2002); In *Re York*, 756 NE 2d 191, 200 (Ohio Ct App 2001).
19. In *Re Bailey*, 150 Ohio App 3d 664b (2002).
20. In *Re Bailey*, 150 Ohio App 3d 668 (2002).
21. Redding R, Frost L. Adjudicative Competence in the modern juvenile court. Va J Soc Pol Law 2001;9:353, 372.
22. Otto RK. Considerations in the assessment of competent to proceed in juvenile court. North KY Law Rev 2007;34:323–42.
23. *Timothy J. v Superior Court of Sacramento County.* 150 Cal App 4th 847 (Ct App 2007).
24. Grisso T. Evaluating juveniles' adjudicative competence. A guide for clinical practice. Sarasota (FL): Professional Resource Press; 2005.
25. Grisso T, Steinberg L, Woolard J, et al. Juveniles' competence to stand trial: a comparison of adolescents' and adults' capacities as trial defendants. Law Hum Behav 2003;27:333–63.
26. Savitsky JC, Karras D. Competency to stand trial among adolescents. Adolescence 1984;74:349–58.
27. Cowden V, McKee G. Competency to stand trial in juvenile delinquency proceedings: cognitive maturity and the attorney client relationship. J Fam Law 1995;33: 629–60.
28. Grisso T, Miller M, Sales B. Competency to stand trial in juvenile court. Int J Law Psychiatry 1987;10:1–20.
29. Redding RE. Adjudicative competence in the modern juvenile court. Va J Soc Policy Law 2002;9:353–410.
30. *Roper v Simmons*, 543 US 551 (2005).
31. Denno DW. The scientific shortcomings of Roper v Simmons. Ohio St J Crim L 2006;3:370 06.
32. *Miller v Alabama*, 567 U. S. ____ (2012).
33. *Atkins v Virginia*, 536 US 304 (2002).
34. *Graham v Florida*, 130 S Ct 2011 (2010).
35. Burrell S, Kendrick C. Blalock B. Incompetent youth in California justice. Stanford Law Pol Rev 2008;19:198–250.
36. Hammond S. Mental health needs of juvenile offenders. Washington, DC: National Conference of State Legislatures; 2007.
37. Va. Code §16.1.358.
38. *Jackson v Indiana*, 406 US 715 (1972).
39. Teplin LA, Abram KM, McClelland GM, et al. Psychiatric disorders in youth in juvenile detention. Arch Gen Psychiatry 2002;59:1133–43.
40. Nicholson R, Kugler K. Competent and incompetent criminal defendants: a quantitative review of comparative research. Psychol Bull 1991;109:355–70.

41. McGaha A, Otto RK, McClaren MD, et al. Juveniles adjudicated incompetent to proceed: a descriptive study of Florida's competence restoration program. J Am Acad Psychiatry Law 2001;29:427–37.
42. Cauffman E, Steinberg L. (Im)maturity of judgment in adolescence: why adolescents may be less culpable than adults. Behav Sci Law 2000;28:741–60.
43. Steinberg L, Cauffman E. Maturity of judgment in adolescence: psychosocial factors in adolescent decision making. Law Hum Behav 1996;20:249–72.
44. Scott ES, Reppucci ND, Woolard JL. Evaluating adolescent decision making in legal contexts. Law Hum Behav 1995;19:221–44.
45. Steinberg L. Risk-taking in adolescence: new perspectives from brain and behavioral science. Curr Dir Psychol Sci 2007;16:55–9.
46. Furby M, Beyth-Marom R. Risk-taking in adolescence: a decision making perspective. Dev Rev 1992;12:1–44.
47. Green A. Future time perspective in adolescence: the present of things future revisited. J Youth Adolesc 1986;15:99–113.
48. Nurmi J. How do adolescents see their future?—a review of the development of future orientation and planning. Dev Rev 1991;11:1–59.
49. Larson K, Grisso T. Developing statutes for competence to stand trial in juvenile delinquency proceedings: a guide for lawmakers. National youth screening and assessment project. 2011. p. 1–104. Available at: http://www.umassmed.edu/uploadedFiles/cmhsr/Products_and_Publications/reports_papers_manuals/developing_statutes.pdf. Accessed April 21, 2012.
50. Berndt TJ. Developmental changes in conformity to peers and parents. Dev Psychol 1979;15:608–16.
51. Hoge SK, Bonnie RJ, Poythress N, et al. MacArthur competence assessment tool-criminal adjudication. Lutz (FL): Psychological Assessment Resources; 2005.
52. Wilson v United States, 391 F2d 460 (DC Cir 1968).

Psychological Testing and the Assessment of Malingering

Barbara E. McDermott, PhD[a,b],*

KEYWORDS

- Malingering • Feigning • Psychological assessment • Criminal and civil evaluations
- Forensic evaluations

KEY POINTS

- Feigning is prevalent in both criminal and civil contexts.
- The prevalence of feigning is often greater in civil forensic evaluations and seems related to financial incentives.
- Feigning of cognitive deficits associated with mild head injury (MHI) is the most prevalent in civil forensic evaluations.
- The most effective method for improving the ability to detect feigning is to use multiple psychological tests with differing assessment paradigms.

INTRODUCTION

The feigning of mental illness for external incentive has been recognized for centuries. Odysseus feigned madness to avoid going to the Trojan War and Hamlet feigned madness to avenge the murder of his father. More recently, Randle McMurphy, the protagonist in *One Flew Over the Cuckoo's Nest*, feigned insanity to serve his sentence for statutory rape in a psychiatric hospital. In 1838, the Drs Beck noted, "Diseases are generally feigned from one of three causes—fear, shame, or hope of gain."[1(p3)] They described motivations commonly viewed as external incentives when they wrote,

> ...the individual ordered on service, will pretend being afflicted with various maladies, to escape the performance of military duty; the mendicant, to avoid labour, and to impose on public or private beneficence; and the criminal, to prevent the infliction of punishment. The spirit of revenge, and the hope of receiving exorbitant damages, have also induced some to magnify slight ailments into serious and alarming illness.[1(p3)]

[a] Division of Psychiatry and the Law, Department of Psychiatry and Behavioral Sciences, University of California, Davis Medical Center, 2230 Stockton Boulevard, Sacramento, CA 95817; [b] Napa State Hospital, Forensic Psychiatry Research Division, 2100 Napa Vallejo Highway, Napa, CA 94558, USA
* Division of Psychiatry and the Law, Department of Psychiatry, UC Davis School of Medicine, 2230 Stockton Boulevard, Sacramento, CA 95817.
E-mail address: bemcdermott@ucdavis.edu

Psychiatr Clin N Am 35 (2012) 855–876
http://dx.doi.org/10.1016/j.psc.2012.08.006

Beck and Beck also noted that the most easily feigned illnesses are those with few to no physical manifestations or those based on self-report. In particular, they suggested that the diseases most amenable to feigning include "insanity, epilepsy, and pain."[1(p26)] They presented 5 suggestions for the detection of feigning, summarized in **Box 1**.

Many of these guidelines, 175 years later, continue to hold true and are a necessary component of a good clinical evaluation when considering malingering. Some of the original detection strategies noted by the Becks have been incorporated into more recently developed structured assessments to detect feigning.

Feigning is often used interchangeably with malingering although the 2 concepts are different. According to the *American Heritage Dictionary*, feigning means "to represent falsely; to imitate so as to deceive."[2] Other than deception, there is no inherent motivation contained in the definition. The oft-quoted definition of malingering as provided by the *Diagnostic and Statistical Manual of Mental Disorders* (Fourth Edition, Text Revision) (*DSM-IV-TR*)[3(p739)] states, "malingering is the intentional production of false or grossly exaggerated physical or psychological symptoms motivated by external incentives." These external incentives can vary greatly, depending on the context. Some investigators[4,5] discuss the distinction between feigning and malingering in terms of the difference between detection and diagnosis. A clinician may know that a symptom is falsely produced (detection), but in order to diagnose (malingering), the external incentive for that production must be elucidated.

Only 2 disorders in the *DSM-IV-TR* involve the conscious production of symptoms: factitious disorder and malingering. The *DSM-IV-TR* states that factitious disorder is "characterized by physical or psychological symptoms that are intentionally produced or feigned in order to assume the sick role."[3(p513)] Although both disorders involve the intentional production of symptoms, either physical or psychological, the definitions imply that clinicians must be able to distinguish between a primary gain (that is, being a patient and the intrinsic benefit that provides) versus secondary gain, which involves some type of external incentive.[6] In the psychiatric setting, external incentives can include the procurement of financial compensation (legal settlements or verdicts, workers' compensation, or disability benefits), the obtainment of prescription medications, or commitment to a psychiatric facility in lieu of incarceration. In *DSM* nosology, factitious disorder is a mental illness, whereas malingering is classified in V codes— other conditions that may be the focus of clinical attention.

In order to accurately diagnose malingering, a comprehensive evaluation is required to verify that feigning is occurring and an external incentive exists. This evaluation must consist of extensive interviewing, contact with collateral informants, and adjunctive psychological testing. For a comprehensive and detailed review of conducting these

---

Box 1
Suggested Beck and Beck guidelines for considering feigning

1. An external incentive is present.

2. No causative factor is present or the illness has a sudden onset.

3. The individual is resistant to receiving treatment.

4. Symptom complaints are inconsistent with the true illness.

5. The course of the disorder is inconsistent with the true illness.

Data from Beck TR, Beck JB. Elements of medical jurisprudence. Philadelphia: Thomas, Cowperthwait, & Co.; 1838.

evaluations, readers are directed to a chapter written by Scott and McDermott,[7] which focuses on the various psychological assessments available to assist clinicians in making a determination of whether or not an individual is feigning; few if any assessments directly assess the external incentive associated with malingering.

EPIDEMIOLOGY

Estimates of malingering vary greatly depending on the evaluation context. Recent research suggests that malingering is substantially more prevalent in the civil arena where financial gain may be significant.[8–10]

Malingering in the Criminal Setting

Malingering in the medicolegal context of the criminal courts is generally for 1 of 2 purposes:

1. To successfully present as incompetent to stand trial
2. To plead not guilty by reason of insanity

In both contexts, feigning a psychotic disorder is the most likely method of success, although intellectual deficits can meet the requirement for a qualifying mental disorder in both competency and criminal responsibility evaluations. Estimates for malingering in incompetence to stand trial evaluations have varied from a low of 8%[11] to a high to 17.4%.[12] A group of forensic psychologists estimated that malingering occurred in almost 16% of forensic patients and more than 7% of nonforensic patients.[13] Additionally, almost 21% of defendants undergoing evaluations of criminal responsibility engaged in or were suspected of engaging in malingering.[14] The author and colleagues' data, presented at an American Academy of Psychiatry and the Law annual meeting,[15] indicated that more than 18% of patients found incompetent to stand trial were malingering their psychiatric symptoms on admission to an inpatient facility for restoration.

The prevalence of malingering increases dramatically in a general offender sample, where the external incentive is substantially different. For example, in a medium-security prison unit, investigators found a malingering rate of 32% based on psychological testing data.[16] Norris and May[17] found that between 45% and 56% of jail inmates requesting psychological services were malingering, depending on the version of the assessment administered. In a study of male prison inmates, 46% of those who claimed psychiatric symptoms were determined malingering.[18] The malingering rate for inmates was 20% in a sample of emergency psychiatric referrals from a large metropolitan jail.[19] In another study, the malingering rate of jail inmates receiving psychological services was 66%, although this number is likely inflated, because only inmates suspected of malingering were referred for assessment.[20] Although not directly studied, the motivation for malingering may contribute to these vastly different prevalence rates. In general, inmates malinger for 1 of 2 reasons: to secure desired medication or to transfer to a more desirable environment.[20,21]

Malingering in the Civil Setting

In civil proceedings, estimates are generally higher than in criminal medicolegal contexts and financial incentives seem to drive this difference. One study found that the rate of malingering was directly related to the monetary reward sought[9] although another study found that other factors, such as revenge, were also relevant.[22]

There is substantial literature indicating high rates of exaggeration of cognitive impairment in patients with MHI seeking compensation. Binder[23] found that 33% of patients with MHIs exaggerated deficits on the Portland Digit Recognition Test. Greiffenstein and Baker[24] found a 37% base rate of malingering in individuals with MHI who were seeking compensation of some sort. Larrabee,[25] in a review of 11 studies, found a prevalence rate of malingering of 40% in 1363 patients who were seeking compensation for an MHI. Larrabee opined that the incidence of exaggeration of deficits in MHI patients seeking compensation was 10 times higher than the base rate for actual deficits.[26] In support of this finding, Green and colleagues[27] found that the evaluee's effort explained 53% of the variability seen on neuropsychological testing of head-injured patients. The evaluee's level of education explained only 11% of the variance and age explained only 4%. Patients with MHIs scored significantly lower on effort tests than patients with more severe injuries. When the MHI patients who demonstrated no effort were removed from the study sample, however, scores on neuropsychological testing for this group (MHIs) were higher than for patients with severe head injuries, as expected.

Although prominent in the literature, MHI is not the only disorder malingered for financial gain. In a study of more than 30,000 cases referred to 144 neuropsychologists, the most likely ailment to be malingered was MHI, but other disorders, such as fibromyalgia, chronic fatigue syndrome, pain, neurotoxic disorders, electrical injury, or seizure disorders, were also reportedly feigned.[28] In a study surveying 105 board-certified orthopedic surgeons and neurosurgeons from 6 states, estimates of the percentages of their patients with low back pain who were malingering varied widely, from a low of 1% to a high of 75%.[29] The majority of the surgeons, however, made low estimates, with 78%, indicating that 10% or fewer of their patients malingered their pain. In contrast, other studies suggest that the incidence of malingered pain is significantly higher. For example, estimates of malingering range from 25% to 30% for fibromyalgia cases,[30] with similar results found for patients malingering chronic pain.[31] Greve and colleagues[32] found a malingering rate of between 20% and 50% for 508 patients complaining of chronic pain who were also seeking financial compensation. Schmand and colleagues[33] found exaggeration of memory deficits in 61% of postwhiplash patients involved in litigation compared with 29% in an outpatient clinic.

Recent reports indicate that the number of veterans receiving disability payment for posttraumatic stress disorder (PTSD) increased by 222% between 1999 and 2010.[34] Gold and Frueh[35] found that either 14% or 22% of veterans referred for an evaluation for PTSD were classified as "extreme exaggerators" on the Minnesota Multiphasic Personality Inventory (MMPI)-2, depending on the criteria used. A more recent study conducted by Frueh and colleagues[36] indicated that approximately 30% of veterans seeking disability compensation for PTSD feign the disorder. In other types of disability claims, Griffin and colleagues[37] found that nearly 1 in 5 social security disability claimants was malingering. Wierzbicki and Tyson[38] determined that 43.5% of college students seeking a diagnosis of attention-deficit/hyperactivity disorder (ADHD), learning disability, or both in order to receive special accommodations under the American with Disabilities Act did not meet criteria for either diagnosis, suggesting that money is not the only incentive for malingering in disability evaluations.

Regardless of the context, when conducting a forensic evaluation, in both the criminal and civil arenas, an identifiable external incentive is always present and, as such, assessments of malingering must be conducted.

MALINGERING ASSESSMENT METHODS

As discussed previously, the optimal assessment of malingering is multimodal and involves a clinical interview, a review of relevant collateral information, and psychological testing. Psychological testing can provide valuable information regarding effort and any response bias adopted by the examinee. McGrath and colleagues[39] provide an informative review of response bias, defined as patients responding in a manner unrelated to the item content. One type of response bias most relevant for malingering is negative impression management, which McGrath and colleagues define as "responding in an excessively aberrant manner."[39 (p451)] Response bias can include, however, styles that are independent of intentional effort. For example, inconsistent responding, acquiescence, and negativism (yea-saying or nay-saying) are examples of response biases that may not necessarily be purposeful. A final type of response bias not often seen in forensic evaluations, with the exception of custody evaluations, is positive impression management, which McGrath and colleagues describe as "the failure to report aberrant tendencies."[39 (p451)]

There are several methods of evaluating response bias with psychological testing, as summarized in part by Larrabee[40] and outlined in this article.

Ombudsmen Tests of Psychological Functioning

Perhaps the most researched strategy in the detection of response bias is to use self-report tests of general psychological functioning that also include validity scales. The 2 instruments most often used in this regard are the MMPI[41] or the more recent version, the MMPI-2,[42] and the Personality Assessment Inventory.[43]

Minnesota Multiphasic Personality Inventory

The MMPI-2 is a 567-item self-report instrument designed as a measure of general psychopathology. It has been cited as "the mostly widely administered objective personality test in forensic evaluations"[44(p1)] largely because of the extensive research conducted on its ability to detect response bias via the embedded validity scales. The 3 original validity scales from the MMPI are the

1. Lie (L) scale
2. Infrequency (F) scale
3. Defensiveness (K) scale

Various configurations of these scales were extensively researched to detect both positive and negative impression management.[45] Further research with the MMPI led to the development of many more validity scales, including variable response inconsistency (the tendency to respond inconsistently to item content), true response inconsistency (the tendency to respond mostly true [or false] to items regardless of content), back infrequency (Fb) (the infrequency items contained on the latter half of the test), and infrequency psychopathology scale (Fp) (items rarely endorsed by psychiatric patients).

As Larrabee describes,[46] the MMPI-2 is efficient at measuring at least 2 types of feigning: feigned severe psychopathology (ie, psychosis) and feigned somatic/neuro-cognitive complaints. Severe psychopathology is most often revealed in a pattern of elevations on the family of F scales and is often associated with the feigning of psychosis in criminal cases. The feigning of somatic and/or neurocognitive complaints, often seen in civil litigation, has led to the development of other composite validity scales, including the Fake Bad Scale (FBS)[47] and the Response Bias Scale (RBS).[48]

Fake bad scale

Larrabee describes the FBS as a measure of "somatic malingering"[49] although other investigators have described it as a measure of general maladjustment.[50] The majority of items on the FBS assesses physical functioning and overlaps with scales 1 (hypochondriasis) and 3 (hysteria). The use of the FBS scale has generated some controversy, with opponents asserting that its scale development was not rigorous and therefore may be inadmissible in court.[51,52]

Response bias scale
The RBS was developed empirically by examining the endorsement of items in individuals both passing and failing cognitive symptom validity tests. The investigators suggest that the RBS improves accuracy above the F scales or the FBS.[44]

Personality Assessment Inventory
The Personality Assessment Inventory (PAI) is a 344-item self-report instrument designed to assess general psychopathology. As with the MMPI, inclusion of validity scales to assess response bias was a critical component of its development. The original validity scales included inconsistency (pairs of items with similar content), infrequency (items expected to be answered by both clinical and nonclinical populations in a similar fashion), negative impression management (the endorsement of bizarre or unlikely symptoms), and positive impression management (items that are rarely endorsed by both clinical and nonclinical respondents but frequently endorsed by those attempting to place themselves in a positive light). A supplementary validity scale was added later—defensiveness, designed to detect underreporting.[53]

More recently, 2 additional scales have shown promise in the detection of malingering:

- The Malingering Index[54] was constructed based on profile characteristics often associated with the feigning of psychiatric disorders.
- The Rogers Discriminant Function[55] was constructed using 3 groups: a clinical group (patients with schizophrenia, major depression, and generalized anxiety disorder) and nonclinical participants categorized as either naïve or sophisticated.

The results of the discriminant analysis indicated that the weighted combination of scales produced a hit rate (accurately detecting a malingerer) of 92%. Furthermore, the Rogers Discriminant Function performed well even with the sophisticated malingerers, with a hit rate of 73%.

Floor Effect
The concept known as the floor effect involves the incorporation of easy questions or tasks in the testing methodology. Such items generally involve overlearned information or simple skills that are easily retained, even in those with limited intellectual functioning. Examples of such items include requests to perform simple arithmetic calculations (eg, $2 + 2 = ?$), questions about basic common information (eg, Who is the President of the United States?), queries regarding basic autobiographic information (such as age or birthday), requests to complete a simple sequence (eg, a, b, _; 3, 4, _), or instructions to copy or recall simple diagrams or designs. The Rey 15-Item Test (FIT)[56] is an example of such an assessment. This test requires that individuals remember a set of 15 letters, numbers, and geometric shapes that are simple because of their redundancy. Various cut scores (the scores that separate malingerers from nonmalingerers) have been suggested although any score less than 10 is generally accepted as indicating a lack of effort. A meta-analysis of the FIT indicated that its specificity (correctly identifying a person as not feigning) was higher than its sensitivity (correctly identifying a person as feigning) (92% vs 43%), with an overall hit rate of 70%.[57] In an effort to improve the sensitivity, Griffin and colleagues[58] modified the

FIT by increasing its redundancy, providing standardized administration instructions, and outlining a method of qualitative scoring. In a clinical population and using the qualitative scoring method, they estimated the sensitivity at 71% although the specificity dropped to 75% with this scoring system. **Table 1** provides a listing of several floor effect tests.

Symptom Validity Testing

Pankratz[59] initially discussed the concept of symptom validity testing (SVT) in the context of the assessment of sensory loss. He described a procedure wherein an individual is presented with a stimulus and instructed to guess whether or not the stimulus was present. Over several trials, if individuals performed worse than chance, it was presumed that they knew the correct response and chose not to report it. In a 2-alternative forced-choice task, below-chance performance is less than 50%, although exact probabilities can be obtained using the normal approximation to the binomial theorem.[40] In assessments of feigning, most SVT assessments incorporate feedback regarding the accuracy of the response.

Multiple assessments of feigned memory and cognitive deficits have been developed using this paradigm, often coupled with the floor effect paradigm. One example is the Test of Memory Malingering (TOMM).[60] The TOMM is a visual recognition test that involves presenting an individual with 50 different picture drawings. Two learning trials are presented followed by a retention trial. Scores below chance or based on

Table 1
Select assessments using the floor effect paradigm

Name	Content	Scoring
FIT	• 15 Redundant items grouped 3 in 5 rows	• Score less than 9 suggestive of feigning
Rey Dot Counting test	• 12 Cards with different numbers of dots • First 6 cards dots random • Last 6 dots grouped	• Responses and response time recorded • Response time of grouped dots equal to ungrouped suggestive of feigning
The b Test	• Circle all lowercase *b*'s in a 15-page booklet • Requires distinguishing between *q*'s, *p*'s, and *d*'s	Malingering suggested by any one of the following: • Greater than 40 *omission* errors (not circling *b*'s) • Greater than 2 *commission* errors (circling *q*'s, *p*'s, or *d*'s) • Greater than 12 minutes to complete
Coin-in-hand test	• Examiner shows evaluee coin in hand for 2 seconds • Evaluee asked to close eyes and count backward from 10 to 1 • Evaluator clenches both hands (hiding coin) • Evaluee asked to tap which evaluator's hand is holding the coin • 10 Trials of evaluee tapping evaluator's hand with coin presented	Less than 9 accurate identifications of hand holding coin suggests feigning

criteria developed from head-injured or cognitively impaired individuals are indicative of feigned memory impairment. **Table 2** presents several of the SVT assessments cited most frequently as useful in the detection of feigning, primarily of memory or cognitive deficits.

Performance Curve Analysis

The performance curve analysis strategy is less widely used in psychological tests developed to assess malingering, perhaps in part because of the complexity of the development of such assessments. This strategy is based on the supposition that malingerers do not distinguish between easy and difficult items when providing inaccurate responses. With nonmalingering individuals, there is an expectation that accuracy of responses decrease as item difficulty increases. Individuals exhibiting a lack of effort or random responding are as likely to respond inaccurately to easy as to difficult items. One test that uses this strategy, coupled with SVT, is the Validity Indicator Profile (VIP).[61] The VIP consists of verbal and nonverbal subtests, both using a 2-alternative forced-choice paradigm. Item difficulty is randomly distributed throughout the test to prevent a test taker from adopting a strategy of answering easy items accurately. After scoring, response styles are categorized as compliant, careless, irrelevant, and malingered. One concern with the VIP is that in order to be classified as malingering, the examinee has to exert effort; otherwise, responses are classified as either careless or irrelevant.

Table 2
Symptom validity tests

Name	Description	Area Assessed
Victoria Symptom Validity Test	• Computer administered • Forced-choice paradigm • 24 Easy and 24 difficult items • Response time recorded	Memory
TOMM	• 2 Alternative forced-choice paradigm • 50 Target pictures presented • Evaluee must recognize previously presented picture from 2 pictures shown	Memory
Portland Digit Recognition Test	• 72 Items, 26 easy and 36 hard • Verbal presentation of 5-digit number • 5-s, 10-s, and 30-s delays for memory recall	Memory
Digit Memory Test	• 3 Blocks of 24 5-digit numbers • Forced choice with 5-s, 10-s, and 15-s delays	Memory
WMT	• 20 Linked word lists • Oral and computerized version	Memory
VIP	• 100 Problems assessing nonverbal abstraction • 78 Word definition problems • 2 Alternative forced-choice paradigm	General cognitive functioning
Computerized Assessment of Response Bias	• Computer administered • 25 Trials of 5-digit string • Response time also recorded	Memory
21-Item test	• 21 Object nouns • 7 Rhyming pairs, 7 semantically similar, 7 unrelated • Free recall and forced-choice recognition	Memory

Unusual Patterns or Responses

Several psychological tests evaluate if an examinee is providing atypical responses to questions about mental health symptoms. Examples of such atypical responses include symptoms rarely presented by those with a genuine mental disorder, an unusual combination of symptoms, highly improbable or absurd symptoms, or an inconsistency in reported symptoms compared with actual behavior observed during the evaluation or with prior reported symptoms on the test. The most widely used assessment for the detection of feigned psychiatric symptoms using this paradigm is the Structured Interview of Reported Symptoms (SIRS).[62] The SIRS was developed to assess a broad range of strategies in the detection of feigning. It is a 172-item structured interview, which requires approximately 30 to 45 minutes to administer. The original SIRS contained 8 primary and 5 supplementary scales. The supplementary scales were used only if a respondent did not endorse symptoms in sufficient quantity to make a definitive determination. Responses on the primary scales were classified as honest, indeterminate, probable, or definite. Individuals were considered feigning psychiatric symptoms if they scored in the definite range on at least 1 primary subscale or in the probable range on 3 or more primary subscales. Studies indicated that these criteria optimized both sensitivity and specificity.[62] The SIRS has been shown a valid and reliable method for detecting malingering[63,64] with low false-positive rates,[65] although other investigators have found the false-positive rate extremely high.[66] Despite this criticism, the SIRS has been reported to have general acceptance among forensic experts in evaluations[67] and is often cited as the gold standard[68] or benchmark[69] in the detection of feigned psychiatric symptoms. The SIRS has recently been revised (SIRS-2),[70] although the primary scales remain unchanged. A new supplementary scale was added, which was developed to assess feigned cognitive deficits. The SIRS-2 provides an algorithm for decision making that includes the use of composite scores as well as the primary scales. No information has yet been provided on the likelihood of feigning based on this algorithm. **Table 3** provides a list of structured assessments developed to assess the feigning of psychiatric symptoms using the unusual patterns or responses paradigm.

MALINGERING ASSESSMENT OF SPECIFIC DISORDERS

Although it is beyond the scope of this article to summarize the literature regarding the structured assessment of all potentially malingered symptoms, key psychological assessments to evaluate malingering in the following disorders are reviewed:

- Psychotic disorders
- PTSD
- Neurocognitive impairment, which can include both intellectual and memory deficits
- Depressive disorders

Malingered Psychosis

Readers are directed to comprehensive articles by Resnick[71,72] for clinical assessment of malingered psychosis. Prior to the development of tests specifically designed to detect feigned psychosis, the MMPI was the instrument used most extensively in this regard. Although not initially developed for this purpose, the family of F scales, in particular, F, Fb, and Fp, have been shown to have validity in detecting feigned psychosis (discussed previously). The Gough Dissimulation Index (F-K)[73] also has evidenced utility in detecting symptom exaggeration. This index was developed by

Table 3
Unusual patterns of response tests

Name	Description	Scoring
SIRS	• 172-Item structured interview • Scores classified as honest, indeterminate, probable, definite • Eight primary scales: ○ Rare symptoms ○ Symptom combinations ○ Improbable/absurd symptoms ○ Blatant symptoms ○ Subtle symptoms ○ Selectivity of symptoms ○ Severity of symptoms ○ Reported versus observed symptoms	• Feigning if score 1 (or more) in the definite range OR 3 (or more) in the probable range • Supplementary scales are only used to aid in the interpretation when the results on the primary scales are NOT definitive for malingering
SIRS-2	• Same as SIRS with new supplementary scale to assess feigned cognitive deficits (improbable failure)	• New algorithm for decision making regarding malingering
SIMS	• 75-Item true/false self-report test • Five subscales: ○ Low intelligence ○ Affective disorders ○ Neurologic impairment ○ Psychosis ○ Amnestic disorders	• Varies for each subscale • Greater than 14 total score indicative of feigning
M-FAST	• 25-Item structured interview • Yields scores relevant to 7 strategies	• Total score of 6 or greater suggestive of feigning

combining 2 of the 3 original validity scales. In original development studies of this index, if the raw score of F minus the raw score of K was greater than +9, the validity profile was designated as over-reporting. Subsequent research has been mixed regarding this cut point, with some investigators suggesting lower cut scores[74] and others suggesting higher ones.[75]

The SIRS (discussed previously) can be extremely valuable in the detection of feigned psychosis. Three of the 8 primary scales on the SIRS are most likely elevated in feigned psychotic symptoms:

1. Rare symptoms
2. Improbable/absurd symptoms
3. Blatant symptoms

Each of these scales includes symptoms many laypersons associate with severe mental illness.

Miller Forensic Assessment of Symptoms Test
The Miller Forensic Assessment of Symptoms Test (M-FAST)[76] was developed as a screening instrument designed to identify malingered psychopathology. It is a 25-item structured interview administered in approximately 5 minutes. It consists of items rationally derived from the literature on constructs useful in identifying malingerers and yields scores relevant to 7 strategies: unusual hallucinations, reported

versus observed, rare combinations, extreme symptomatology, negative image, unusual symptom course, and suggestibility. A score of 6 or higher is suggested by the manual as indicating a need for more extensive assessment. Research indicates that it is effective in identifying feigning in a variety of settings.[77,78]

Structured Inventory of Malingered Symptomatology

The Structured Inventory of Malingered Symptomatology (SIMS)[79] is a 75-item true/false self-report test developed as a screening tool. One advantage of the SIMS is that it contains 5 subscales that assess malingering in areas other than psychopathology. The subscales are low intelligence, amnestic disorders, neurologic impairment, affective disorders, and psychosis. Research has been mixed regarding its effectiveness in discriminating psychiatric patients from malingerers.[80,81]

Malingered Posttraumatic Stress Disorder (PTSD)

PTSD is especially easy to malinger because the diagnosis is based primarily on a person's self-report. Information about PTSD criteria is readily available; more than 2 million citations describing PTSD were found in a recent Google search.[82] Furthermore, many of the standard assessment instruments to assess PTSD use a structured interview format with questions that are obviously directed toward possible PTSD symptoms. Questioning in this suggestive manner may actually teach specific PTSD symptoms to an examinee thereby enhancing the possibility of successful feigning. PTSD is the only diagnosis in the *DSM-IV-TR* that specifically states, "Malingering should be ruled out in those situations in which financial remuneration, benefit eligibility, and forensic determinations play a role."[82(p467)]

Recently, there has been an abundance of research examining the utility of the MMPI-2 in detecting feigned PTSD. The detection of malingered PTSD is complicated by individuals with genuine PTSD who may experiencing substantial distress and legitimately elevate some validity scales. The Fp scale has evidenced an ability above the standard F and Fb scales to distinguish individuals with genuine psychopathology from those asked to feign disorders. More recently, the FBS has shown promise in identifying malingered PTSD in personal injury claims[83] although further research was mixed in this regard. For example, Butcher and colleagues[50] asserted that because of the "unacceptably high" false-positive rates, the FBS should not be used in disability evaluations.

Infrequency posttraumatic stress disorder scale

Elhai and colleagues[84] developed a scale specifically to detect feigned PTSD—the Infrequency-Posttraumatic Stress Disorder scale, which includes items infrequently endorsed by veterans with legitimate PTSD. In the development sample, this scale was found to improve the accuracy of detection of feigned PTSD above other F scales, although subsequent research failed to replicate that finding. For example, in a study of veterans seeking disability compensation who were instructed to feign, the family of F scales, in particular, F, Fb, and Fp, was most effective in discriminating between honest reporters and feigners. Fp in particular was superior in discriminating the 2 groups. The investigators suggest using a cut score of Fp greater than 99 (T score) for identifying individuals feigning PTSD. They also reported that the Infrequency-Posttraumatic Stress Disorder scale did not improve the accuracy of detection and that the FBS scale "produced unacceptable positive predictive power" and should not be used.[85]

Morel Emotional Numbing Test

The Morel Emotional Numbing Test (MENT)[86] has been described as an SVT specific to PTSD. This instrument assesses affect recognition in a 2-alternative forced-choice format. Although many of the SVTs commonly used are measures of malingered memory deficits, the MENT assesses primarily PTSD malingering. Using a 2-alternative format, the MENT is designed to give test takers the impression that deficits in affect recognition are pathognomonic of PTSD. Evaluees are told, "Some individuals with PTSD may have difficulty recognizing facial expressions" and they are then asked to note the emotion associated with the facial expression they are shown. The MENT consists of 20 photographs of 10 facial expressions for both genders. Three trials are presented. In the first trial, 1 photo is presented with 2 words; the subject is asked to circle the word that describes the emotion. In the second trial, 2 photos are shown with 1 word; the subject is asked to select the photo that matches the word. In the third and final trial, 2 photos and 3 words are presented and the task is to match the appropriate photo with the word. According to Morel,[86] adults who put forth a reasonable amount of effort (except for the visually impaired or those with less than a third-grade reading level) can complete the task with 90% to 100% accuracy even if they have PTSD, recommending that more than 9 errors is suggestive of malingering. In a study investigating the use of the MENT with Croatian war veterans (who have been shown to evidence symptom over-reporting when seeking compensation), using a cut score of 9 produced a sensitivity of 92% and specificity of 96%.[87] This suggests that the MENT may be useful as one component of an assessment of malingered PTSD.

Atypical response scale

The Atypical Response (ATR) scale of the Trauma Symptom Inventory, Second edition (TSI-2) has also been described as useful in distinguishing genuine symptoms of PTSD from simulated PTSD.[88] In their study of 75 undergraduate students trained to simulate PTSD and 49 undergraduate students with genuine PTSD, Gray and colleagues[89] determined that the ATR correctly classified 75% of genuinely distressed individuals and 74% of PTSD simulators. This scale is a revised version of the ATR from the original TSI, which had evidenced unimpressive classification rates.[90,91]

Malingered Cognitive Impairment

The diagnosis of most psychiatric disorders relies on a patient's accurate self-report of symptoms. As discussed previously, with the exception of factitious disorder and malingering, the presumption is that most patients are not consciously attempting to misrepresent their symptoms. When they are, there is ample opportunity via the Internet to become well versed in specific symptoms to report. In contrast to the production of psychiatric symptoms, feigning cognitive impairments often requires a demonstration of absence of functioning. Slick and colleagues[92] coined the term, malingering of neurocognitive dysfunction, which is characterized by the intentional exaggeration or fabrication of cognitive dysfunction for the purpose of obtaining some external incentive or avoiding responsibility. Many investigators have attempted to put forth guidelines regarding when to suspect this type of malingering. Greiffenstein and colleagues[93] indicated that examiners should suspect malingered memory deficits under the following circumstances:

1. Poor performance on 2 or more standard neuropsychological assessments
2. Complete disability in a social role
3. Inconsistency between reported symptom history and other sources of information
4. Remote memory loss

Pankratz and Binder[94] suggested 7 behaviors that are indicative of malingering and require further exploration. The first and foremost is dishonesty: if patients misrepresent details of their lives, they also may be misrepresenting their symptoms. Additionally, the following 6 are suggestive of malingering:

1. Inconsistency between reported and observed symptoms
2. Inconsistency between physical and neuropsychological findings
3. Resistance to or avoidance of standardized tests
4. Failure on measures designed to detect malingering
5. Functional findings on medical examination
6. Delayed cognitive complaints after trauma

Faust and Ackley[95] also suggest 6 behaviors that are indicative of feigned cognitive deficits:

1. Poor effort
2. Exaggerated symptoms
3. Production of nonexistent symptoms
4. Distortion of history regarding symptoms
5. Distortion of premorbid functioning
6. Denial of strengths

Slick and colleagues[92] have proposed a more complicated schema for the detection of malingered cognitive deficits, which includes 4 criteria, designated as criteria A through D. Criterion A is the presence of financial incentive. Criterion B includes evidence of exaggeration on neuropsychological tests. Criterion C includes evidence of false or exaggerated self-report, and criterion D is that both criteria B and C cannot be accounted for by psychiatric, neurologic, or developmental factors. An individual is considered a probable malingerer when criterion A is met and 2 or more items (of a list of 6) are met from criterion B or 1 from criterion B and 1 from criterion C (of a list of 5). Possible malingering is defined as the presence of criterion A plus 2 (or more) items from criterion C. More simply put, these investigators believe that self-report evidence (other than an admission of malingering) is only suggestive of malingering; evidence of malingering on standard neuropsychological testing is necessary to be more definitive. One component of this schema is the presence of an external incentive. **Table 4** provides the components of each criterion.

The National Academy of Neuropsychology issued similar guidelines regarding possible feigned performance on neurocognitive tests[96]:

1. Inconsistencies in various domains (eg, symptoms inconsistent with known pattern of brain function)
2. Performance on neuropsychological assessments suggestive of feigning
3. Evidence of exaggeration on psychological testing
4. Poor performance on SVT
5. Below-chance performance on forced-choices assessments

Although these guidelines vary in complexity, one consistency in all is the use of structured, standardized assessments. Such assessments are a critical component when evaluating the validity of neurocognitive dysfunction. In a meta-analysis of 32 studies of the most commonly used testing, Vickery and colleagues[57] found that individuals feigning cognitive deficits achieved scores more than 1 SD below that of honest responders. They found that the Digit Memory Test,[97] the Portland Digit Recognition Test,[98] the FIT,[56] and the 21-item test[99] all evidenced high specificity, although the Digit Memory Test evidenced the highest sensitivity (83%). The Portland Digit Recognition Test and FIT had comparable sensitivities (44% and 43%, respectively) whereas the 21-item test performed the worst in this regard (22%). Each of these tests is briefly described in **Tables 1** and **2**.

Table 4
Slick criteria for malingered neurocognitive deficits

Criterion	Definition
A. Presence of substantial external incentive	At least one clearly identifiable and substantial external incentive present at the time of the examination

B. Evidence from neuropsychological testing	• Definite or probable response bias
	• Discrepancy between test data and the following:
	  o Known patterns of brain functioning
	  o Observed behavior
	  o Reliable collateral reports
	  o Documented background history

C. Evidence from self-report	• Self-reported history is discrepant with the following:
	  o Known patterns of brain functioning
	  o Behavioral observations
	  o Information obtained from collateral informants
	• Evidence of exaggerated or fabricated dysfunction

D. Behaviors noted in criteria B and C are the product of an informed, rational, volitional effort aimed to achieve an external incentive	Behaviors noted in criteria B and C are not fully accounted for by psychiatric, neurologic, or developmental factors

In a direct comparison of the TOMM and the Word Memory Test (WMT), Greiffenstein and colleagues[100] found that although the WMT evidenced a slight advantage over the TOMM, they expressed concern about the high failure rate on the WMT in patients with severe traumatic brain injury. They concluded that the WMT may have a false-positive rate higher than the TOMM and suggested that further research is necessary using a known groups design.

Unfortunately, individuals can successfully feign deficits on tests designed to measure intelligence. For example, Graue and colleagues[101] showed that community volunteers were able to feign a lowered IQ on the Wechsler Adult Intelligence Scale–Third Edition when instructed to do so, and embedded tests of malingering (Digit Span scaled score and Reliable Digit Span) did not reliably identify such feigning. Likewise, measures of adaptive behavior, such as the Adaptive Behavior Assessment System–Second Edition,[102] are also susceptible to manipulation.[103]

Unlike abundant studies examining characteristics of feigned cognitive impairment, there is limited research on appropriate testing methods for feigned intellectual disabilities and/or mental retardation. In their survey of 50 forensic psychology diplomats, Victor and Boone[104] determined that 64% reported using the TOMM, 50% reported used the VIP,[61] and 44% reported using the FIT[56] to assess malingered intellectual disabilities, despite few data on the use of these measures with this population. In a survey of neuropsychologists who consistently practice in the area of compensation claims,[105] more than 45% indicated that they routinely use the TOMM,[60] and more than 33% indicated that they use the FIT.[56]

Of particular concern are individuals with intellectual disabilities, who may be falsely identified as not providing adequate effort on many of the effort tests commonly used to assess feigned cognitive impairment.[106] Evaluators should use caution in incorporating the same symptom validity tests and neurocognitive test indicators for malingering when evaluating individuals with intellectual disabilities. A similar phenomenon may be true with instruments designed to detect feigned psychopathology. To evaluate the utility of the SIRS-2 in this population, Weiss and colleagues[107] administered this instrument to a sample of 43 persons diagnosed with intellectual disabilities with no incentive to feign psychiatric symptoms. They found that 23.3% of the sample was misclassified as feigning psychiatric symptoms using the original SIRS scoring system. When the modified scoring algorithm described in the SIRS-2 manual was implemented, only 7.0% of the sample was incorrectly identified as feigning. Although this represents a significant improvement, the high percentage of potential false-positive results raises particular concern. Those individuals with a comorbid psychiatric diagnosis were at particular risk for being misclassified as malingering.[107]

In an attempt to address limitations of current effort tests and structured interviews administered to individuals claiming low cognitive functioning during their social security disability evaluation, Chafetz and colleagues[108] developed the Symptom Validity Scale (SVS) for low-functioning individuals. The SVS uses 11 embedded indicators validated for use in low cognitive functioning individuals. The embedded indicators use a variety of strategies to assess effort, including missing simple arithmetic calculations, performing simple sequences, not knowing or being able to pick the US President from a list of names, missing personal information, providing Ganser-like answers (ie, near misses to easy questions), a variety of target items from the Wechsler scales, providing a highly improbable response to questions (eg, What is the shape of a ball? "A triangle"), and claiming improbable pathology (such as seeing a ghost).

Malingered Depression

As with PTSD symptoms, a diagnosis of depression relies primarily on individual self-report. Unlike PTSD however, depression is more ubiquitous; the results of the National Comorbidity Survey indicate a lifetime prevalence of 20% for women and 10% for men.[109] This suggests that the general public may be more familiar with the symptoms of depression. Moreover, Griffin and colleagues[37] found that a substantial percentage of disability applicants reported depression as their primary complaint. Additionally, many standard assessments of depression contain questions about symptoms easily identified as associated with depression (eg, the Beck Depression Inventory)[110] and rarely contain embedded validity scales. As such, detecting feigned depression has been problematic. Although the assessment of response styles in forensic evaluations has led to the proliferation of methods, scales, and procedures for the detection of feigning of many disorders, until recently, little has been published on the detection of feigned depression using psychological assessments.

MMPI-2

The MMPI-2 is perhaps the most researched instrument regarding the feigning of severe psychopathology and somatic/neurocognitive deficits. As discussed previously, it has evidenced impressive validity in this regard. Unfortunately, the MMPI-2 is less effective in the detection of feigned depression. There may be several reasons for this. In a recent meta-analysis, Rogers and colleagues[111] found that patients with legitimate depression often produced elevations on the standard validity scales. Bagby and colleagues[112] found that the MMPI-2 validity scales were more successful in detecting feigned schizophrenia compared with feigned depression in a group of college students instructed to simulate one or the other disorder. Viglione and colleagues[113] showed that when simulators were educated to avoid extreme exaggeration of depression, the MMPI-2 was unable to detect feigning on the standard validity scales.

Malingered depression scale

Because of the limited ability of the standard validity scales on the MMPI-2, Steffan and colleauges[114] developed a validity scale (malingered depression [Md]) specific to the feigning of depressive symptoms. They selected items based on effect sizes that discriminated between participants instructed to feign depression and those with legitimate depression. The resultant scale included 32 items. Receiver operator characteristic analyses based on a cut score of 15 evidenced impressive specificity and sensitivity in the development sample, with an area under the curve (AUC) of 0.969. To place this in context, an AUC of .50 is like flipping a coin. The closer the AUC is to 1.0, the higher the predictive power. The cross-validation sample suggested that a cut score of 22 was most effective in distinguishing simulators from individuals with depression. Unfortunately, further research suggested that the Md scale was not effective in distinguishing patients presenting for a neuropsychological evaluation seeking compensation from those who were not.[115] Henry and colleagues[116] revised the Md, reducing the number of items from 32 to 15, and found that using a cut score of 8 they obtained no false-positive errors.

Assessment of Depression Inventory

Mogge and LePage[117] attempted to overcome the limitations of most depression assessments by developing an instrument with embedded validity scales, the Assessment of Depression Inventory (ADI). The ADI is a 39-item, self-report instrument that assesses symptoms of depression and contains 2 validity scales—feigning and random. The ADI has shown impressive correlations with other standard measures of depression in both inpatients[118] and outpatients.[119] In addition, in both studies, the ADI feigning scale correlated with the validity scales of the PAI. The investigators suggest that future research with the ADI should be conducted with more sophisticated feigners.

SUMMARY

Psychological testing is a critical component in assessing the validity of an individual's reported mental health and/or cognitive symptoms. Poor performance on any one test may not be definitive for malingering, because an evaluee may have other reasons that explain suboptimal performance outside of a deliberate intent to mislead the examiner for secondary gain. Poor performance on multiple symptom validity tests increases the likelihood that individuals are deliberately feigning or exaggerating their reported symptoms.[120] As this article describes, there are many psychological tests of malingering available that use a variety of strategies for detecting malingering. Selecting tests appropriate to the type of malingering and specific to the disorder that is malingered is crucial. A comprehensive assessment of feigning should include multiple tests using varying strategies of detection. In this way, forensic clinicians can augment a thorough assessment and go beyond detection to provide a definitive diagnosis of malingering.

REFERENCES

1. Beck TR, Beck JB. Elements of medical jurisprudence. Philadelphia: Thomas, Cowperthwait & Co.; 1838.

2. Feigning. American heritage dictionary of the English language. 4th edition. Available at: http://dictionary.reference.com/browse/feigning. Accessed March 30, 2012.
3. American Psychiatric Association. Diagnostic and statistical manual of mental disorders. 4th edition, text revision. Washington, DC: American Psychiatric Association; 2000.
4. Heilbronner RL, Sweet JJ, Morgan JE, et al. American Academy of Clinical Neuropsychology consensus statement on the neuropsychological assessment of effort, response bias and malingering. Clin Neuropsychol 2009;23:1093–129.
5. McCullumsmith CB, Ford CV. Simulated illness: the factitious disorders and malingering. Psychiatr Clin North Am 2011,34.621–41.
6. Scott CL, McDermott BE. Malingering and mental health disability evaluations. In: Gold LH, Vanderpool D, editors. Clinical guide to mental disability evaluations. New York: Springer Science and Business Media, in press.
7. Scott CL, McDermott B. Malingering. In: Buchanan A, Norko M, editors. The psychiatric report, principles and practice of forensic report writing. New York: Cambridge University Press; 2011. p. 240–53.
8. Bianchini KJ, Curtis KL, Greve KW. Compensation and malingering in traumatic brain injury: a dose-response relationship? Clin Neuropsychol 2006;20: 831–47.
9. Rohling ML, Binder LM, Langhinrischen-Rohling J. Money matters: meta-analytic review of the association between financial compensation and the experience and treatment of chronic pain. Health Psychol 1995;14:537–47.
10. Binder LM, Rohling ML. Money matters: meta-analytic review of the effects of financial incentives on recovery after closed-head injury. Am J Psychiatry 1996;153:7–10.
11. Cornell DG, Hawk GL. Clinical presentation of malingerers diagnosed by experienced forensic psychologists. Law Hum Behav 1989;13:375–83.
12. Rogers R, Salekin RT, Sewell KW, et al. A comparison of forensic and nonforensic malingerers: a prototypical analysis of explanatory models. Law Hum Behav 1998;22:353–67.
13. Rogers R, Sewell KW, Goldstein AM. Explanatory models of malingering: a prototypical analysis. Law Hum Behav 1994;18:543–52.
14. Rogers R, Seman W, Clark CR. Assessment of criminal responsibility: initial validation of the R-CRAS with the M'Naghten and GBMI standards. Int J Law Psychiatry 1986;9:67–75.
15. McDermott BE, Rabin A, Scott CL, et al. Triaging the IST patient: a brief screen to reduce LOS. Proc Am Psych Law. Baltimore; 2009.
16. Pollock P, Quigley D, Worley K, et al. Feigned mental disorder in prisoners referred to forensic mental health services. J Psychiatr Ment Health Nurs 1997;4:9–15.
17. Norris MP, May MC. Screening for malingering in a correctional setting. Law Hum Behav 1998;22:315–23.
18. Walters GD, White TW, Greene RL. Use of the MMPI to identify malingering and exaggeration of psychiatric symptomatology in male prison inmates. J Consult Clin Psychol 1988;56:111–7.
19. Rogers R, Ustad KL, Salekin R. Convergent validity of the personality assessment inventory: a study of emergency referrals in a correctional setting. Assessment 1998;5:3–12.
20. McDermott BE, Sokolov G. Malingering in a correctional setting: the use of the structured interview of reported symptoms in a jail sample. Behav Sci Law 2009; 27:753–65.

21. Walters GD. Coping with malingering and exaggeration of psychiatric symptom-atology in offender populations. Am J Forensic Psychol 2006;24:21–40.
22. Peace KA, Masliuk KA. Do motivations for malingering matter? Symptoms of malingered PTSD as a function of motivation and trauma type. Psychol Inj Law 2011;4:44–55.
23. Binder LM. Assessment of malingering after mild head trauma with the Portland digit recognition test. J Clin Exp Neuropsychol 1993;15:170–82.
24. Greiffenstein MF, Baker WJ. Miller was (mostly) right: head injury severity inversely related to simulation. Legal and Criminological Psychology 2006;11:131–45.
25. Larrabee GJ. Detection of malingering using atypical performance patterns on standard neuropsychological tests. Clin Neuropsychol 2003;17:410–25.
26. Larrabee GJ. Forensic neuropsychological assessment. In: Vanderploeg AD, editor. Clinician's guide to neuropsychological assessment. 2nd edition. Malwah (NJ): Lawrence Erlbaum; 2000. p. 301–35.
27. Green P, Rohling ML, Lees-Haley PR, et al. Effort has a greater effect on test scores than severe brain injury in compensation claims. Brain Inj 2001;15:1045–60.
28. Mittenberg W, Patton C, Canyock EM, et al. Base rates of malingering and symptom exaggeration. J Clin Exp Neuropsychol 2002;24:1094–102.
29. Leavitt F, Sweet JJ. Characteristics and frequency of malingering among patients with low back pain. Pain 1986;25:357–64.
30. Gervais RO, Russell AS, Green P, et al. Effort testing in patients with fibromyalgia and disability incentives. J Rheumatol 2001;28:1892–9.
31. Gervais RO, Green P, Allen LM, et al. Effects of coaching on symptom validity testing in chronic pain patients presenting for disability assessments. J Forensic Neuropsychol 2001;2:1–19.
32. Greve KW, Ord JS, Bianchini KJ, et al. Prevalence of malingering in patients with chronic pain referred for psychologic evaluation in a medico-legal context. Arch Phys Med Rehabil 2009;90:1117–26.
33. Schmand B, Lindeboom J, Schagen S, et al. Cognitive complaints in patients after whiplash injury: the impact of malingering. J Neurol Neurosurg Psychiatr 1998;64:339–42.
34. Marx BP, Holowka DW. PTSD disability assessment. PTSD Research Quarterly 2011;22:1–6.
35. Gold PB, Frueh BC. Compensation-seeking and extreme exaggeration of psychopathology among combat veterans evaluated for PTSD. J Nerv Ment Dis 1999;187:680–4.
36. Frueh BC, Hamner MB, Cahill SP, et al. Apparent symptom overreporting in combat veterans evaluated for PTSD. Clin Psychol Rev 2000;20:853–85.
37. Griffin GA, Normington J, May R, et al. Assessing dissimulation among social security disability income claimants. J Consult Clin Psychol 1996;64:1425–30.
38. Wierzbicki MJ, Tyson CM. A summary of evaluations for learning and attention problems at a university training clinic. Journal of Postsecondary Education and Disability 2007;20:16–27.
39. McGrath RE, Mitchell M, Kim BH, et al. Evidence for response bias as a source of error variance in applied assessment. Psychol Bull 2010;136:450–70.
40. Larrabee GJ. Assessment of malingering. In: Larrabee GJ, editor. Forensic neuropsychology: a scientific approach. Oxford (United Kingdom): University Press; 2011. p. 116–59.
41. Hathaway SR, McKinley JC. MMPI manual. New York: Psychological Corporation; 1967.

42. Butcher JN, Dahlstrom WG, Graham JR, et al. MMPI-2: manual for administration and scoring. Minneapolis (MN): University of Minnesota Press; 1989.

43. Morey LC. Personality assessment inventory: professional manual. Odessa (FL): Psychological Assessment Resources; 1991.

44. Wygant DB, Sellbom M, Gervais RO, et al. Further validation of the MMPI-2 and MMPI-2-RF Response Bias Scale: findings from disability and criminal forensic settings. Psychol Assess 2010;22:745–56.

45. Greene RL. The MMPI: an interpretive manual. New York: Grune & Stratton, Inc; 1980.

46. Larrabee GJ. Forensic neuropsychology. New York: Oxford University Press; 2005.

47. Lees-Haley PR, English LT, Glenn WJ. A fake bad scale for the MMPI-2 for personal injury claimants. Psychol Rep 1991;68:203–10.

48. Gervais RO, Ben-Porath YS, Wygant DB, et al. Development and validation of a Response Bias Scale (RBS) for the MMPI-2. Assessment 2007;14:196–208.

49. Larrabee G. Somatic malingering on the MMPI and MMPI-2 in litigating subjects. Clin Neuropsychol 1998;12:179–88.

50. Butcher JN, Arbisi PA, Atlis MM, et al. The construct validity of the Lees-Haley Fake Bad Scale Does this scale measure somatic malingering and feigned emotional distress? Arch Clin Neuropsychol 2008;23:855–64.

51. Gass CS, Williams CL, Cumella E, et al. Ambiguous measures of unknown constructs: the MMPI-2 Fake Bad Scale. Psychol Inj Law 2010;3:81–5.

52. Butcher JN, Gass CS, Cumella E, et al. Potential for bias in MMPI-2 assessments using the Fake Bad Scale. Psychol Inj Law 2008;1:191–209.

53. Morey LC. Defensiveness and malingering indices for the PAI. Paper presented at the meeting of the American Psychological Association. Toronto, 1993.

54. Morey LC. An interpretive guide to the personality assessment inventory (PAI). Odessa (FL): Psychological Assessment Resources; 1996.

55. Rogers R, Gillard ND, Wooley CN, et al. The detection of feigned disabilities: the effectiveness of the Personality Assessment Inventory in a traumatized inpatient sample. Assessment 1996;19:77–88.

56. Rey A. L'examen Clinique en psychologie (the clinical examination in psychology). Paris: Presses Universitaire de France; 1964.

57. Vickery CD, Berry DTR, Inman TH, et al. Detection of inadequate effort on neuropsychological testing: a meta-analytic review of selected procedures. Arch Clin Neuropsychol 2001;16:45–73.

58. Griffin GAE, Glassmire DM, Henderson EA, et al. Rey II: redesigning the Rey corooning toot of malingering. J Clin Psychol 1997;53.757–66.

59. Pankratz L. Symptom validity testing and symptom retraining: procedures for the assessment and treatment of functional sensory deficits. J Consult Clin Psychol 1979;47:409–10.

60. Tombaugh TN. Test of memory malingering (TOMM). New York: Multi-Health Systems; 1996.

61. Frederick RI, Foster HG. The validity indicator profile. Minneapolis (MN): National Computer Systems; 1997.

62. Rogers R, Bagby RM, Dickens SE. Structured interview of reported symptoms: professional manual. Odessa (FL): Psychological Assessment Resources; 1992.

63. Gothard S, Viglione DJ, Meloy JR, et al. Detection of malingering in competency to stand trial evaluations. Law Hum Behav 1995;19:493–505.

64. Hayes JS, Hale DB, Gouvier WD. Malingering detection in a mentally retarded forensic population. Appl Neuropsychol 1998;5:33–6.

65. Rogers R. Handbook of diagnostic and structured interviewing. New York: Guilford Press; 2001.
66. Pollock PH. A cautionary note on the determination of malingering in offenders. Psychol Crime Law 1996;3:97–110.
67. Lally SJ. What tests are acceptable for use in forensic evaluations? A survey of experts. Prof Psychol Res Pr 2003;34:491–8.
68. Green D, Rosenfeld B. Evaluating the gold standard: a review and meta-analysis of the structured interview of reported symptoms. Psychol Assess 2011;23:95–107.
69. Kocsis RN. The structured interview of reported symptoms 2nd edition (SIRS-2): the new benchmark towards the assessment of malingering. J Forensic Psychol Pract 2011;11:73–81.
70. Rogers R, Sewell KW, Gillard ND. Structured interview of reported symptoms professional manual. 2nd edition. Odessa (FL): Psychological Assessment Resources; 2010.
71. Resnick PJ. Malingered psychosis. In: Rogers R, editor. Clinical assessment of malingering and deception. 2nd edition. New York: Guilford; 1997. p. 47–67.
72. Resnick PJ. The detection of malingered psychosis. Psychiatr Clin North Am 1999;22:159–72.
73. Gough HG. The F minus K dissimulation index for the MMPI. J Consult Clin Psychol 1950;14:408–13.
74. Sivec HJ, Lynn SJ, Garske JP. The effect of somatoform disorder and paranoid psychotic role-related dissimulations as a response set on the MMPI-2. Assessment 1994;1:69–81.
75. Graham JR, Watts D, Timbrook RE. Detecting fake-good and fake-bad MMPI-2 profiles. J Pers Assess 1991;57:264–77.
76. Miller H. Miller forensic assessment of symptoms test (MFAST) professional manual. Odessa (FL): Psychological Assessment Resources; 2001.
77. Guy LS, Miller HA. Screening for malingered psychopathology in a correctional setting: utility of the miller-forensic assessment of symptoms test (M-FAST). Crim Justice Behav 2004;31:695–716.
78. Jackson RL, Rogers R, Sewell KW. Forensic applications of the Miller Forensic Assessment of Symptoms Test (MFAST): screening for feigned disorders in competency to stand trial evaluations. Law Hum Behav 2005;29:199–210.
79. Widows MR, Smith GP. Structured inventory of malingered symptomatology professional manual. Odessa (FL): Psychological Assessment Resources; 2005.
80. Edens JF, Otto RK, Dwyer T. Utility of the structured inventory of malingered symptomatology in identifying persons motivated to malinger psychopathology. J Am Acad Psychiatry Law 1999;27:387–96.
81. Rogers R, Jackson RL, Kaminski PL. Factitious psychological disorders: the overlooked response style in forensic evaluations. J Forensic Psychol Pract 2005;5:21–41.
82. Hall CW, Hall CW. Malingering of PTSD and diagnostic considerations, characteristics of malingerers and clinical presentations. Gen Hosp Psychiatry 2006; 28:525–35.
83. Lees-Haley PR. Efficacy of MMPI-2 validity scales and MCMI-II modifier scales for detecting spurious PTSD claims: F, F-K, fake bad scale, ego strength, subtle-obvious subscales, DIS and DEB. J Clin Psychol 1992;48:681–9.
84. Elhai JD, Ruggiero KJ, Frueh BC, et al. The infrequency-posttraumatic stress disorder scale (Fptsd) for the MMPI-2: development and initial validation with veterans presenting with combat-related PTSD. J Pers Assess 2002;79:531–49.

85. Elhai JD, Naifeh JA, Zucker IS, et al. Discriminating malingered from genuine civilian posttraumatic stress disorder a validation of three MMPI-2 infrequency scales (F, Fp, and Fptsd). Assessment 2004;11:139–44.

86. Morel KR. Development and preliminary validation of a forced-choice test of response bias for posttraumatic stress disorder. J Pers Assess 1998;70:299–314.

87. Geraerts E, Kozaric-Kovacic C, Merckelbach H. Detecting deception of war-related posttraumatic stress disorder. J Forens Psychiatry Psychol 2009;20: 278–85.

88. Briere J. Trauma symptom inventory (TSI-2) professional manual. 2nd edition. Odessa (FL): Psychological Assessment Resources, 2010.

89. Gray MJ, Elhai JD, Briere J. Evaluation of the atypical response scale of the trauma symptom inventory-2 in detecting simulated posttraumatic stress disorder. J Anxiety Disord 2010;24:447–51.

90. Elhai JD, Gray MJ, Naifeh JA, et al. Utility of the trauma symptom inventory's atypical response scale in detecting malingered post-traumatic stress disorder. Assessment 2005;12:210–9.

91. Efendov AE, Sellbom M, Bagby RM. The utility and comparative incremental validity of the MMPI–2 and trauma symptom inventory validity scales in the detection of feigned PTSD. Psychol Assess 2008;20:317–26.

92. Slick DJ, Sherman EM, Iverson GL. Diagnostic criteria for malingered neurocognitive dysfunction: proposed standards for clinical practice and research. Clin Neuropsychol 1999;13:545–61.

93. Greiffenstein MF, Baker WJ, Gola T. Validation of malingered amnesia measures with a large clinical sample. Psychol Assess 1994;6:218–24.

94. Pankratz L, Binder LM. Malingering on intellectual and neuropsychological measures. In: Rogers R, editor. Clinical assessment of malingering and deception. 2nd edition. New York: Guilford Press; 1997. p. 223–38.

95. Faust D, Ackley MA. Did you think it was going to be easy? Some methodological suggestions for the investigation and development of malingering detection techniques. In: Reynolds CR, editor. Detection of malingering during head injury litigation. New York: Plenum Press; 1998. p. 1–54.

96. Bush SS, Ruff RM, Troster AI, et al. Symptom validity assessment: practice issues and medical necessity NAN Policy & Planning Committee. Arch Clin Neuropsychol 2005;20:419–26.

97. Hiscock M, Hiscock C. Refining the forced-choice method for the detection of malingering. J Clin Exp Neuropsychol 1989;11:967–74.

98. Binder LM. Malingering following minor head trauma. Clin Neuropsychol 1990;4: 25–36.

99. Iverson G, Franzen M, McCracken L. Evaluation of an objective assessment technique for the detection of malingered memory deficits. Law Hum Behav 1991;15:667–76.

100. Greiffenstein MF, Greve KW, Bianchini KJ, et al. Test of memory malingering and word memory test: a new comparison of failure concordance rates. Arch Clin Neuropsychol 2008;23:801–7.

101. Graue LO, Berry DTR, Clark JA, et al. Identification of feigned mental retardation using the new generation of malingering instruments: preliminary findings. Clin Neuropsychol 2007;21:929–42.

102. Harrison PL, Oakland T. Adaptive behavior assessment system. 2nd edition. San Antonio (TX): The Psychological Corporation; 2003.

103. Doane B, Salekin KL. Susceptibility of current adaptive behavior measures to feigned deficits. Law Hum Behav 2009;33:329–43.

104. Victor TL, Boone KB. Identification of feigned mental retardation. In: Boone KB, editor. Assessment of feigned cognitive impairment: a neuropsychological perspective. New York: Guilford Press; 2007. p. 310–45.

105. Slick DJ, Tan JE, Strauss EH, et al. Detecting malingering: a survey of experts' practices. Arch Clin Neuropsychol 2004;19:465–73.

106. Salekin KL, Doane B. Malingering intellectual disability: the value of available measures and methods. Appl Neuropsychol 2009;16:105–13.

107. Weiss RA, Rosenfeld B, Farkas MR. The utility of the structured interview of reported symptoms in a sample of individuals with intellectual disabilities. Assessment 2011;18:284–90.

108. Chafetz MD, Abrahams JP, Kohlmaier J. Malingering on the social security disability consultative exam: a new rating scale. Arch Clin Neuropsychol 2007;22:1–14.

109. Kessler RC, McGonagle KA, Zhao S, et al. Lifetime and 12-month prevalence of DSM-III-R psychiatric disorders in the United States: results from the National Comorbidity Survey. Arch Gen Psychiatry 1994;51:8–19.

110. Beck AT, Ward CH, Mendelson M, et al. An inventory for measuring depression. Arch Gen Psychiatry 1961;5:462–7.

111. Rogers R, Sewell KW, Martin MA, et al. Detection of feigned mental disorders: a meta-analysis of the MMPI-2 and malingering. Assessment 2003;10:160–77.

112. Bagby RM, Rogers R, Buis T. Detecting feigned depression and schizophrenia on the MMPI-2. J Pers Assess 1997;68:650–64.

113. Viglione DJ, Wright DM, Dizon NT, et al. Evading detection on the MMPI-2: does caution produce more realistic patterns of responding? Assessment 2001;8: 237–50.

114. Steffan JS, Clopton JR, Morgan RD. An MMPI-2 scale to detect malingered depression (Md scale). Assessment 2003;10:382–92.

115. Sweet JJ, Malina A, Ecklund-Johnson E. Application of the new MMPI-2 malingered depression scale to individuals undergoing neuropsychological evaluation: relative lack of relationship to secondary gain and failure on validity indices. Clin Neuropsychol 2006;20:541–51.

116. Henry GK, Heilbronner RL, Mittenberg W. Empirical derivation of a new MMPI-2 scale for identifying probable malingering in personal injury litigants and disability claimants: the 15-item malingered mood disorder scale (MMDS). Clin Neuropsychol 2008;22:158–68.

117. Mogge NL, LePage JP. The assessment of depression inventory (ADI): a new instrument used to measure depression and to detect honesty of response. Depress Anxiety 2004;20:107–13.

118. Mogge NL, Steinberg JS, Fremouw W. The assessment of depression inventory (ADI): an appraisal of validity in an outpatient sample. Depress Anxiety 2008;25: 64–8.

119. Mogge NL. The assessment of depression inventory (ADI): an appraisal of validity in an inpatient sample. Depress Anxiety 2006;23:434–6.

120. Chafetz MD. Malingering on the social security disability consultative exam: predictors and base rates. Clin Neuropsychol 2008;22:529–46.

Forensic Aspects and Assessment of School Bullying

Bradley W. Freeman, MD[a],*, Christopher Thompson, MD[b],
Cory Jaques, MD[c]

KEYWORDS

- Bullying • School bullying • Aggression • Children and adolescents
- Forensic evaluation

KEY POINTS

- There are at least 4 distinct categories of bullying, including physical, verbal, social (relational), and cyberbullying.
- Forensic assessments of victims are usually done in civil torts in which the client is seeking intentional or negligent infliction of emotional distress, emotional effects of a physical injury, stress as a result of discrimination or harassment, and emotional harm from defamation or libel.
- When performing assessments for the juvenile court, recommendations for treatment are usually appreciated if applicable to the matter at hand.
- The evaluator must be aware of his or her biases during the course of the evaluation and should be careful to present alternative hypotheses and discuss limitations of the opinions expressed at the conclusion of the report.
- Case and statutory law is evolving rapidly in this area, and the evaluator should be aware of legislation applicable to his or her jurisdiction.
- Schools' responsibilities to protect students and provide a safe learning environment have expanded over the past 20 years as their obligation has transformed from *duty to care* to *duty to protect*.
- Case and statutory law is rapidly evolving and changing, particularly with regard to non–school-based (but possibly school-related) bullying (eg, cyberbullying). At the federal court level, both First Amendment (freedom of speech) and Fourteenth Amendment (equal protection) issues are involved.
- Some bullying behaviors may be delinquent or criminal offenses.
- Prosecution of school bullies via the juvenile or adult courts is a relatively new phenomenon and likely to increase as changes to the delinquency code and criminal statutes are implemented.

Drs Freeman, Thompson, and Jaques have nothing to disclose.
[a] Child Adolescent Division, Department of Psychiatry, Vanderbilt University School of Medicine, 1601 23rd Avenue South, Suite 3023, Nashville, TN 37212, USA; [b] Child & Adolescent Division, Department of Psychiatry and Biobehavioral Sciences, David Geffen School of Medicine at UCLA, 10850 Wilshire Blvd., Suite 850, Los Angeles, CA 90024, USA; [c] Department of Psychiatry, UCLA Semel Institute for Neuroscience and Human Behavior, 760 Westwood Plaza, Los Angeles, CA 90095, USA
* Corresponding author.
E-mail address: bradley.w.freeman@vanderbilt.edu

Psychiatr Clin N Am 35 (2012) 877–900
http://dx.doi.org/10.1016/j.psc.2012.08.007
0193-953X/12/$ – see front matter © 2012 Elsevier Inc. All rights reserved.

psych.theclinics.com

INTRODUCTION

School bullying is a common, problematic behavior among children. Bullying is, of course, not a new phenomenon, but national attention was drawn to the problem in the 1990s after several highly publicized incidents of school violence (eg, Columbine). Bullying is a pervasive, cross-cultural, cross-gender phenomenon that seems to peak in early to midadolescence[1,2] and affects approximately half of school-aged youth worldwide.[3,4] The definition of school bullying includes several key elements: physical, verbal, or psychological attack or intimidation that is intended to cause fear, distress, or harm to the victim; an imbalance of power (psychological or physical) with a more powerful child (or children) oppressing less powerful ones; and repeated incidents between the same children over a prolonged period of time.[5–7] This article assists evaluators when assessing youth who are involved in bullying behavior, either as victims or perpetrators. Key areas highlighted include an overview of bullying behaviors, legal issues related to a school's responsibility in preventing or curtailing bullying behaviors, important components of a bullying assessment, and proposed interventions to minimize bullying.

OVERVIEW OF BULLYING BEHAVIORS

There are different categories of bullying behaviors. Volk and colleagues[8] identified 5 distinct types of bullying:

1. Racial/ethnic
2. Sexual
3. Physical
4. Verbal
5. Indirect/social

They also noted that new forms of bullying were developing, such as cyberbullying. Other researchers have identified 4 main categories of bullying,[3,9,10] which are highlighted in **Box 1**:

1. Physical
2. Verbal
3. Relational
4. Cyberbullying

Regardless of the typology system used, the same roles exist. Traditionally, bullying does not occur between individuals of equal power, although with cyberbullying, the power differential may not be significant. A bully is an individual who has power over his or her victim. The victims are those individuals who are less powerful than the bully. The bully-victims are individuals who have assumed the roles of both bully and victim at different times. Bystanders are individuals who learn about the bullying behavior either by witnessing the incident (eg, seeing a schoolyard fight) or by being exposed indirectly to the behavior (eg, reading a blog about an attack).

Volk and colleagues[11] questioned the maladaptive nature of the behavior and framed the phenomenon in an evolutionary perspective. Additionally, Sugden and colleagues[12] described the role of genes in the moderation of the effects of bullying on victims. Research has also shown that bullying is not just a problem of the present but that bullying behaviors can affect an individual into his or her adulthood. After adjusting for age, race, and educational attainment, Falb and colleagues[13] reported that frequent victims of bullying had a higher risk of perpetrating intimate partner violence as adults. Perhaps more disturbingly, Meltzer and colleagues[14] reported

---

Box 1
Bullying terminology

Bullying is a repetitive behavior over a long period of time in which an individual with greater power attacks, humiliates, or intimidates a less powerful individual with the intent to cause harm or psychological distress.

Physical bullying is behavior in which a more powerful individual intentionally uses physical contact or significant threat of physical contact to bully a less powerful individual (ie, a student threatening to fight a less powerful student after school hours).

Verbal bullying is behavior in which a student intentionally uses direct, deliberate language to cause psychological distress in another student for the purposes of humiliation, intimidation, or other deprecating reason (ie, a student continually calls another student names in front of their peers).

Social bullying occurs when individuals use social status and/or interpersonal relationships to cause intentional psychological distress in another individual (ie, a group of students spread rumors and gossip, alienate from social activities, and create a general hostile environment for another student).

Cyberbullying is the use of information technology to repeatedly and intentionally try to humiliate, embarrass, degrade, or otherwise harm a specific individual or group of individuals (ie, a student posts derogatory comments and pictures of another student on social networking site to cause embarrassment and humiliation). There does not need to be a power differential present between the bully and the victim.

---

that even after controlling for other suicide risk factors, those adults who reported being bullied in childhood were more than twice as likely as controls to attempt suicide later in life.

As with many human behaviors, the cause of bullying seems to be multifactorial. Humans are a product of both their genes and their environment and each helps determine their physical and psychological phenotype, likely through a dynamic interplay (see later discussion). For example, from a genetic standpoint, Sugden and colleagues reported that a specific genotype of the serotonin transporter can place an individual at risk for future emotional problems if they are bullying victims.[12] From an environmental standpoint, it is common knowledge that children often model their behavior after their parents. In addition to these discrete variables, other researchers have suggested that behavior (eg, aggression) is mediated via a gene x environment interaction. This interaction is hypothesized to occur when an individual with a specific genetic makeup is subjected to a particular environmental stressor. By way of example, Blazei and colleagues[15] examined the father-child transmission of antisocial behavior in a primarily Caucasian sample from the Minnesota Twin Family Study. They determined that the father's antisocial behaviors significantly predicted the child's externalizing behaviors, although it was not clear whether this association was based on genetic or environmental factors.

SCHOOL'S RESPONSIBILITY AND BULLYING BEHAVIORS
Origins of a School's Duty to Care

Education plays a central role in our society. The common law doctrine of in loco parentis (Latin for "in the place of a parent") vests the teacher with the responsibility of protecting the interests of a child in the school environment. Understanding the relationship between the school and student in public schools today is increasingly important. Policymakers have created numerous laws and rules to ensure equality in educational opportunities and safeguard students from discriminatory practices and dangerous actions. As an evolving legal concept, in loco parentis has taken on a new and more definitive meaning.[16] Public schools are responsible for providing students with instruction and supervision and for properly maintaining school grounds, facilities, and equipment. These multiple requirements essentially establish a *duty to care* for student safety. This evolution of the legal duty of school officials marks a major shift in both educational law and school system policy.

Legal Standards Governing a School's Duty to Protect

The various public school systems in the United States have often struggled to keep pace with evolving social mores. In the post-Columbine era (ie, after April 1999), with heightened public awareness about new potential dangers in the schools, educators are struggling to keep pace with increasing public expectations and evolving legal standards regarding their role in keeping students safe. Since Columbine, school officials increasingly have been expected not only to create and maintain safe schools but also to protect children from harm. *Safety in schools* has expanded far beyond the traditional scope of the *duty to care* owed to students and effectively has become an affirmative *duty to protect*.[17] The alleged breach of the school's *duty to protect* is often the impetus for litigation against school officials.

Before the early 1990s, the typical student injury case that found its way into a court of law took the form of a negligence tort. A tort is defined as the legal mechanism in civil court to make an injured party whole again, usually through financial compensation. To receive damages in a negligence case, the plaintiff must establish the existence of a duty owed to the student by the school, a breach of that duty by the public school officials, and an injury to the student proximately caused, or directly resulting from, that breach. The duty of care can arise either from state law or from the Due Process Clause of the Fourteenth Amendment to the US Constitution, which protects citizens from state action that results in the loss of or injury to life, liberty, or property. Cases filed in federal court frequently allege a constitutional violation of due process by the state (ie, school officials) under Section 1983 of the Civil Rights Act.

Before 1989, the United States Supreme Court had consistently held that, under most circumstances, government officials or employees have no constitutional obligation to protect citizens from harm caused by a third party. In *DeShaney v Winnebago County*, the Court ruled, "Nothing in the language of the Due Process Clause itself requires the state to protect life, liberty, and property of its citizens against the invasion of private actors."[18] However, the Court also held that when "[t]he state takes a person into custody and holds him there against his will, the Constitution imposes on it a corresponding duty to assume responsibility for his safety and general well-being…" After the *DeShaney* ruling, some courts began to impose liability on schools, finding that state-imposed compulsory attendance places students in the functional custody of the state.[19] By expanding the scope of school officials' *duty to protect,* this decision established a basis for holding school officials liable for harm caused when that duty is breached.

Today, most courts have ruled that the functional custody theory of liability alone is insufficient to establish a *duty to protect* for school officials. Legal responses to emerging demands for additional student protections have created a generally accepted rule that there must be a *special relationship* or other factors present in the school setting to create a duty.[20]

Courts have considered what type of special relationship or unique factors could create a constitutional duty to protect. Since the mid 1990s, courts have increasingly required the following elements to be present before imposing liability[17]:

1. *Imminent danger* to students
2. *Deliberate indifference* by school officials to that danger

In other words, plaintiffs must demonstrate that school officials deliberately ignored actual notice or knowledge of the circumstances that were likely to lead (and did indeed lead) to the injury.[16] Although this change might seem to limit schools' liability, operationally, it has created a requirement for school officials to respond swiftly to students who report being threatened or harassed, thereby mitigating the potential risk to the student.

In 1996, Jamie Nabozny won a landmark lawsuit against officials at his former high school in Ashland, Wisconsin, because of their failure to intervene in antigay verbal and physical abuse by fellow students.[21] Jamie's classmates regularly referred to him as "faggot" and subjected him to various forms of physical abuse, including striking and spitting on him, urinating on him, and performing a mock rape in a classroom while other students watched. Over a several-year period, both Nabozny and his parents reported these incidents (including the names of the perpetrators) to the school's guidance counselor, principal, and district officials, asking for protection from the harassment and assaults. No action was taken. Twice during high school Jaime attempted suicide. He was eventually diagnosed with posttraumatic stress disorder (PTSD).

Nabozny filed suit claiming school officials violated his constitutional right to due process as well as a violation of his right to equal protection. Nabozny's claim of a due process violation relied on the fact that school officials "failed to act" in response to repeated pleas for help.[21] The Court found that Nabozny presented sufficient evidence to show that the defendants failed to act and that their failure to act was intentional. However, relying on *J.O. v Alton Community*, the Court found that the defendants had no affirmative duty to act (and therefore had not violated Nabozny's right to due process) because Nabozny was unable show that the defendants' failure to act created a risk of harm or exacerbated an existing one. The Court noted, "However untenable it may be to suggest that under the Fourteenth Amendment a state can force a student to attend a school when school officials know that the student will be placed at risk of bodily harm, our court has concluded that local school administrations have no affirmative substantive due process duty to protect students."[22] In *J.O. v Alton Community,* the Court held that state actors have a duty to care for citizens if the state actors' conduct "creates, or substantially contributes to the creation of, a danger or renders citizens more vulnerable to a danger than they otherwise would have been."[22] Although the defendants' failure to act left Nabozny in a position of danger, nothing suggested that their failure to act placed him in the danger or increased the preexisting threat of harm. In addition, because Nabozny did not allege that a special relationship existed, the court did not consider this factor in their decision. Importantly, however, the Court did conclude that school officials violated his rights under the Fourteenth Amendment's Equal Protection Clause by discriminating against him because of his sexual orientation, setting a precedent for claiming civil rights violations based on sexual orientation.

In 1999, the US Supreme Court, in *Davis v Monroe,* established the current judicial standard for deciding whether or not school officials should be held liable for harm caused by student-on-student harassment. In this case, the petitioner sought damages under a violation of Title IX of the Education Amendments of 1972, which prohibit a student from being "excluded from participation in, be[ing] denied the benefits of, or be[ing] subjected to discrimination under any education program or activity receiving Federal financial assistance."[23] The petitioner alleged that a fellow student repeatedly harassed her over a 5-month period and that, despite her reporting the misconduct to school officials on numerous occasions, these officials failed to investigate or to attempt to put an end to the harassment. The petitioner alleged the harassment was severe enough to limit her access to educational opportunities (specifically, her previously high grades allegedly dropped as she became unable to concentrate on her studies), a finding of which is essential to a claim of a Title IX violation. Moreover, the petitioner alleged that, at the time of the events, the Monroe County Board of Education had not instructed its personnel on how to respond to peer sexual harassment and had not established a policy on the issue.

In an opinion written by Justice Sandra Day O'Connor, the Court held that school officials may be liable for student (peer) harassment when they are "deliberately indifferent to known acts of student-on-student sexual harassment," the alleged harassment is "so severe, pervasive, and objectively offensive that it effectively bars the victim's access to an educational opportunity," and when "the student harasser is under the school's disciplinary authority."[18] In applying the deliberate indifference standard, the Court acknowledged the practical realities of the school officials' ability to respond to student behaviors. Holding school officials potentially liable for failure to act when made aware of the harassment has expanded the *duty to care* into a more proactive *duty to protect* students in school settings.[24] This decision emphasizes the importance of documenting the following when working with schools and parents to evaluate claims of damages because of peer-on-peer harassment: the dates and times of each offense; exactly what was said or done during each offense; which school personnel was notified of each offense; and all formal and informal interventions implemented for each offense and their respective outcomes.

In addressing the dissent written by Justice Kennedy, Justice O'Connor outlines clear limitations on school liability for Title IX violations. She stressed that a single instance of harassment, unless "sufficiently severe," is unlikely to have an appreciable effect on a student's access to education.[18] She also emphasized the importance of considering the ages of both the victim and the harasser in limiting liability "for simple acts of teasing and name-calling among school children."[18] Because young children are still learning how to interact appropriately with their peers, the Court thought it reasonable and expected that they would engage in "insults, banter, teasing, shoving, pushing, and gender-specific conduct that is upsetting to the students subjected to it"[18] and that such behavior was not necessarily actionable.

State Bullying Laws and Policies

In recent years, several states have taken dramatic and affirmative steps to reduce bullying in schools. In many states, antibullying legislation was preceded by the adoption of model policies that focused on managing bullying behaviors. These model policies provide guidance to school districts and individual schools as well as apprising them of changes in state educational codes and other legislation involving bullying, cyberbullying, and related behaviors.

In 1999, Georgia became the first state to pass antibullying legislation. Since then, 48 other states have also adopted antibullying policies or legislation. As of April 2012, Montana is the only state without antibullying legislation; however, that state recently adopted its own model policies. Of note, although Hawaii passed antibullying legislation in November 2011, the legislation is not slated to take effect until July 1, 2030.[25]

As an example of how state policy often precedes formal legislation, California first addressed bullying in its state educational code.[26] Education Code §35,294.2 (2001) requires the California Department of Education to develop model policies both on the prevention of bullying and on conflict resolution. Education Code §48,900 (2008) permits a student to be suspended from school or recommended for expulsion for engaging in acts of bullying, including bullying committed by electronic means. Education Code §32,261 encourages "school districts, county offices of education, law enforcement agencies, and agencies serving youth to develop and implement inter-agency strategies, in-service training programs, and activities that will improve school attendance and reduce school crime and violence."[26] This crime and violence includes all forms of bullying and cyberbullying.

In October 2011, Governor Jerry Brown signed into law Assembly Bill 9 Ch. 723 (known as Seth's Law), which strengthened the existing California antibullying law. As a result, schools were required to establish policies to prevent bullying, to be responsive to complaints about bullying, to train personnel how to recognize and inter-vene in bullying, and to make resources available to bullying victims.[27]

In December 2010, the United States Department of Education (USDE) reviewed existing state laws. In their report to Congress, they recommended that antibullying legislation include 11 common components[28]:

- Purpose and definition (components 1–4): purpose, scope, definition of pro-hibited behavior, and enumeration of protected groups
- District policy development and review (components 5–6): implementation of policies and review for compliance
- School district policy components (component 7): assignment of responsibility to carry out the law
- Additional components (components 8–11): communication of policies, moni-toring and accountability, actions and interventions to prevent bullying behav-iors, legal remedies for victims

Each state addresses bullying behavior differently, which has resulted in inconsis-tent state laws and policies. Only Maryland and New Jersey have adopted legislation that covers all key components outlined by the USDE.[25] Four of the 49 states with existing antibullying legislation have laws that prohibit bullying without defining specific prohibited behaviors. Only 35 of the 49 states enumerate protected groups; most of these do not include language that establishes bullying based on actual or perceived sexual orientation as harassment of a protected group.

Federal Involvement in Antibullying Efforts

Currently, no federal statute directly addresses bullying, although federal laws do address particular kinds of harassment based on race, national origin, and sex. In the last several years, congressional efforts to address school bullying concerns have increased. In 2011, the Safe Schools Improvement Act of 2011 (SSIA) was intro-duced in both the House of Representatives and the Senate.[29] The SSIA amends the Elementary and Secondary Education Act of 1965. The bills have had hearings in the House of Representatives and the Senate and await a floor vote, which has yet to be scheduled.

If passed, the SSIA will require schools that receive federal funding to establish codes of conduct that explicitly prohibit bullying and harassment. In addition, schools will be required to adopt effective prevention strategies and professional development programs designed to help school personnel meaningfully address issues associated with bullying and harassment. Finally, the bill will require states to collect data on inci-dents of bullying and report the information to the USDE.

Importantly, this legislation addresses the lack of uniformity among the 50 different state legal approaches to bullying. The bill directs states to adopt state policies covering all of the 11 recommendations identified by the USDE (specified earlier). The SSIA clearly defines what constitutes bullying and includes *electronic communi-cation* in that definition. In addition, the bill fully enumerates the groups protected. Current federal laws do not include sexual orientation as a protected group under the civil rights laws; SSIA expands protections for students specifically by including gay and lesbian students as a protected group. This expansion of protections remains controversial and is a major reason for opposition to the bill. Some federal legislators oppose SSIA because they view it as an example of federal encroachment on local control of public schools. The SSIA was introduced in other forms in previous sessions of Congress; it never received a floor vote. Although President Obama has endorsed the legislation and Michelle Obama has made school bullying one of her signature issues, passage of the bill remains uncertain.

Federal involvement has also been triggered by civil lawsuits against a school district. For example, in 2011, a lawsuit was filed against the Anoka-Hennepin School District, claiming the district failed adequately to respond to reports of persistent physical and verbal harassment of 6 students, which they claimed was based on their actual or perceived sexual orientation. The suit was recently settled after a 5 to 1 school board vote, which agreed to award the 6 students a lump sum of $270,000. In addition, the settlement established a 5-year partnership between the school district and the US Department of Justice and the USDE to help create programs and procedures to improve the learning environment for all students.[30] This partnership is unprecedented and sets a new standard for antibullying efforts nationwide.

Cyberbullying and Free Speech

A school's duty to protect students from harm has been previously applied only to students in their physical custody (eg, on school grounds or during school field trips). Cyberbullying presents a unique problem because the actions often occur off of school grounds, although they may be viewed as school related. One readily can see from newspaper headlines the rapidly increasing popularity of social networking sites and their use as a platform for bullying. This situation poses a challenge to the traditional views of a school's duty to protect and adds an expanding geographic scope to the problem of bullying.

Many states continue to assess their antibullying laws. As a component of this assessment, some states have begun to craft (or even implement) anticyberbullying legislation, which would (or does) codify a requirement for school districts to update their policies to include cyberbullying or other types of electronic harassment in their definitions of prohibited behavior. Today, only 14 states include cyberbullying in their statutory definition of bullying, although 38 states include electronic harassment. Thirteen states allow schools to have jurisdiction over off-campus behavior that creates a "hostile school environment."[25] If passed, the SSIA would also set a minimum standard for all states because it includes cyberbullying in its definition.

This expansion of jurisdiction has created a new dilemma that is currently being decided in the courts and debated by legal scholars. As school officials are attempting to comply with mandates requiring them to monitor and respond to off-campus behaviors, the courts are consistently ruling that doing so violates students' civil rights.

Cyberbullying legislation, in particular, has been criticized for seeking to regulate behavior that is considered free speech. Courts are often called on to determine the types of behaviors states may constitutionally regulate and whether school districts, in attempting to protect students from bullying activities, can interfere with the behavior or speech of students that occurs on or off campus. One of the most influential US Supreme Court cases involving school regulation of student speech remains *Tinker v Des Moines School District* (1969). In *Tinker,* the Court ruled that the suspensions of 3 public school students for wearing black armbands to protest the Vietnam War violated the Free Speech Clause of the First Amendment. This case established that school personnel have the burden of demonstrating that the speech or behavior resulted in a "substantial interference with school discipline or the rights of other students"[31] before limiting lawful student speech. The courts have consistently applied the Tinker standard when deciding cases involving alleged violations of student free speech.

In *Layshock v Hermitage School District* (2007), a student brought suit against the school district claiming a violation of his free speech rights. Layshock was punished by the school district for posting on the Internet from his home computer a nonthreatening, nonobscene parody profile that made fun of the school principal. A US District Court ruled in favor of Layshock, finding that the speech did not result in an "actual disruption of the day-to-day operation" of the school.[32] In a similar case, *J.S. v Blue Mountain School District* (2007), student J.S. filed suit against the school claiming a free speech violation after the school suspended her for creating a parody profile of her principal on MySpace.com on her home computer. The US District Court found in favor of the school, finding that the "off-campus speech had an effect on-campus" and that the student was, therefore, subject to disciplinary action.[33] These cases eventually came before the US Third Circuit Court of Appeals in 2010, and decisions in both cases were handed down on the same day in 2011. The appellate court affirmed the decision in *Layshock* and overruled the District Court decision in *J.S.*, finding that the speech did not affect the school environment in a substantial way.[34,35] When the US Supreme Court was petitioned, both cases were denied certiorari.

In December 2005, high school senior Kara Kowalski was suspended from school for 5 days for creating and posting to a MySpace.com Web site called "S.A.S.H.," which Kowalski claims stood for "Students Against Sluts Herpes" and which was largely dedicated to ridiculing a fellow student. Kowalski filed suit against the school district claiming, in part, a violation of her First Amendment rights. The district court ruled in favor of the defendants, concluding that school officials were authorized to punish Kowalski because her Web site was "created for the purpose of inviting others to indulge in disruptive and hateful conduct," which caused an "in-school disruption."[36] The US Fourth Circuit Court of Appeals affirmed this decision.[37] The US Supreme Court also denied certiorari in this case.

The US Supreme Court has yet to rule on the issue of whether a school violates a student's free speech rights by punishing them for creating, on their own time and using their own computers, electronic material that mocks or insults school officials or classmates. Until they do, lower courts and school officials will continue to struggle with this issue. The trend among lower courts, consistent with *Tinker*, has been to allow schools to punish off-campus cyberbullying only when such actions cause a material and substantial interference with on-campus school administration. But that standard relies on sets of particular facts, which often cannot take into account inventive mischief of technology savvy students.

EVALUATING BULLYING VICTIMS AND BULLIES
Clarifying the Referral

Forensic evaluations typically begin with a referral from an attorney, a guardian ad litem (a guardian appointed by the court to represent the interests of infants, the unborn, or incompetent persons in legal actions), the court, a family, or another nonmedical entity. In some circumstances, a school district may refer a student for an evaluation. Before accepting the referral, the evaluator must determine if he is qualified to address the issue presented. The evaluator must have the referring agency delineate the specific questions or issues at hand. The evaluator may want to ask the referring source to provide a cover letter that outlines their needs. Inexperienced attorneys or naive school districts may need the evaluator to educate them about the services they are able to provide, which can assist them in developing well-informed questions for the evaluation.

The logistics of the evaluation also need to be considered. These logistics include the availability of the individuals involved and relevant documentation; the time frame for the evaluation, report, and potential testimony; potential conflicts of interest; and compensation. The evaluator and referral source should determine the type of work product needed (eg, verbal consultation, brief letter, full report, deposition, testimony). Although some of these needs are fluid and may change in the future, they help estimate the time needed and expense likely to be incurred. The individuals or entities to which the findings should be distributed should also be discussed with the referring source. If the evaluation is for juvenile court, whose focus generally is rehabilitative, the evaluator should provide diagnosis and treatment recommendations (if applicable).

Initial Meeting with the Client and Family

The next step in the evaluation process is to meet with the family of the referred youth to organize the evaluation. The family should be informed about the lack of confidentiality that normally exists in a doctor-patient relationship. Then the client assents to the evaluation and the family gives written consent to the evaluation before proceeding. Releases of information are obtained for collateral sources of information. If needed, psychological testing and additional meetings should be scheduled. Before ending the meeting, the evaluator should ask if there are additional questions or concerns.

Reviewing Relevant Records

Reviewing records is a necessary component to a comprehensive evaluation. The evaluator should ask for medical, mental health, school, and legal records. Mental health records include counseling and medication management documentation. The school records should include the child's grades, attendance, class schedule, behavior history, accommodations, such as an Individualized Educational Plan (IEP), and available information from the school guidance counselor and nurse. Importantly, the school should also provide incident reports of bullying behavior as well as all formal and informal attempts by the school to remedy the situation.

The evaluator should maintain a secure, organized file and add records as they arrive. Spending some extra time keeping the files organized will lead to more efficient use of time and a less costly evaluation overall. Additionally, keeping the files organized is immensely helpful when called to provide expert testimony either at a deposition or in court, especially given the length of time between record review and potential testimony. Before conducting interviews, it is helpful to have reviewed the case material. The background information will help to focus on missed details, determine the consistency of the report, and assess for malingering. The objective of a bullying victim evaluation is more akin to a personal injury case (civil) rather than a child abuse investigation (criminal).

Interviewing the Parents

Interviewing the parents before meeting with the child has advantages. The adults can discuss their anxieties and concerns, information about which can be used during the interview with the child. Having this knowledge before the child interview allows the evaluator to ask more appropriate probing questions. The evaluator can also ask the parents how the legal system became involved, the purpose of the litigation, and the parents' expectations regarding the evaluation.

Additionally, the child may be more willing to participate in the interview with the understanding that the interviewer already has some information regarding what has happened to the youth. For example, a child may be more likely to discuss an embarrassing case of harassment if he knows that the interviewer is already aware of the details. The evaluator must remain objective despite being exposed to often emotional, biased, or misleading information from the adults.

The nature of the forensic evaluation sets the meeting with the parents apart from a clinical interview. The evaluator must maintain a degree of skepticism about the information provided. The data collected should have internal consistency with the other information provided and external consistency with collateral sources. For example, a parent might report that their child was so tormented by her classmates that she could barely attend school, yet school records indicate very few missed days during the school year. A useful way of checking for consistency is to interview the parents individually on the same day, thereby limiting their ability to coordinate reports. The main goals of the parent interviews are to elicit information about the child's functioning, behavior, relationships, strengths, and weaknesses.

During the course of the parent interview, the evaluator should ask about the bullying in a free-narrative style. A general, nonleading question (eg, why is your child being evaluated?) is posed first, followed by other open-ended questions. When specific information is needed, focused questions (eg, has your child ever been suicidal?) are helpful. In addition to the alleged bullying behavior, the evaluator will need to inquire about past episodes of bullying (either as the victim or bully), aggressive behavior, trauma exposure, developmental problems, psychosocial stressors, family structure, treatment/counseling, and the family's reaction to the situation at hand. The evaluator should also ask the family how this situation escalated to the point that a forensic evaluation was required. Their answer to this question will provide the evaluator with some sense of the family's intentions.

Speaking with Collateral Sources

When talking with collateral sources, it is important to identify your role, the purpose of your contact with the collateral source, and to provide them with a signed release of information (if required). The evaluator should ask the source about the nature and duration of their relationship with the person being evaluated. Similar to the interview with the parents and the evaluation of the child, the evaluator should begin with free narrative questions and then move to more focused questions to help supply the necessary missing details. Internal and external consistency remains important. In selecting collateral sources, it generally is most useful to interview those individuals that can give an objective observation of the child and his or her behaviors. For example, the child's schoolteacher (or other school staff) is generally interviewed. Additional helpful collateral sources may include religious leaders, coaches, activity directors, or others that know the child well. The most helpful sources tend to be those individuals that have known the child and family before and after the alleged bullying behaviors, for obvious reasons.

Conducting Psychological Testing

In some cases, the evaluator will want to use psychological testing as part of the comprehensive assessment. This testing usually is best done and interpreted by a mental health professional who has experience working with children and is familiar with the assessment instruments. The evaluation might include general screening tools (completed both by the child and the parent), specific aptitude measures, intelligence assessments, and assessments for particular psychiatric disorders, such as attention-deficit/hyperactivity disorder (ADHD), autistic disorder, PTSD, and anxiety disorders. In some cases, the child already may have had testing completed through the school system. If so, this testing should be requested and reviewed.

With regard to the assessment of bullying, some psychological tools purport to provide a more objective measurement of the behavior. The California Bullying Victimization Scale was developed by Felix and colleagues[38] to address the limitations of self-report measures. Other tools have also been developed to assess bullying behaviors among youth; these are highlighted in **Table 1**.

Both bullying victims and bullies may benefit from completing either psychological screening tools (designed to identify a broad range of potential psychiatric conditions [see **Table 1**]) or more specialized testing (eg, Structured Assessment of Violence Risk in Youth [SAVRY], Hare Psychopathy Checklist–Youth Version [PCL-YV]). The labeling of a youth as a psychopath is controversial and the evaluator should be familiar with the pros and cons of using psychopathy measures in this population. Jones and Cauffman[39] found that youth who were labeled psychopaths and were reported to have psychopathic traits were viewed as less treatable and more dangerous and were more likely to be recommended for restrictive placement than youth not described as such in judicial decisions. Boccaccini and colleagues[40] reported that jurors thought that youths labeled as psychopaths posed greater risk for future crime and deserved greater punishment compared with youth described as meeting diagnostic criteria for psychopathy or conduct disorder. The results of psychological testing should be considered in the child's psychosocial and developmental context. Additional testing may be needed to help determine the violence risk or necessary interventions (eg, intelligence testing to help determine if a child has an intellectual disability and might benefit from more specialized services).

Table 1	
Examples of areas to explore when evaluating an alleged victim of bullying	
General information	• Establish if a power differential exists between the child and the alleged bully • Check for external and internal consistency, malingering • When and where does the bullying occur • What has the child's relationship been with the alleged bully • How has the behavior affected the child • Why does the child think he or she is being bullied • Does the child have a solution in mind
Physical bullying	• Obtain a history about the alleged incidents, injuries, and persons involved • Review documentation about physical injuries
Verbal bullying	• What is the content of the bullying behavior • Is there a theme (ie, physical appearance, family, academic performance, cultural) • Quote the child's words exactly
Social bullying	• The most difficult type to evaluate and substantiate • Examine the child's own social skills • Have the child give examples of changes in their social life or relationships • Are other types of bullying also occurring, especially verbal or cyberbullying
Cyberbullying	• What types of communications are involved (ie, texting, social networks, blogs) • Review the alleged bullying if available (ie, printouts, text message logs)

General Principles of the Child/Adolescent Interview

Mental health professionals may be asked to evaluate a reported bully victim, an alleged bully, or both. The evaluator should clarify with the youth the limits of confidentiality specific to the evaluation/case. At the outset of the evaluation and in an age-appropriate manner, the evaluator should review with the child the following areas:

1. The child's understanding of the evaluation's purpose
2. What the child has been told about the evaluation process
3. Whether the child has been instructed about what to say or not to say (and if so, by whom)
4. The child's thoughts and feelings about the evaluation
5. What the child hopes (or fears) the evaluation will accomplish

The evaluator should attempt to build rapport at the start of the interview, especially in children who seem anxious or unwilling to participate. The evaluator should ask the child about his or her family, school, friends, daily routine, sleep, and so forth in a developmentally appropriate manner. Open-ended questions (eg, tell me about your family) are used because they produce more accurate information[41] than closed-ended questions. However, closed-ended questions are often needed to elicit specific information (eg, suicidality). The evaluator should also screen the child or adolescent for symptoms of mental illness, such as depression, anxiety, and ADHD.

Evaluation of a Reported Bullying Victim

In the evaluation of an alleged bullying victim, the referral question usually concerns potential psychiatric disorders or symptoms (ie, damages) to the bullied child and the causal nexus (or lack thereof) of the bullying and the psychiatric disorders or symptoms.

Taking a lifetime trauma history

During the evaluation, the evaluator needs to take a trauma inventory in which the child is asked about the bad things that may have happened to them during their life. Placing the potentially traumatic events in chronologic order is important because this order may impact the evaluator's opinion regarding the effects of the alleged bullying on the child. Nonbullying-related traumatic events (and their sequelae) that occurred around the time of the reported bullying are particularly critical to investigate thoroughly. The evaluator needs to collect details of each trauma's impact on the child. Common components of the trauma history include the frequency, duration, and perceived intensity of the trauma itself and the residual symptoms. Typical trauma-related symptoms include sleep disturbance, anxiety, depression, and difficulty with concentration. Some children are understandably hesitant to discuss prior traumatic events. Therefore, the evaluator may need to rely heavily on collateral sources in order to accurately perceive the impact the trauma had on the child.[42–44]

Reviewing bullying history

The evaluator should screen for each type of bullying and, if bullying reportedly has occurred or is occurring, then elicit a more detailed description of the particular type of bullying behavior, as outlined in **Table 2**. Although the referral source usually will relay the type of bullying to which the child reportedly has been subjected, the child may also have experienced other forms of bullying. The most obvious types of bullying are physical and verbal. Social bullying is not always readily apparent; electronic bullying can be even more discrete.

Table 2	
Psychological tools that may be useful for forensic evaluations	
Client Type	**Psychological Tool**
Victim	• California Bullying Victimization Scale • Reynolds Bulling Victimization Scales for Schools • Olweus Bully/Victim Questionnaire • The Bully Surveys • School Connectedness Scale • Students' Life Satisfaction Scale • Peer Relations Assessment Questionnaires-Revised
Bully	• SAVRY • PCL-YV • Early Assessment Risk Lists for Boys • Early Assessment Risk Lists for Girls • Youth Level of Service/Case Management Inventory

After building rapport with the child, the evaluator should inquire about the alleged bullying. The evaluator should attempt to use open-ended questions when asking about all types of bullying, particularly during the initial part of the interview. The evaluator should avoid introducing emotionally charged terms, such as bullying. Instead, asking the child to identify any alleged aggressors (if possible), the context of the bullying, and specific bullying behavior may be helpful.

During the course of the evaluation, questions should focus on the who, what, why, where, when, and how of the reported bullying (ie, conventional journalistic style). The child should be asked about their perception of the bullying behavior. Questions might include

- How do the other students treat you at school?
- Why do you think they do that to you?
- What does your family think about this?
- Has the school (ie, school personnel) done anything to help you?

The evaluator should also inquire about the specific time and school area in which the bullying occurs (eg, between classes, after school, on certain school days, in a poorly supervised area of the school); this information can be extremely helpful in identifying potential interventions at the school.

Examples of open-ended questions regarding verbal bullying include

- Do you ever feel sad/hurt/angry about what people say to you?
- Do other people say mean things to you?
- Can you tell me more about that?

Identifying a bullying theme may assist the evaluator in better understanding the nature of the behavior, its cause, and potential successful interventions. As an ancillary benefit, allowing the child to provide a free narrative likely will improve the evaluator's rapport with the child and assist with information gathering. Some children prefer to write down the verbal remarks rather than say them out loud.

As with verbal bullying, social bullying is more likely to involve girls. This type of bullying tends to be more covert, and the target may not be able to identify all of those involved. Because social bullying does not cause physical injury, it can be more difficult to substantiate and assess. Verbal aggression is typically involved, as is alienation of the bullying victim. Substantiating claims of social bullying may prove difficult without a comprehensive investigation by the school.

A more recent form of bullying is electronic bullying, also known as cyberbullying. Cyberbullying has evolved along with emerging forms of social media. Cyberbullying does not require proximity between the bully and the victim; therefore, the power differential between the victimizer and victim may not be significant. In some cases, forensic computer experts review electronic interchanges, including texts, emails, and social media postings. If a forensic computer expert has conducted an evaluation, the psychiatric evaluator should carefully review the content and context of his or her findings.

Evaluating level of functioning

A decrease in the bullied child's level of functioning is an important indicator that the bullying behavior may have had a significant negative impact on the child. The evaluator needs to determine if a child's level of functioning has worsened, quantify the change, and determine if the decreased level of functioning is related to the bullying behavior. Quantifying the change obviously requires a comparison of the child's level of functioning before and after the alleged bullying. The evaluator needs to compare domains of functioning, such as family and peer relationships, academic performance, behavioral problems (eg, presence/absence, degree), mood symptoms, and involvement in social activities. The evaluator also needs to assess premorbid and postevent domains, such as sleep, appetite, energy level, anxiety, and somatic symptoms. The evaluator should also consider how other changes in the child's psychosocial environment may have impacted the child's level of functioning.

Assessing psychological impact

The evaluator needs to determine if the reported bullying has had a negative impact on the mental health of the child and, if so, to what degree. Lemstra and colleagues[45] used data from a Canadian school survey that asked about physical bullying over the previous 4 weeks to examine more than 4000 youths in grades 5 through 8. He determined that children who were repeatedly physically bullied were more likely to have poor health outcomes, including depression. Lemstra also reported that children who were ever physically bullied were 80% more likely to have a depressed mood.[45] Nansel and colleagues[46] evaluated the relationship between bullying and psychosocial adjustment in a cross-national section of 113 200 students representing 25 countries. They reported that across all countries, involvement in bullying, either as victim, bully, or bully-victim, was associated with poorer psychosocial adjustment. Klomek and colleagues[47] reported that the association between bullying behavior at 8 years of age and subsequent suicidal behavior later in life differs between males and females. After controlling for conduct and depression symptoms, girls maintained the association with later suicide attempts and completions but this was not true of boys.[47] Assessing the psychological strengths and weaknesses of the child will aid the evaluator in providing appropriate recommendations to the child's caregivers and school.

Various investigators have reported a multitude of psychiatric symptoms in bullying victims that are attributable to the bullying. These symptoms include suicidal thinking; depression; sleep disturbances; anxiety; enuresis; and somatic symptoms, including headaches and abdominal pain.[48–51] Such problems tend to manifest themselves according to the role that the child has in the bullying behavior. These roles include the bully, the victim, the bully-victim, and the bystander (which can include noninvolved observers and/or the general culture/milieu in which the behavior occurs).

Some investigators have noted that victims of bullying may become suicidal. Studies of middle and high school students show an increased risk of suicidal behavior among bullies and their victims.[52] Cyberbullying victims are almost twice as likely to attempt suicide as youths who have not been cyberbullying victims.[53] Although suicide is one of the most serious sequelae of bullying, it is also rare. There are many other ways in which bullying can harm a student. Bullying can impair seriously the physical and psychological health of its victims and create conditions that negatively affect learning, undermining the bullied students' ability to achieve their full academic potential.[54]

Evaluation of a Reported Bully

Evaluations of suspected bullies are usually conducted to assess the child's risk of violence or to determine what interventions might be helpful for the child (eg, improve the mental health of the child, decrease the child's risk of continuing bullying behavior). Frequently, the person being evaluated will not report engaging in bullying behavior. Occasionally, the child will admit that he or she has bullied others at school. In these cases, the evaluator then should ask the child what he or she means by the word *bully*, what behaviors he or she thinks constitute bullying, and why he or she thinks this behavior is occurring. The evaluator should attempt to gather more information about the child's motivation for engaging in this behavior. This type of questioning may help elicit symptoms of a psychiatric illness (depression, anxiety, trauma, and so forth) in the child that may not be disclosed during more direct questioning. This information will aid the evaluator in offering helpful recommendations for treatment and/or other interventions, as will identifying the particular type of bullying behavior in which the youth is engaging.

Risk evaluations for children involve collecting biopsychosocial information (both via collateral records and the face-to-face evaluation) and, if necessary, conducting psychological testing (see later discussion). The child should be asked specifically about risk factors, such as prior violent behavior, violent thoughts or fantasies, pervasive anger, symptoms of conduct disorder, substance abuse, trauma, abuse or maltreatment, or psychotic symptoms.[55,56] Parents should be asked about their concerns about their child's behavior, socioeconomic status, exposure to trauma, environmental stressors, abuse or maltreatment, developmental concerns (eg, prenatal alcohol or drug exposure), and relationships with peers. Legal problems and behavior problems at school should also be investigated. The parents should be asked what, if any, previous interventions have been used and their perceived effectiveness.

Making a Diagnosis

In general, forensic evaluations should use accepted diagnostic schemas, such as the *Diagnostic and Statistical Manual of Mental Disorders*. The forensic evaluator must be able to support the diagnosis with the data collected. Because the forensic evaluation assesses the youth's current symptoms and functioning, historical diagnoses alone are not recommended. Unless there is strong evidence of a personality disorder, the evaluator should use extreme caution in making this type of diagnosis in a child or adolescent.

Providing an Opinion

The opinion section of the report first and foremost should address the referral question. The evaluator should state the conclusions to a reasonable degree of medical certainty, which is colloquially defined as *more likely than not*. Each conclusion generally is followed by an explanation and supportive data are provided. The examiner should strive to provide the clearest conclusions possible. For instance, if a victim develops major depressive disorder because of bullying behavior, the evaluator could opine that (1) the child has a diagnosis of major depressive disorder, (2) the child was a target of bullying behaviors, and (3) the bullying behaviors caused the major depressive disorder. Breaking opinions down into smaller pieces clarifies the points being made and assists the reader in understanding the evaluator's thought process.

In a civil suit, the assessment of emotional damages is often an important component of the evaluation. The evaluator must focus on current symptoms and attempt to determine what caused those symptoms. In personal injury litigation, claims generally include intentional or negligent infliction of emotional distress, emotional effects of a physical injury, stress as a result of discrimination or harassment, and emotional harm from defamation or libel. The data collected during the evaluation should aid the evaluator in reaching an objective opinion related to whether and, if so, how reported and observed symptoms relate to the purported conduct. As noted previously, the evaluator should consider the life history of the child and attempt to determine whether the bullying behavior or other experiences caused or contributed to the damages.

In delivering the final opinion, the evaluator should consider alternative explanations to the child's current level of functioning. The evaluator should acknowledge gaps in the data, understand the limitations of the evaluation, consider malingering, and remain objective throughout the process. Treating providers generally rely on the child's self-report and often do not have access to all collateral information. Therefore, they should appreciate their limitations in offering an opinion regarding any causal relationships of alleged bullying to self-reported symptoms and potential ethical conflicts in doing so (eg, dual agency).

Providing accurate opinions about prognosis can be especially difficult. The evaluator should be familiar with the extant literature related to the long-term outcomes of individuals subjected to particular types of bullying behavior.[57-59] Some psychological effects include difficulty with social adjustment, depression, anxiety, eating disorders, suicidal ideation, and suicide attempts. Bullying can also place individuals at risk for somatic problems, including sleep disturbances, abdominal pain, fatigue, headaches, and fatigue.[60] The evaluator also needs to consider a child's psychosocial environment and the potential efficacy of interventions. When asked about prognosis, this is an excellent opportunity to discuss the various interventions that might be helpful to the child.

RECOMMENDING INTERVENTIONS TO DECREASE BULLYING

The evaluator, when asked, should provide and review interventions that may assist the referral party in addressing the bullying behavior. Bullying behaviors have been difficult for schools to control despite the currently available interventions.[61] Rigby suggested 6 different types of intervention, including a traditional disciplinary approach, strengthening the victim, mediation, restorative practice, a support group, and a method of shared concern.[62] Others have suggested that school-based intervention programs can be a meaningful and successful form of intervention but that they need to include parent meetings, firm disciplinary methods, and improved playground supervision to maximize their chances of success.[63]

Generally speaking, there are 3 main areas of intervention with regard to bullying behaviors. The victims and bullies can be involved directly in individual treatment programs to assist with their psychological adjustment, decision making, anger management, and other psychological aspects related to the bullying behavior. At a slightly broader level, an intervention that incorporates the family systems of a bully and/or a victim can be used. Lastly, a school-wide, systems-based approach can be used in which the culture of the student body surrounding bullying behavior is addressed. This approach has shown the most effectiveness in decreasing bullying behaviors.

There are no universally accepted interventions for victims, bullies, or bystanders. The United States Department of Health and Human Services maintains the Web site www.stopbullying.gov in an effort to educate the public about this problematic behavior. The American Academy of Pediatrics comments on the pediatrician's role with regard to youth violence prevention.[64] The American Academy of Child and Adolescent Psychiatry has issued a policy statement related to the prevention of bullying-related morbidity and mortality.[65] President Obama has also spoken out against bullying in a documentary entitled "Stop Bullying-Speak Up," which airs on the Cartoon Network.[66] Additionally, the courts continue to seek out professional guidance for recommendations on interventions that may decrease these behaviors.

Potential Interventions for the Student

The most obvious mental health intervention for an individual involved in bullying behavior (either as victim or bully) is to address any comorbid psychiatric symptoms. Research supports the idea that bullying causes both short- and long-term effects on both bullies and victims. These effects include academic problems, relationship problems, and psychological problems.[14,67,68] Although Ttofi and Farrington[57] did not appreciate a significant effect from individual treatment in their meta-analysis, they were quick to acknowledge that this avenue of intervention should not be ignored. Children who are victimized can suffer from significant mental health repercussions, including school avoidance, severe depression, and even completed suicide. With regard to bullies, Volk and colleagues[11] reported that students who were identified as pure bullies (ie, never victims of bullying) tend to have equal or better mental health than uninvolved adolescents and victims. Merrell and colleagues[61] noted that most bullies do not have mental health problems and that they are able to interact with peers in a positive manner. Volk noted that theory-of-mind research does not support the idea that bullies lack social understanding and that this is not a driving force of their antisocial behavior; they seem to understand that others have beliefs, desires, and intentions that are unique from their own.

Individual interventions for children need to be tailored to both the context of the bullying or victimization and the child's developmental level. Evaluators should have a conversation with the child's family about the bullying. The parents need to take responsibility for supporting their child through this potentially difficult time period. It is not unreasonable for the evaluator to recommend that the child and his or her family be involved in family therapy. The goal might be to improve the family's communication and to assess the family system for patterns of behavior that may be detrimental to the child. Additionally, it is recommended that the child (especially if they are an adolescent) have a separate therapist. Adolescents are generally very concerned about privacy, and having both an individual and family therapist is likely to be more beneficial to them than having a shared family therapist alone.

Bostic and Brunt[69] offers interventions for victims, bullies, and bystanders according to their school level/grade. There interventions are highlighted in **Box 2**.

Interventions for victims that do not seem to be effective include having the child ignore the bullying behavior, having the child fight back physically with the aggressor, and having the child's parents contact the other student's parents directly.

Recommended interventions for bullies include the following:

- Set strict limits and appropriate discipline by both the school and the parents.
- Increase parental supervision.

Box 2
Recommended interventions for victims of bullying

- Regenerate the child's sense of safety.
- Assess for child maltreatment and provide assistance as necessary.
- Improve deficient social skills and encourage socialization because individuals with fewer friends tend to be targeted more frequently by bullies.
- Educate the child on how to confront the aggressor effectively.
- Identify and treat comorbid psychiatric illnesses or symptoms, including anxiety, depression, and anger.
- Educate the child about safety measures.
- Involve the parents in supporting the child.
- Talk about sex at home to decrease the stigmatization surrounding sexual topics in social settings.
- Provide a go-to person at the school whom the child can access for assistance at any time.

- Screen for, and treat, psychiatric disorders, such as anxiety and depression.
- Use consequences to teach empathy (eg, have the bully role play a scenario in which he or she is the victim).

As with victims, there are strategies to avoid with bullies. The zero-tolerance policy does not work to reduce bullying behaviors. Suspending or expelling students acts as a barrier to communication about the behaviors and sets up a hostile environment for students and staff. Mediation and conflict resolution with peers has not proved effective. Using student groups to attempt to police bullying behavior seems to worsen these behaviors. Additionally, group treatments, such as anger management groups, do not seem to be effective in reducing bullying behavior because the members tend to reinforce the negative behavior in each other.

Potential interventions for the system
To date, there is little evidence of systems-based approaches being especially effective in reducing bullying behavior. Still, school systems are tasked with identifying and implementing systems-based approaches for addressing and reducing bullying behavior (for safety, educational, and political concerns). The most well-known intervention, the Olweus Bullying Prevention Program (OBPP), was developed by Dan Olweus, PhD, a Swedish psychologist. This intervention has been implemented in numerous settings, both in the United States and internationally, and has been the model for many of the new and innovative antibullying programs that have been developed. The OBPP focuses on the individuals involved, classroom teaching, and school-wide cultural changes to reduce and eventually eliminate the bullying behaviors. Ttofi and colleagues[63] noted that in addition to the intensity of the program, the components most strongly correlated with a decrease in bullying were

- Parent meetings with the teachers
- Improved playground supervision
- Presence of disciplinary methods
- Classroom management for behavioral control
- Teacher training about bullying and how to manage bullying behavior
- Explicit classroom rules regarding acceptable and unacceptable behavior
- A whole-school antibullying policy

- Frequent school conferences
- Information for parents about the identification of and interventions for bullying
- Cooperative group work to build social skills

When asked to provide recommendations for intervention or treatment in a particular case, the evaluator will need to learn about the interventions and policies that presently exist in the child's school. This knowledge will allow the evaluator to tailor specific recommendations based on the available resources. It would be simple, yet wholly impractical, for an evaluator to recommend implementing a program, such as the OBPP, if the school infrastructure and/or resources could not support such an intervention. Research has shown, however, that the whole-school–based approach has better outcomes than other interventions. Fonagy and colleagues[70] followed 9 elementary schools for 3 years. Three were introduced to the manualized Creating A Peaceful School Learning Environment (CAPSLE) intervention, 3 were provided with manualized school psychiatric consultation (SPC), and 3 were given treatment as usual (TAU). The study found that the CAPSLE approach, which was based on the Olweus model, decreased student victimization and aggression significantly when compared with the TAU schools but only modestly when compared with the SPC schools.[70] This research supports the contention that an antibullying approach needs to be system wide to be effective.[71] Yet not all research supports the efficacy of system-wide programs, such as OBPP.[61,72]

Similarly, Johnson examined the existing literature related to school-violence interventions and noted 5 significant factors that were associated with a decrease in violence[73]:

1. Students' positive relationships with teachers
2. Students' belief that the school has fair rules
3. Students' ownership in their school
4. Students' having positive classroom and overall school environments that focus on student comprehension
5. Students' having access to school interventions that focus on the safety of the physical environment

Merrell[61] noted that to implement change, the following must occur: there must be increased social costs to the bully; more prosocial alternatives to bullying need to be developed and promoted; and antibullying interventions must be tailored to each student and flexible enough to adapt to the student's growth and his or her changing environment.

Of note, if a child meets criteria for an IEP, accommodations may be offered to the student to decrease their exposure to situations in which they are at high-risk of bullying. These accommodations may include allowing the student to leave class 5 minutes early to avoid bullies in the hallway; granting the student use of a bathroom in a more supervised location, such as the administration office; and seating the student in certain areas of the bus or classroom to decrease the risk of being bullied. Additionally, social skills training might be offered to improve the child's social relatedness, which seems to decrease an individual's likelihood of being bullied.

School systems should appreciate that bullying is pervasive and not necessarily isolated to a particular school within their system. As students move from one grade to the next and one school to another (and absent effective intervention), bullying is likely to continue. Focusing on vertical and horizontal integration of the antibullying policy and plan is critical. Good communication among school personnel about problematic students and targeted children can be very helpful in combating bullying.

SUMMARY

The focus on bullying behavior has become increasingly prominent in the popular media and has helped heighten public awareness of the phenomenon. Bullying has also become an important policy agenda item, as evidenced by President Obama's promoting anti-bullying legislation. Parents and school systems are attempting to find extrajudicial solutions, although courts increasingly becoming more involved in the process as schools' responsibilities to protect students have increased (see later discussion).

Mental health providers, particularly those who work with children, are in a good position to assist schools and parents with assessments and intervention planning designed both to decrease bullying behavior and to mitigate the mental health impact of bullying. Unfortunately, because there are few longitudinal studies regarding the impact of bullying behaviors, it is difficult to determine a long-term prognosis with any degree of certainty for victims or bullies themselves. Additional research is needed related to the potential long-term comorbidities associated with specific types of bullying. These findings can help us better tailor effective interventions. Based on the extant literature, systems-based approaches aimed at changing the culture of the school are the best general interventions to decrease bullying behavior.

REFERENCES

1. Smith PK, Cowie H, Olafsson RF, et al. Definitions of bullying: a comparison of terms used, and age and gender differences, in a fourteen-country international comparison. Child Dev 2002;73(4):1119–33.
2. Craig W, Harel-Fisch Y, Fogel-Grinvald H, et al. A cross-national profile of bullying and victimization among adolescents in 40 countries. Int J Public Health 2009; 54(Suppl 2):216–24.
3. Wang J, Iannotti RJ, Nansel TR. School bullying among adolescents in the United States: physical, verbal, relational, and cyber. J Adolesc Health 2009;45(4): 368–75.
4. Mishna F, Cook C, Gadalla T, et al. Cyber bullying behaviors among middle and high school students. Am J Orthopsychiatry 2010;80(3):362–74.
5. Farrington DP. Understanding and preventing bullying. Crime and justice a review of research, vol. 17. Chicago: University of Chicago Press; 1993. p. 381–458.
6. Olweus D. Bullying at school: what we know and what we can do. Oxford (United Kingdom); Cambridge: Blackwell; 1993.
7. Glew G, Rivara F, Feudtner C. Bullying: children hurting children. Pediatr Rev 2000;21(6):183–9 [quiz: 190].
8. Volk A, Craig W, Boyce W, et al. Adolescent risk correlates of bullying and different types of victimization. Int J Adolesc Med Health 2006;18(4):575–86.
9. Crick NR, Grotpeter JK. Relational aggression, gender, and social-psychological adjustment. Child Dev 1995;66(3):710–22.
10. Raskauskas J, Stoltz AD. Involvement in traditional and electronic bullying among adolescents. Dev Psychol 2007;43(3):564–75.
11. Volk AA, Camilleri JA, Dane AV, et al. Is adolescent bullying an evolutionary adaptation? Aggress Behav 2012;38(3):222–38.
12. Sugden K, Arseneault L, Harrington H, et al. Serotonin transporter gene moderates the development of emotional problems among children following bullying victimization. J Am Acad Child Adolesc Psychiatry 2010;49(8):830–40.
13. Falb KL, McCauley HL, Decker MR, et al. School bullying perpetration and other childhood risk factors as predictors of adult intimate partner violence perpetration. Arch Pediatr Adolesc Med 2011;165(10):890–4.

14. Meltzer H, Vostanis P, Ford T, et al. Victims of bullying in childhood and suicide attempts in adulthood. Eur Psychiatry 2011;26(8):498–503.

15. Blazei RW, Iacono WG, McGue M. Father-child transmission of antisocial behavior: the moderating role of father's presence in the home. J Am Acad Child Adolesc Psychiatry 2008;47(4):406–15.

16. Alexander K, Alexander M. Student rights: common law, constitutional due process, and statutory protections. American Public School Law. 6th edition. Belmont (CA): Thompson West; 2005. p. 433.

17. See, e.g., Walton v. Alexander (5th Cir. 1997), holding that liability will attach "[w]here a school official knows, or willfully avoids knowing about the possibility of serious harm to a student, fails to take appropriate action, and the student is harmed." Also, Doe v. Oyster River (D.N.H. 1997), holding that school officials may be held liable for student-on-student sexual harassment "if (1) school officials knew or should have known of the matter but failed to correct the problem, (2) a special relationship existed to protect students from harm, and (3) the harassment was severe and pervasive."

18. Davis v. Monroe City Board of Education, 526 U.S. 629 (1999).

19. See, e.g., Lichtler v. County of Orange, 813 F. Supp. 1054 (S.D. N.Y. 1993), where the court held that "[a] state imposing compulsory attendance on school children must take reasonable steps to protect those required to attend from foreseeable risks of personal injury or death."

20. See, e.g., Shrum v. Muck, 249 F. 3d 773 (8th Cir. 2001), holding: "there is no constitutional duty of care for school districts, as state mandated school attendance does not entail so restrictive a custodial relationship as to impose a duty upon the state."

21. Nabozny v Podlesny, 92 F. 3d 446. (7th Circuit, 1996).

22. J.O. v. Alton Community Unit School Dist. 11, 909 F.2d 267 (7th Cir. 1990).

23. U.S.C. § 1681(a).

24. Vacca R. The duty to protect students from harm. CEPI Education Law Newsletter 2002;1-3. Available at: http://www.cepi.vcu.edu/newsletter/2002-2003/2002_November.html. Accessed April 1, 2012.

25. United States Department of Health and Human Services. Available at: http://www.stopbullying.gov/laws/index.html. Accessed April 1, 2012.

26. California Education Code. Available at: http://www.leginfo.ca.gov/cgi-bin/calawquery?codesection=edc&codebody=&hits=20. Accessed April 15, 2012.

27. California Assembly Bill No. 9, Chapter 723. Available at: http://www.leginfo.ca.gov/pub/11-12/bill/asm/ab_0001-0050/ab_9_bill_20111009_chaptered.pdf. Accessed April 15, 2012.

28. U.S. Department of Education, Office of Planning, Evaluation and Policy Development, Policy and Program Studies Service. Analysis of state bullying laws and policies, Washington, DC. 2011. Available at: http://www.ed.gov/about/offices/list/opepd/ppss/index.html. Accessed April 1, 2012.

29. Safe Schools Improvement Act of 2011, S.506 and H.R. 1648. 112th Congress.

30. Bacca M. Anoka-Hennepin School District settles bullying lawsuit. Available at: http://www.startribune.com/local/north/141427303.html?page=1&c=y. Accessed April 21, 2012.

31. Tinker V. Des Moines Independent Community School Dist., 393 U.S. 503 (1969).

32. Layshock v. Hermitage School District 496 F.Supp.2d 587 (WD PA 2007).

33. J.S. v. Blue Mt. Sch. Dist., 2007 U.S. Dist. LEXIS 23406 (M.D. Pa., Mar. 29, 2007).

34. Layshock v. Hermitage School District, 593 F.3d 249 (3rd Cir. 2010).

35. J.S. ex rel. Snyder v. Blue Mountain School Dist., 593 F.3d 286 (3rd Cir. 2010).

36. Kowalski V. Berkeley County Schools, U.S.D. C. ND of WVa., 2009. (3:07-cv-00147-JPB).

37. Kowalski V. Berkeley County Schools, 652 F.3d 565 (4th Cir. 2011).

38. Felix ED, Sharkey JD, Green JG, et al. Getting precise and pragmatic about the assessment of bullying: the development of the California Bullying Victimization Scale. Aggress Behav 2011;37(3):234–47.

39. Jones S, Cauffman E. Juvenile psychopathy and judicial decision making: an empirical analysis of an ethical dilemma. Behav Sci Law 2008;26(2):151–65.

40. Boccaccini MT, Murrie DC, Clark JW, et al. Describing, diagnosing, and naming psychopathy: how do youth psychopathy labels influence jurors? Behav Sci Law 2008;26(4):487–510.

41. Oates K, Shrimpton S. Children's memories for stressful and non-stressful events. Med Sci Law 1991;31(1):4–10.

42. Finkelhor D, Ormrod RK, Turner HA. Polyvictimization and trauma in a national longitudinal cohort. Dev Psychopathol 2007;19(1):149–66.

43. Finkelhor D, Ormrod RK, Turner HA. Re-victimization patterns in a national longitudinal sample of children and youth. Child Abuse Negl 2007;31(5):479–502.

44. Gustafsson PE, Nilsson D, Svedin CG. Polytraumatization and psychological symptoms in children and adolescents. Eur Child Adolesc Psychiatry 2009; 18(5):274–83.

45. Lemstra ME, Nielsen G, Rogers MR, et al. Risk indicators and outcomes associated with bullying in youth aged 9-15 years. Can J Public Health 2012;103(1): 9–13.

46. Nansel TR, Craig W, Overpeck MD, et al. Cross-national consistency in the relationship between bullying behaviors and psychosocial adjustment. Arch Pediatr Adolesc Med 2004;158(8):730–6.

47. Klomek AB, Sourander A, Niemelä S, et al. Childhood bullying behaviors as a risk for suicide attempts and completed suicides: a population-based birth cohort study. J Am Acad Child Adolesc Psychiatry 2009;48(3):254–61.

48. Arseneault L, Walsh E, Trzesniewski K, et al. Bullying victimization uniquely contributes to adjustment problems in young children: a nationally representative cohort study. Pediatrics 2006;118(1):130–8.

49. Williams K, Chambers M, Logan S, et al. Association of common health symptoms with bullying in primary school children. BMJ 1996;313(7048):17–9.

50. Kim YS, Leventhal B. Bullying and suicide. A review. Int J Adolesc Med Health 2008;20(2):133–54.

51. Kim YS, Leventhal BL, Koh YJ, et al. School bullying and youth violence: causes or consequences of psychopathologic behavior? Arch Gen Psychiatry 2006; 63(9):1035–41.

52. Klomek A, Sourander A, Gould M. Bullying and suicide: detection and intervention. Psychiatric Times 2011;28(2).

53. Hinduja S, Patchin JW. Bullying, cyberbullying, and suicide. Arch Suicide Res 2010;14(3):206–21.

54. Hinduja S, Patchin J. Offline consequences of online victimization: school violence and delinquency. J Sch Violence 2007;6(3):89–112.

55. Borum R. Assessing violence risk among youth. J Clin Psychol 2000;56(10): 1263–88.

56. Vincent GM. Psychopathy and violence risk assessment in youth. Child Adolesc Psychiatr Clin N Am 2006;15(2):407–28, ix.

57. Ttofi MM, Farrington DP. Risk and protective factors, longitudinal research, and bullying prevention. New Dir Youth Dev 2012;2012(133):85–98.

58. Roeger L, Allison S, Korossy-Horwood R, et al. Is a history of school bullying victimization associated with adult suicidal ideation? A South Australian population-based observational study. J Nerv Ment Dis 2010;198(10):728–33.

59. Arseneault L, Bowes L, Shakoor S. Bullying victimization in youths and mental health problems: 'much ado about nothing'? Psychol Med 2010;40(5):717–29.

60. Sansone RA, Sansone LA. Bully victims: psychological and somatic aftermaths. Psychiatry (Edgmont) 2008;5(6):62–4.

61. Merrell KW, Gueldner BA, Ross SW, et al. How effective are school bullying intervention programs? A meta-analysis of intervention research. Sch Psychol Q 2008; 23(1):26–42.

62. Rigby K. New perspectives on bullying. London; Philadelphia: J. Kingsley; 2002.

63. Ttofi MM, Farrington DP, Losel F, et al. The predictive efficiency of school bullying versus later offending: a systematic/meta-analytic review of longitudinal studies. Crim Behav Ment Health 2011;21(2):80–9.

64. Committee on Injury VaPP. Policy statement - role of the pediatrician in youth violence prevention. Pediatrics 2009;124(1):393–402.

65. American Academy of Child & Adolescent Psychiatry Task Force for the Prevention of Bullying. Prevention of bullying related morbidity and mortality. 2012. Available at: http://www.aacap.org/cs/root/policy_statements/policy_statement_prevention_of_bullying_related_morbidity_and_mortality. Accessed April 30, 2012.

66. Deshishku S. President Obama says "stop bullying – speak up" – the 1600 report - CNN.com Blogs. 2012. Available at: http://whitehouse.blogs.cnn.com/2012/03/13/president-obama-says-stop-bullying-speak-up/. Accessed April 30, 2012.

67. Swearer S, Espelage D, Vaillancourt T, et al. What can be done about school bullying? Educational Researcher 2010;39(1):38–47.

68. Renda J, Vassallo S, Edwards B. Bullying in early adolescence and its association with anti-social behaviour, criminality and violence 6 and 10 years later. Crim Behav Ment Health 2011;21(2):117–27.

69. Bostic JQ, Brunt CC. Cornered: an approach to school bullying and cyberbullying, and forensic implications. Child Adolesc Psychiatr Clin N Am 2011;20(3): 447–65.

70. Fonagy P, Twemlow SW, Vernberg EM, et al. A cluster randomized controlled trial of child-focused psychiatric consultation and a school systems-focused intervention to reduce aggression. J Child Psychol Psychiatry 2009;50(5):607–16.

71. Vreeman RC, Carroll AE. A systematic review of school-based interventions to prevent bullying. Arch Pediatr Adolesc Med 2007;161(1):78–88.

72. Bauer NS, Lozano P, Rivara FP. The effectiveness of the Olweus Bullying Prevention Program in public middle schools: a controlled trial. J Adolesc Health 2007; 40(3):266–74.

73. Johnson SL. Improving the school environment to reduce school violence: a review of the literature. J Sch Health 2009;79(10):451–65.

Psychiatric Consultation in Problem Employee Situations

Ronald Schouten, MD, JD

KEYWORDS

- Occupational psychiatry • Americans with Disabilities Act • Violence risk assessment
- Fitness for duty evaluations • Workplace violence • Disability discrimination

KEY POINTS

- Psychiatric consultations in the workplace that involve potential adversarial issues follow the same general principles, structure, and format as other forensic evaluations. These represent a subset of the broader array of psychiatric consultations that may be beneficial to the workplace.
- Familiarity with the Americans with Disabilities Act and the Family and Medical Leave Act is important for psychiatrists providing consultation in the occupational setting.
- Clinical information gathered in the course of these consultations should only be shared on a need-to-know basis and with authorization from the evaluee.
- Treating clinicians are a valuable source of information in workplace-related consultations, but should not be expected to be able to provide objective assessments because of the usual biases that arise in the treatment relationship.

INTRODUCTION

Occupational psychiatry is a subspecialty of psychiatry that focuses on workplace behavioral health issues, including conflicts that arise between employees and employers. This article discusses some of the clinical and consultative roles that psychiatrists may be asked to fill with regard to problematic employee situations. In keeping with the theme of this issue, this article focuses on roles that are primarily forensic in nature (ie, dealing with issues that involve or could lead to adversarial proceedings). Many other important issues that fall under the rubric of occupational psychiatry, such as treatment of workplace-related conditions, workers compensation evaluations, consultation on employee health issues and organizational behavior matters, disability management, executive coaching, and team building, are not covered as part of this discussion.

The author has no financial disclosures to make.

Department of Psychiatry, Law and Psychiatry Service, Massachusetts General Hospital, Harvard Medical School, 15 Parkman Street, WAC 812, Boston, MA 02114, USA

E-mail address: rschouten@partners.org

Psychiatr Clin N Am 35 (2012) 901–913
http://dx.doi.org/10.1016/j.psc.2012.08.010　　　　　　　　**psych.theclinics.com**

Successful employers know how to handle routine employee problems. Absenteeism, poor productivity, insubordination, failure to follow instructions, sexual harassment, and a host of other problematic behaviors are bread and butter issues for human resource professionals. However, when those behaviors raise the specter of mental illness or violence, employers often seek consultation from psychiatrists or other mental health professionals. The reasons for this include the expertise of mental health professionals with abnormal behavior, psychopathology, and interpersonal conflict, and the public's long-held presumption of a strong link between mental illness and violence.

This article focuses on psychiatric consultation to employers, because that is the most common scenario in which a psychiatrist's consultation is requested regarding problematic employee behavior. However, an employee may seek consultation himself or herself, especially when a disagreement has arisen and the prospects for adversarial proceedings arise. The principles described here apply in both sets of circumstances.

COMMON PRINCIPLES IN FORENSIC OCCUPATIONAL PSYCHIATRY EVALUATIONS

Before turning to examples of situations in which psychiatric expertise may be sought, it is useful to consider the following 10 underlying and unifying concepts that apply to these consultations.

1. Employer concern about transgressing disability discrimination laws
2. Recognition of the workplace as a complex system made up of individuals in an organization that has its own unique structure and culture
3. Differential diagnosis for problematic employee behaviors
4. "Fitness for duty evaluations"
5. Obligation of the psychiatrist to be objective and honest and to protect confidentiality
6. Fulfillment of a successful consultation meets three important aspects
7. Goal of workplace evaluations is to answer a specific question or questions
8. Psychiatrists' awareness of situations in which employer is trying to solve a managerial problem by referring an employee for a psychiatric evaluation
9. Role of the psychiatrist in workplace evaluations is that of consultant, not ultimate decision maker
10. Role of the treating psychiatrist is to provide clinical information relevant to the evaluation of workplace issues, not expert opinion

1. **Employers are appropriately concerned** about transgressing disability discrimination laws when addressing behavioral health issues that arise in the workplace. The Americans with Disabilities Act (ADA)[1] and analogous state statutes prohibit disparate treatment of individuals who have or have had physical or mental disabilities, or who are perceived as having a disability. These statutes and their associated regulations prohibit discrimination against covered individuals with regard to employment so long as they can perform the essential functions of the job, with or without reasonable accommodations. What constitutes a "reasonable" accommodation depends on multiple factors, including the nature of the position, the uniqueness of the employee's skills required for it, and the size and resources of the employer.[2] Although consulting mental health professionals may opine as to what accommodations are necessary or helpful in making it possible for a disabled employee to work, the determination of whether a specific accommodation is "reasonable" is up to the employer, at least until that determination is challenged.

Fear of triggering a disability discrimination claim causes many employers to avoid noticing, considering, or responding to potential mental health issues among employees, a phenomenon this author refers to as "litigation-induced paralysis." The result is that these employers often miss an opportunity to assist an employee with issues that may have a substantial negative effect on employee wellness, productivity, and workplace safety. A knowledgeable psychiatrist can help an organization address these issues and minimize the risk of disability discrimination claims. We revisit this issue later, in connection with case examples.

2. Although the focus in these matters tends to be on the employee, it is important to recognize that the **workplace is a complex system made up of individuals functioning within an organization that has its own unique structure and culture.** Whatever characteristics an individual employee may bring to the workplace, they must be considered in this broader context if the problem in question is to be correctly understood and managed optimally.[3] As such, the "problem employee" may be thought of as analogous to the identified patient in family therapy.

3. **There is a differential diagnosis for problematic employee behaviors.** Behavior that is presumed to be a function of the employee's personality may prove to be the product of an underlying illness, substance abuse, medications or toxins, exacerbation of illnesses because of extreme stress, cultural differences, or general life stress. The opposite also may be true: behavior that is presumed to be related to some specific condition or substance may be a function of an employee's personality traits and how the employee has learned to function in the workplace and personal life.

4. **Many workplace forensic evaluations fall under the heading of "fitness for duty evaluations."** Broadly defined, these are comprehensive evaluations designed to determine if an employee is capable of performing the essential functions of his or her job. Like other forensic evaluations, a thorough fitness for duty evaluation requires consideration of collateral sources of information, such as personnel records, information from coworkers or supervisors, and background investigations.[4] The report and its contents should be tailored to the party receiving it, as discussed later in #7.

5. As in all other forensic evaluations, **the psychiatrist has an obligation to be objective and honest and to protect confidentiality to the extent possible,** even where the evaluation is being conducted on behalf of a third party and there is no doctor-patient relationship with the evaluee. In addition, the evaluator has an obligation to make sure that the evaluee's agreement to undergo the evaluation is informed with regard to the limitations on confidentiality, the role of the evaluator, and the inability to guarantee any particular outcome. In many situations, the evaluee's participation is not fully voluntary because he or she may be required to undergo the evaluation as a condition of any prospect of continued employment. Although there is an element of coercion in this, the employee has the option of forgoing the evaluation, albeit with the potential loss of his or her job as a result. Despite this, the employee's participation can still be considered voluntary, so long as there is full disclosure of the terms and conditions of the evaluation.

6. **A successful consultation of any type requires that the consultant (1) understand the questions being asked, (2) know who is asking the question and how the information will be used, and (3) have sufficient knowledge and skill to answer the questions posed.** Special populations of employees (eg, law enforcement, firefighters, members of the intelligence community, and certain industries) have specific behavioral health issues unique to the nature

of their work. The psychiatric consultant should be aware that these unique characteristics may exist and become familiar with them before undertaking the consultation.

7. **The goal of these evaluations is to answer a specific question or questions, not to provide unnecessary details of the evaluee's diagnosis, personal and medical history, and life circumstances to the employer.** Most employers prefer to receive a direct answer to the question at hand (eg, "Is the employee fit to return to work?" or "Does this employee pose a risk of violence?") rather than detailed personal medical information, because it can increase the risk of a disability discrimination allegation. Similarly, evaluees generally do not want their personal health information shared with supervisors and possibly coworkers. In light of this, when presenting findings to an employer, it is best for the psychiatrist to answer the specific question posed (eg, "Fit for duty?" "Need for accommodations?" "What type?") and to disclose only essential clinical information on a need-to-know basis. Indeed, a California case held that the evaluating psychiatrist and the employer could be held liable for violation of privacy under the California Constitution and violation of the Confidentiality of Medical Information Act where, among other things, clinical information was shared with an employee's managers.[5] Clinical information can be shared with management personnel with the employee's consent, but even then the disclosure should be limited to a need-to-know basis. Ideally, that information is shared only with occupational health personnel; however, this also requires employee consent.

8. **Psychiatrists who undertake these evaluations should be mindful of situations in which the employer is trying to solve a managerial problem by referring the employee for a psychiatric evaluation.** For example, a supervisor who is having difficulty managing an employee or has concerns about the employee's performance may request a fitness for duty evaluation with the hope or expectation that the psychiatrist will declare the employee unfit for duty. This author advises clients that an employee should not be sent for a fitness for duty evaluation if the employer is planning to terminate the employee anyway, because there is an even chance that the employee will be found fit to perform the essential functions of the job.

9. **The role of the psychiatrist in these evaluations is that of consultant, not ultimate decision maker.** As noted, certain matters, such as what constitutes a reasonable accommodation, are business decisions that may or may not include consideration of clinical issues. Consultants' opinions and recommendations may be rejected outright, or may be subjected to requests for modification or reconsideration. Psychiatrists who consult on workplace issues are well-advised to think of themselves as members of a team, each member of which brings unique skills and experiences to the process. In some cases, the team may look to the psychiatrist for leadership, whereas in other cases, the psychiatrist takes a more peripheral role. In all cases, an essential role of the psychiatrist is to help make clinical concepts understandable and useful to the rest of the team.

10. **Although treating clinicians have an important role in providing clinical information relevant to the evaluation of workplace issues,** the task of providing an objective expert opinion to a third party or in the course of litigation is best left to an independent expert with whom the employee has not had a treatment relationship. As in other forensic evaluations, an objective assessment requires consideration of information from records and collateral sources not normally reviewed in the course of treatment, and a degree of objectivity that threatens the therapeutic alliance, which itself injects a level of bias that prevents full objectivity.[6,7]

CASE EXAMPLES

The following cases, drawn from real events but with identifying details obscured, are just four examples of situations in which psychiatrists can play a role in addressing problematic issues in the workplace. Each of them involves a psychiatrist consulting to the employer, because that is the most common scenario in which a psychiatrist's consultation is requested regarding problematic employee behavior. However, employees may seek consultation when a disagreement has arisen and the prospects for adversarial proceedings increase.

Sick or Sick of Working? Assessing the Legitimacy of Family and Medical Leave Act Leave

This first example focuses on the Family and Medical Leave Act (FMLA).[8] The FMLA was passed in 1993 to protect employees' jobs when they needed to take time off to care for a newborn, adopted child, or foster child, or to be away from work to deal with a health-related matter for themselves or a family member. The FMLA provides for up to 12 weeks of unpaid leave annually in such situations. The leave may be intermittent (eg, half a day off for regularly scheduled doctor's appointments) or periodic (eg, absences caused by exacerbation of migraine headaches).

To qualify for FMLA leave, an employee or the family member must be suffering from a serious health condition, inform his or her employer of the need for leave, and comply with any requirement the employer may have for certification by a qualified healthcare professional. Qualified professionals include psychologists, social workers, chiropractors, and other licensed practitioners; Christian Science practitioners; and any healthcare provider accepted by the employee's health insurance plan as eligible to certify a health condition. In most cases, an employee's treating clinician is asked to write a note indicating that the employee qualifies for FMLA leave, in conjunction with the employee filing an application for such leave.

When an employee wishes to return from FMLA leave, the employer is obligated to accept the treating clinician's opinion that the employee is able to return. If the employer wishes to challenge the leave itself or the return to work, the employer can require that the employee undergo an independent evaluation, a task often performed by psychiatrists when mental health issues are the basis for the leave. If the independent evaluator disagrees with the treating clinician's opinion, a mutually agreed on third evaluator is brought in as a tie-breaker, as this case example demonstrates.

Serious medical condition vs. difficulty managing conflict?

Sheila, age 55, is an assembler at Electro, Inc., an electronic parts company in the Midwest. Originally trained as an electrician, she went to work at Electro after she was laid off from her nonunion electrician's job. Sheila came to Electro with "an attitude," reminding everyone (including her supervisors) that she was a "real" electrician and not just another assembly line worker. She frequently contradicted her supervisor about how and why things needed to be done. When she made mistakes, she blamed them on her supervisor's inability to explain things. On several occasions, Sheila left work early after an argument with her supervisor over some assigned task, claiming that she was sick. One day, Sheila left work mid-afternoon after another argument with her supervisor. She returned with a note from her social worker therapist that she would require intermittent time off under FMLA to manage her medical condition, which the social worker listed as "stress." When asked to complete a more detailed form, the social worker indicated diagnoses of anxiety disorder not otherwise specific (NOS) with prominent posttraumatic stress disorder symptoms. Somewhat skeptical of this diagnosis and the basis for the absences, the employer referred Sheila for an independent medical evaluation (IME) by a forensic psychiatrist.

The IME psychiatrist conducted a thorough evaluation, which included a review of Sheila's personnel file and her medical and mental health records, and an in-person evaluation of Sheila and a telephone interview with the social worker. During the evaluation, Sheila described her superior knowledge and skills, expressed dismay that her supervisor did not listen to her, and recounted several examples of how she had been mistreated by management and how this upset her. She told the evaluator that she was fed up with how the company mistreated her and that the stress of it made her physically ill. Asked to elaborate on what she meant by stress, Sheila described being angry and frustrated, and indicated that her "stress" was strictly limited to work; everything else in her life was "fine." She denied specific symptoms of any anxiety disorders, including panic disorder, generalized anxiety disorder, social phobia, or obsessive-compulsive disorder, although she was worried that her boss was trying to set her up to be laid off. The only "trauma" in her life was her conflict with her supervisor. There was no evidence of a psychotic disorder or mood disorder. In a telephone conversation, the social worker explained that Sheila was suffering from anxiety disorder NOS as a result of the stress of the job, and that the workplace was extremely stressful. Asked how she knew this, she explained that Sheila had told her so. She acknowledged that she had not visited the workplace or interviewed others, and did not really know much about what Sheila's job entailed.

On the basis of the examination, the medical records, and the absence of symptoms anywhere but the workplace, the IME psychiatrist concluded that Sheila did not suffer from an anxiety disorder, and pointed out that "stress" is not a diagnosis. He concluded that Sheila was leaving work out of anger and frustration because of difficulty resolving conflict with her supervisor, rather than because of a serious health condition. Sheila and her attorney disagreed and asked for a tiebreaker evaluation by another psychiatrist. The third psychiatrist concluded that Sheila suffered from adjustment disorder with anxiety and recommended that Sheila and her supervisor use the services of the company employee assistance program to work through their conflict; she did not believe that Sheila suffered from a condition that required her to have periodic medical leave. On learning this, Sheila requested and was given a severance package and left the company.

The FMLA provides an important benefit to employees and their families. Like other benefits, however, it can be abused and presumptions of eligibility may be erroneous. This example shows the challenges faced by treating clinicians when asked to certify a patient's eligibility for FMLA medical leave. Sheila's therapist completed the paperwork and offered an opinion based on the information available to her from Sheila and tried to assist her, consistent with her role as an advocate for her patient. In doing so, she attempted to construct a clinical disorder, rather than identifying the problem as one of poor conflict management skills and maladaptive personality traits.

It is the experience of this author that treating clinicians routinely yield to the patient's preferences with regard to leave or return to work, except in the most extreme of clinical circumstances, and may resist alternative explanations for the problems other than what the patient offers. In some cases, an employee/patient may pressure his clinician to clear his return to work when he is not ready. The result may be suboptimal performance that leads to discipline or termination. Moreover, the treating clinician is unlikely to rely on collateral sources of information, including review of other records or discussions with the employer. This is because of logistical (eg, insufficient time allotted in the clinical practice schedule) and clinical considerations (eg, damage to the treatment relationship as a result of coming to a conclusion that differs from the patient's view).

An independent psychiatrist consulted by the employer can help the employer understand the problems inherent in relying on the treating clinician's opinion. Treating clinicians who are uncomfortable certifying the patient for leave or return to work may also raise this issue with the requesting patient or employer, and suggest that an opinion be obtained from an independent evaluator. The independent evaluation can be of great benefit to the employee and employer, especially in return to work situations where there are safety issues or premature return might threaten the patient's continued employment.

The Problem Professional

Psychiatrists may also be asked to bring their clinical skills to bear in the assessment of executives and professionals whose problematic behavior gets them into difficulty with their organizations, practices, licensing boards, or other agencies. These third parties may instruct the executive or professional to obtain an evaluation as part of an investigative or disciplinary process. Alternatively, third-party organizations may engage the psychiatrist directly to conduct the evaluation. In the former situation, the executive or professional is generally required to pay for the evaluation personally. In the latter situation, the third party generally covers the cost. The former situation is somewhat problematic, given that a dissatisfied evaluee (ie, one who is displeased with the results of the evaluation) may refuse to pay. As a practical matter and a way to limit the possible actual or implied bias such a financial link may cause, evaluators should work against a retainer in such cases. Ideally, the consultant's professional relationship should be with the evaluee's attorney, rather than with the evaluee himself or herself. However, in many of these cases, the evaluee is not represented by counsel, because adversarial proceedings have not yet begun.

Considering alternative explanations for problematic behavior

Fred was one of the founding partners of a group medical practice. Well-regarded in the community and a high earner, he was a key member of the group. Fred did not suffer fools gladly. And "fools" included anyone or anything he believed was interfering with the care he wanted to provide to his patients—a list that had grown quite long as medicine changed over the course of his career. And as it did, Fred became more and more irritable—with clinic and hospital staff, and particularly with administrators. Nurses and other physicians began to comment about his irritability and episodes of forgetfulness. One day, Fred blew up at a nurse who could not answer a question about one of his patients, shouting at her and slamming the chart down on the nursing station desk. The head nurse filled out an incident report and the situation was referred to the chief of the medical staff.

Because of his seniority and previously good record, Fred was allowed to take a voluntary leave of absence and self-report to his state medical society's physician health program (PHP) for an evaluation. The director of the PHP interviewed Fred and concluded that he needed a thorough evaluation before a decision as to whether PHP programs might be appropriate. According to the PHP's standard practice, he gave Fred the names of three different psychiatrists from whom to choose for the evaluation, to be paid for by Fred. All three had conducted evaluations for PHP in the past. Fred chose Dr Smith based on cost and availability.

Dr Smith conducted a thorough evaluation consistent with the guidelines provided by the Federation of State Medical Boards (FSMB).[9] This included review of a physical examination, laboratory tests including toxicology screen, a review of Fred's medical records and the complaint against him, and a thorough psychiatric evaluation that revealed poor short-term memory. Dr Smith also got permission from Fred to talk with Fred's office staff about what he was like in the office. He learned that Fred's staff had been covering up for significant memory deficits for over a year. Out of devotion to Fred, and their ability to cover for him and protect the patients, they had not said anything to anyone. Dr Smith referred Fred to a neuropsychologist for testing and to a neurologist, both of whom confirmed his diagnosis of early dementia, consistent with Alzheimer disease. Eventually, Fred was persuaded to retire from practice and file for disability.

Disruptive behavior by physicians has received considerable attention in recent years, with the recognition that it is causally related to poor patient care, increased errors, and bad outcomes.[10] The American Medical Association defines disruptive behavior as "a style of interaction with physicians, hospital personnel, patients, family members, or others that interferes with patient care."[11] As Pastner[12] has pointed out, neither the American Medical Association nor the Joint Commission for the Accreditation of Healthcare Organizations provides specific examples of such behavior. Both acknowledge that defining the behavior is subjective and suggest that institutions arrive at their own definitions. He notes:

> *Thus, there is no "standard" procedure for handling disruptive behavior per se, and no firm guidance to differentiate between righteous indignation on the part of a frustrated physician and the rude, disruptive behavior which potentially threatens patient safety and about which all parties are justifiably concerned.*

The American Medical Association and FSMB, and the Joint Commission for the Accreditation of Healthcare Organizations, have all emphasized that disruptive behavior can be the result of a wide range of conditions: addictions of various types, substance abuse, other Axis I disorders, Axis II disorders, and several medical conditions that would be listed on Axis III. Nevertheless, many of these referrals for evaluations are made with the assumption that the behavior in question is the result of the physician acting out in response to the stress of modern medicine (ie, the product of individual personality traits and the environment). In my experience as an evaluator and copresenter at a course for physicians entitled "Managing Workplace Conflicts," that is often the case. However, as this example shows, it is essential that the evaluator conduct a thorough psychiatric evaluation, with an open mind regarding the differential diagnosis.

Although this example concerns a physician, the same principles apply, albeit with varying degrees of regulatory overlay, to evaluations of business people, lawyers, nurses, accountants, and every other type of worker.

The Potentially Violent Employee

No workplace issue raises as much concern as the potential for violence by a current or former employee. In addition to the fear that an act of violence will occur, with its many adverse consequences, management of these situations gives rise to multiple legal concerns. Employers confronted with potentially violent behavior in the workplace face the risk of liability if a violent event occurs and they have failed to act. They also face potential liability for disability discrimination if they handle the situation in a way that results in disparate treatment of employees with disabilities, as this example demonstrates.

Disability discrimination and the potential for workplace violence

Mary had repaired equipment for XYZ Corporation for 10 years. It was a rough and tumble organization, with occasional fistfights and verbal threats between the employees. On one occasion, an employee was suspended for a week after bringing a loaded gun to the workplace. One year after she started, Mary went out on sick leave for several months. Unknown to her employer, during that time she had been psychiatrically hospitalized and treated for schizoaffective disorder. Mary did well after her discharge and was compliant with her medications for 8 years. She did so well that her outpatient psychiatrist began to question the diagnosis. Eventually, the psychiatrist suggested that they taper off the antipsychotic medication and monitor for the emergence of symptoms.

Mary did well for a year after she stopped her medication. One day, however, she showed up at work ranting about Satan, and how she was on an assignment from the CIA to protect the factory equipment from being possessed by demons. She began waving a loaded pistol when police approached her, warning them not to interfere with her mission on behalf of the federal government. After the police talked her into giving up the gun, Mary was arrested, arraigned on charges of unlawful possession of a concealed weapon, assault with a dangerous weapon, and resisting arrest, and immediately sent to the state forensic hospital. Her medications were resumed and she recovered quickly.

After being found not guilty by reason of mental illness, Mary was hospitalized briefly and discharged to outpatient care, at which point she asked her employer about returning to work. Although her supervisor was sympathetic to her situation and was willing to have Mary return if she were fit to do so, her coworkers expressed concerns about Mary's ongoing risk of violence and fitness to return to work. Some threatened to quit if she were allowed to return.

On the advice of its employment attorney, XYZ referred Mary for a fitness for duty evaluation, hoping that the forensic psychiatrist would find her unfit and not eligible to return to work. The psychiatrist who evaluated her reviewed her personnel records, the police reports, and medical records from the forensic hospital and subsequent treaters. He also spoke with those treating clinicians and conducted an extended evaluation of Mary. This all revealed the iatrogenic cause of her relapse after many years of compliance, that her psychosis had resolved, her current compliance with treatment, the absence of any history of violence or substance abuse, and her awareness of the link between her mental illness and what had happened.

The evaluating psychiatrist informed XYZ's human resources manager that Mary posed a low risk of violence and was fit to return. After some deliberation, the employer decided to terminate Mary's employment for violating the workplace violence policy, but offered her a severance package. Mary consulted an employment attorney and filed a disability discrimination claim with the Equal Employment Opportunity Commission. The claim alleged that other employees who were not disabled or perceived as disabled, but who committed similar violations of the workplace violence policy, had received little or no punishment and that she had been deemed fit to work by the XYZ's chosen evaluator. After some protracted litigation, XYZ settled Mary's' claim for a sizable amount.

XYZ faced the legal pressures discussed previously: potential liability if a violent incident did occur after Mary returned and charges of disability discrimination if she were not allowed to return. In this case, the latter threat was realized because XYZ had treated Mary differently than it had other employees who violated the workplace violence policy. XYZ's workplace violence policy was typical in that it contained a "zero tolerance" clause calling for potential discipline "up to and including termination" for violations. Mary's actions were in clear violation of the policy, and there were legitimate grounds for terminating or otherwise disciplining her. Indeed, one could argue that XYZ was obligated to respond in accordance with its policy.

Where XYZ ran into difficulty was that it failed in its obligation to treat all individuals equally, with no disparate treatment of those with past, current, or presumed disabilities. Employers are free to treat individual employees differently, so long as the decision to do so is not based on the employee's membership in a protected class (eg, race, religion, ethnicity, gender, disability, or, in some states, sexual orientation). Enforcing the policy with regard to Mary when other employees who had violated the policy received little or no punishment was a powerful indicator that she was treated in a disparate fashion based on her disability.

Some would argue that that the best outcome was reached in this case: XYZ did not have to take Mary back and avoided having to deal with employees who were concerned about her return, and Mary received a substantial settlement. XYZ management miscalculated if they assumed that Mary would not be fit for duty. If a decision had already been made that Mary could not return, XYZ could have offered Mary a retirement package at the outset and avoided the expense of the independent evaluation and, potentially, the litigation and settlement.

From a social policy standpoint, the goal of protecting people with disabilities from discrimination and destigmatizing mental illness clearly were not met. No matter how strong the urge to do so, it is not the responsibility of the psychiatrist to further social policy objectives. However, there were ways in which XYZ could have chosen to use his services to reach a more optimal outcome from a legal, cost, and social policy standpoint. For example, with Mary's permission, XYZ could have asked the psychiatrist to meet with supervisors and even other employees to help them understand mental illness and violence risk assessment, and offer reassurance regarding Mary's safety. XYZ also could have taken a stronger stand in response to the resistance of the coworkers to Mary's return.

This case example demonstrates some of the complexities and concerns that the ADA injects into the assessment of potential workplace violence. A detailed discussion of the workplace violence threat assessment itself is beyond the scope of this article, but is readily available elsewhere.[13–15]

The Paranoid Researcher

The determination of whether an employee is fit for duty becomes especially problematic in the presence of obvious mental illness that does not seem to affect the employee's work itself, but results in the disruption of the workplace overall, as this example demonstrates.

Fitness for duty in the presence of disability

Dr Harris was a physician at a large university medical center who had stopped treating patients to do clinical research in the laboratory of a senior researcher. One day, the director of the laboratory called the chief of occupational health at the hospital to ask for advice about what to do with Dr Harris. Apparently, Dr Harris had been coming to him for the past year complaining that someone was breaking into the laboratory at night, tampering with his research files, and sabotaging his research. Specifically, he accused a former colleague who now primarily worked at another institution, but retained access to their laboratory space because of some joint projects. After a full investigation by hospital security, which found no evidence of break in or loss of files or other materials, Dr Harris had stopped complaining for several months. Recently, however, he had been asserting to the director (and anyone within earshot) that someone must be tampering with his research. Not surprisingly, his allegations had a disruptive effect on work throughout the laboratory, because his fellow researchers and support staff all wondered if he suspected them.

After consultation with the chief of occupational health, a decision was made to refer Dr Harris to a forensic psychiatrist for a fitness for duty evaluation. At the meeting with the psychiatrist, Dr Harris expressed concern that people thought he was crazy. The psychiatrist offered reassurance that she was not making any such judgment, but pointed out that the hospital was concerned about his ability to perform his job because of his continued assertions that someone was sabotaging his work, given the lack of evidence from multiple investigations. The psychiatrist made clear that it was not her job to determine the accuracy of his complaints, but rather to determine if he was able to perform the essential functions of his job despite his ongoing concerns. She pointed out that being fit for duty included the ability to work safely, to not disrupt the workplace, and to be able to work accurately.

Dr Harris provided a detailed personal and medical history, denying any medical or psychiatric problems in himself or family members. This was consistent with the results of a full medical evaluation conducted 1 month earlier. Dr Harris denied any history of violence or legal difficulties, and related an academic and work history that was without problems and consistent with his personnel records. He described how he had concluded that someone was sabotaging his work, explaining in intricate detail what he claimed was the evidence. Asked why he thought the hospital police had failed to turn up any concrete evidence of wrongdoing, Dr Harris stopped short of directly accusing the police of being part of a conspiracy. Instead, he suggested that they must have just missed something, although he alluded to possibility of the hospital security personnel colluding with his tormentors, citing the stature of the former colleague he had first suspected, and noting that the colleague was friends with the president of the hospital and was well-connected in the scientific community.

The psychiatrist reached the conclusion that Dr Harris was suffering from delusional disorder, persecutory type. Although his paranoid delusion increased his risk of violence, the absence of any history of substance abuse, childhood oppositional defiant disorder, or antisocial behavior as an adult, limited his risk.[16] At the psychiatrist's request, the laboratory director conducted a detailed review of Dr Harris' research patient files, interviewed a random assortment of patients about their experiences, and reviewed his research work. No problems were discovered in any of these.

The psychiatrist wrote a letter to the laboratory director and director of Occupational Health outlining what was done in the course of the evaluation and stating her conclusion that "Based upon the information available to me, it is my opinion at this time that Dr Harris is able perform some, but not all, of the essential functions of his job. Specifically, he does not seem to have difficulties in his interactions with patients, record keeping, data analysis, or other research-related activities. At present, he does not seem to pose a significantly elevated risk of harm to himself or others; however, that analysis may change if he continues to hold these beliefs and experiences increased frustration at a lack of resolution of his concerns. Although Dr Harris seems fit to work in these respects, he does pose an ongoing risk of causing significant distress and distraction to coworkers by continuing to express his beliefs regarding workplace events."

The psychiatrist recommended that (1) Dr Harris be referred to the Employee Assistance Program; (2) be encouraged to pursue a full clinical psychiatric evaluation with a goal of better understanding the source of his concerns; and (3) as a condition of his continued employment, be required to discuss any additional concerns about sabotage with the laboratory director or hospital police. In addition she recommended that the laboratory director have a low threshold for contacting Occupational Health should there be changes in Dr Harris' behavior or appearance.

In an expanded version of the report, sent to the director of Occupational Health, the psychiatrist offered a provisional diagnosis of delusional disorder, paranoid type; the time course and treatment difficulties associated with this condition; and emphasized the importance of monitoring Dr Harris' symptoms through reports from any clinicians from whom he sought treatment and through visit with Occupational Health.

Few employees fulfill the term "problematic" as fully as those who exhibit paranoia. They are often distracted by their persecutory beliefs and unable to be fully productive, and they tend to distract others with their complaints and their behavior, frequently inducing anxiety about the potential for violence. In some cases, the paranoia is sufficiently disabling that the employee cannot perform the essential functions of the job. In others, especially those involving highly educated and skilled workers, the employee may be able to perform the technical aspects of his or her duties despite significant paranoia. The latter situation gives rise to much consternation for many managers, and some clinicians, who have difficulty with the idea that someone with an obvious mental illness can be fit to work.

It is important to remember, in working on such matters, that these are exactly the sort of cases that the ADA was meant to address: an individual with a known or suspected disability who can perform the essential functions of the job should not be prevented from working. The main challenges in situations like this are to have a clear understanding of what the essential functions of the job actually are and determining the extent to which the employee can or cannot fulfill them. As an initial step, the essential functions of the position can be determined by reviewing the written job description. A more complete and accurate understanding requires a discussion with employees and management as to what the position truly entails.

Ultimately, it is up to the employer to define the essential functions of the position, and up to the psychiatric consultant to assess whether the employee can fulfill these functions. In this case, the psychiatrist provided additional input, suggesting that if the employer regarded avoidance of disruptive comments and behavior to be essential functions, then that requirement should be enforced with regard to Dr Harris. So long as such a requirement is applied in an equal manner to all employees, disabled or not, the employer should not run into significant difficulties.

Cases such as this commonly end in the employee violating one or more work rules, and either being dismissed or going out on disability. In this case, however, the laboratory director decided to allow Dr Harris to return to the laboratory on the condition that he not discuss his concerns with anyone else. At 1-year follow-up, Dr Harris had consulted with the Employee Assistance Program about stress management, had begun seeing a psychiatrist, and was still working productively in the laboratory.

SUMMARY

The complexities of individual and group behavior provide a seemingly endless number of opportunities for conflicts and disputes between employees and employers. These cases are a small sample of the array of circumstances in which psychiatrists may be asked to contribute their expertise to resolving some of these problematic situations. The problems themselves, and the psychiatric consultations for each of them, share the common features outlined at the beginning of the article. Each calls on the psychiatrist's diagnostic skills, clinical acumen, professional ethics, and ability to think flexibly and creatively in solving these problems, providing an opportunity for significant personal and professional satisfaction.

REFERENCES

1. Americans with Disabilities Act of 1990, 42 USC §12113(b).
2. Equal Employment Opportunity Commission. EEOC enforcement guidance on the Americans with Disabilities Act and psychiatric disabilities. EEOC NOTICE Number 915.002. Washington (DC): U.S. Equal Employment Opportunity Commission; 1997.
3. Unterberg MP. Personality: personalities, personal style, and trouble. In: Kahn JP, Langlieb AM, editors. Mental health and productivity in the workplace. San Francisco (CA): Jossey-Bass; 2003. p. 458–80.
4. Anfang SA, Wall BA. Psychiatric fitness for duty evaluations. Psychiatr Clin North Am 2006;29:675–93.
5. Pettus v Cole, Cal Rptr 2d, 46 (1996).
6. Schouten R. Pitfalls of clinical practice: the treating clinician as expert witness. Harv Rev Psychiatry 1993;1:64–5.
7. Strasburger LH, Gutheil TG, Brodsky A. On wearing two hats: role conflict in serving as both psychotherapist and expert witness. Am J Psychiatry 1997; 154:448–56.
8. Family and Medical Leave Act of 1993, 29 USC §2601.
9. Federation of State Medical Board. Policy on physician impairment. Euless (Texas): FSMB, Inc; 2011.

10. Rosenstein AH, O'Daniel M. Survey of the impact of disruptive behaviors and communication defects on patient safety. Jt Comm J Qual Patient Saf 2008;34: 464–71.
11. American Medical Association. Code of medical ethics, E-9045 physicians with disruptive behavior. American Medical Association; 2000. Available at: http:// www.ama-assn.org/ama/pub/physician-resources/medical-ethics/code-medical-ethics/opinion9045.page. Accessed August 3, 2012.
12. Pastner B. Disruptive behavior by physicians in hospitals: a threat to patient safety? Health Law Perspectives; 2008. Available at: http://www.law.uh.edu/healthlaw/perspectives/homepage.asp. Accessed August 3, 2012.
13. Schouten R. Workplace violence: an overview for practicing clinicians. Psychiatr Ann 2006;36:790–7.
14. Schouten R. Workplace violence and the clinician. In: Simon RI, Tardiff K, editors. Textbook of violence assessment and management. Washington (DC): American Psychiatric Press; 2008. p. 501–20.
15. Schouten R. Workplace violence evaluations and the ADA. In: Gold LH, Vanderpool D, editors. Clinical guide to mental disability evaluations. New York: Springer; in press.
16. Elbogen EE, Johnson SC. The intricate link between violence and mental disorder. Arch Gen Psychiatry 2009;66(2):152–61.

Testamentary Capacity and Guardianship Assessments

Jason G. Roof, MD

KEYWORDS

- Testmentary capacity • Guardianship • Ward • Capacity assessment
- Geriatric psychiatric assessment • Wills • Insane delusion • Undue influence

KEY POINTS

- Under common law, testamentary capacity requires the person to have the following abilities: (1) know the nature and extent of their property; (2) know the natural objects of their bounty; (3) understand how the will disposes of their property; and (4) demonstrate the ability to make a rational plan as to the disposition of their property.
- Allegations of undue influence are common and often successfully challenge the validity of a will.
- Common illnesses affecting testamentary capacity in older individuals include delirium and dementia.
- A person determined to be a ward of the state may lose many fundamental rights including: consent or refusal of medical care, management of their finances, entry into contracts, ability to marry, and self-determination of living arrangements.
- Evaluators should screen for elder abuse in their evaluations. Physical abuse, emotional abuse, financial abuse, and neglect may be present in the lives of evaluees.

INTRODUCTION

As Americans live for longer periods of time and in greater numbers, there is an ever increasing need for mental health professionals to assist civil courts in answering questions related to issues of adult guardianship and distribution of property after an individual's death. The US Department of Human Services reports that Americans older than 65 years numbered 40.4 million in 2010, an increase of 5.4 million since 2000. Since 1900, the number of Americans aged 65 or older has more than tripled. By this definition, 1 in every 8, or 13% of the population, is an older American.

Funding sources: None.

Conflict of interest: None.

Division of Psychiatry and the Law, Department of Psychiatry and Behavioral Sciences, University of California, Davis Medical Center, 2230 Stockton Boulevard, 2nd Floor, Suite 210, TICON II, Sacramento, CA 95817, USA

E-mail address: jason.roof@ucdmc.ucdavis.edu

Psychiatr Clin N Am 35 (2012) 915–927

http://dx.doi.org/10.1016/j.psc.2012.08.011

psych.theclinics.com

Projections indicate that Americans 65 years or older will reach 72.1 million by 2030 and 88.5 million by 2050.[1]

Better financial security, medical advances, greater awareness of medical conditions, and the pursuit of healthier lifestyles have extended and improved the quality of life for people as they age.[2] Unfortunately, while living longer, many of the elderly also live with disabilities. In 2010, nearly 37% of older persons suffered from some type of disability, such as sensory deficits, problems in ambulation, or impairment in self care or independent living. Furthermore, almost 50% of surveyed individuals older than 80 years reported a severe disability and approximately 30% of those older than 80 reported that they needed some form of assistance. In a 2009 study to evaluate older Americans' ability to perform activities of daily living (ADLs), more than 27% of community-resident Medicare beneficiaries older than 65 had difficulty performing 1 or more ADL while 95% of institutionalized Medicare beneficiaries had difficulties with 1 or more ADLs.[1]

This article reviews important factors to consider when assessing the impact of aging and disability on 2 key areas that many older people will face: testamentary capacity and guardianship assessments.

TESTAMENTARY CAPACITY
Overview

Testamentary capacity is a civil competence and involves an individual's ability to make a will. Legally, a person is presumed to have adequate capacity to create a will and in doing so they recognize (1) the natural objects of their bounty, (2) the nature and extent of their estate, and (3) the fact that they are making a plan to dispose of the estate after their death.[3] The modern right to determine who will take ownership of their property after death originates from the eleventh-century Norman principle of primogeniture, which is the passing of the estate to the first-born son. The Statute of Wills, enacted in England in 1540, allowed landowners to pass their land to others who had survived them.[3] The Statute of Frauds, enacted in 1688, required that various documents, including wills, be committed in writing for the contract to be enforceable.[3] The United States adopted a significant portion of English law related to wills. Many consider the act of making a will a fundamental right, although this specific activity is not described as a protected right in the Constitution.[4]

Making a will is not necessarily complicated. In general, creating a will requires a statement of intent to create the will, a witness, a date, and a signature of the will's author. The will's author is also referred to as the "testator."[4] The termination of a will can be significantly more difficult than its creation, and care must be given to clearly resolve any conflicts that exist between different versions of an individual's will. Revocation, and therefore termination, of a will can occur through physical destruction of the original (and any other copies) or by the valid creation of a later dated will that revokes all prior wills. A will cannot be revoked simply by an oral declaration.[4]

Wills are rarely contested. In fact, studies have shown that approximately 99% of wills are executed as written.[5] Only an individual directly affected by the will may contest that will. If contested, a will may be rejected for a variety of reasons. As previously mentioned, many states require a statement of intent, a valid witness or witnesses, a date, and a signature of the testator. In addition, the author of the will must have reached the age of majority accepted by the state and have the mental capacity to compose the will. Individuals are assumed mentally competent to create a will unless it is proven that they are not competent to do so. As a result, those who contest a will bear the burden of proof that the testator lacked mental competency when the document was created.[5]

A historical and illustrative English case regarding testamentary capacity was heard by Chief Justice Cockburn. In the 1870 case of *Banks v Goodfellow*, Mr John Banks' will was contested after his death and the subsequent death of his niece to whom he had passed his estate. Under normal circumstances, Mr Banks' estate would have passed to his niece's descendants. However, medical opinions were submitted opining that Mr Banks was "insane" and incapable of managing his affairs both before and after the time of the creation of his will.[6] Ultimately, Chief Justice Cockburn found that Mr Banks' will was valid and he set forth the following test for testamentary capacity.

It is essential to the exercise of such a power that a testator shall understand the nature of the act and its effects; shall understand the extent of the property of which he is disposing; shall be able to comprehend and appreciate the claims to which he ought to give effect; and with a view to the latter object, that no disorder of the mind shall poison his affections, pervert his sense of right, or prevent the exercise of his natural faculties — that no insane delusion shall influence his will in disposing of his property and bring about a disposal of it which, if the mind had been sound, would not been made.[7]

In summary, Chief Cockburn stated that a testator must understand the nature of a will itself; the general extent of their assets; be able to appreciate the claims of those who might expect to benefit from the will; understand the impact of the distribution described in the will; and not have a disorder of the mind, including delusions, that influenced the creation of the will. If the validity of a will is challenged, it must be proven by the complainant that the testator lacked at least one of the following elements at the time of the creation of the will outlined in **Box 1**.[4]

One may better understand the unwillingness of courts to invalidate wills, even in individuals with chronic mental illness, by considering the "lucid interval" doctrine. When a witness to the signing of the will can provide testimony that the testator had a lucid interval on the signing of the document, despite chronic mental disability, the will is often considered valid.[4] In such circumstances, the burden to prove a "lucid interval" was present at the time the will was created falls to those who wish to have the will survive as written.

Insane Delusion

Mental health professionals may be called on to assess for the presence of delusions affecting the testator's capacity to create a will. A delusion is often defined as a fixed,

---

Box 1
Components required for testamentary capacity

1. Knowledge of the nature and extent of his property

2. Knowledge of the natural objects of his bounty

3. Knowledge of how the will would dispose of his property

4. The ability to make a rational plan as to the disposition of his property

Data from Frolik LA. The strange interplay of testamentary capacity and the doctrine of undue influence. Are we protecting older testators or overriding individual preferences? Int J Law Psychiatry 2001;24(2–3):253–66.

false belief system, which is inconsistent with an individual's culture and has no basis in fact. In testamentary capacity cases, the evaluator may find it necessary to consider if an insane delusion affected the testator's decision-making capacity. According to one legal definition, an insane delusion is an irrational, persistent belief in an imaginary state of facts resulting in a lack of capacity to undertake acts of legal consequence, such as making a will.[3] In the US Supreme Court Case *Mutual Life Insurance Company v Terry* the court examined an insurer's responsibility to pay on a policy whereby an individual committed suicide, legally voiding the policy. The court reasoned that the proviso was valid unless the insured was insane. The court provided a more detailed definition of insane delusion when they wrote:

> If the death is caused by the voluntary act of the assured, he knowing and intending that his death shall be the result of his act, but when his reasoning faculties are so far impaired that he is not able to understand the moral character, the general nature, consequences, and effect of the act he is about to commit, or when he is impelled thereto by an insane impulse, which he has not the power to resist, such death is not within the contemplation of the parties to the contract, and the insurer is liable.[8]

The following hypothetical case illustrates how an insane delusion may be considered as invalidating a will.

Insane delusion

Mr Jones is known to have a history of bipolar disorder. Despite the urgings of his family and psychiatrist he has again discontinued his psychiatric medications. Years earlier, a will was created with the assistance of attorney, which left his estate to his wife and children. His wife observes the onset of alarming behavior such as sleeplessness, rapid speech, increased anger, and paranoia regarding the government. Mr Jones leaves the family home late one night and is found a week later dead in a hotel room. A note beside his hotel bed is titled "Last Will and Testament" and contains language in his hand writing to invalidate the previous will. This new will is signed and dated by an unknown female witness named Sparkles. Mr Jones writes in the document that he will "not provide a single penny" to the "government terrorists who have been disguising themselves as my wife and child all of these years" and instead instructs that all of his property to be given to Sparkles, a female adult entertainer who he claims to have married the day before his death.

The preceding example demonstrates how an insane delusion may affect the testator's reasoning related to making the will. While knowing the nature and extent of his property, the natural objects of his bounty, and that the will would dispose of his property, Mr Jones likely lacked the ability to make a rational plan because of his active mental illness. Sparkles could, however, testify in court that Mr Jones was having a "lucid moment" when he created the document after their marriage ceremony the night before. She will face significant difficulty in prevailing, as the delusional accusations contained in Mr Jones' document are similar to earlier claims made by Mr Jones when known to be manic. However, having a delusional belief system alone may be insufficient to invalidate a will. The party challenging the will must demonstrate that the delusion directly affected the creation of the will.

Undue Influence

One of the most often attempted, and most successful, challenges to the validity of a will involves allegations of "undue influence."[4] In the 1931 Arkansas case of *Hyatt v Wroten*, the court provided the following definition of undue influence: "…the opportunity of the beneficiary of the influenced's bequest to mold the mind of the testator to suit his or her purposes…"[9] Frolik outlines 4 fundamental elements of undue influenced, highlighted in **Box 2**.

The following hypothetical vignette raises questions regarding the presence of undue influence.

Undue influence

Ms Hall is a widowed woman who recently celebrated her 89th birthday. Ms Hall has one surviving daughter and a substantial estate worth at least 1 billion dollars. Ms Hall's daughter has becoming increasingly concerned about the nature of her mother's relationship with a well-known 26-year-old male model named Mr Flash. While the relationship with her mother has always been stormy, she had some comfort in fact that, as Ms Hall's only child, she was the sole heir of the estate. Alarmed to see her mother's face on a popular entertainment magazine she soon discovers, through her mother's attorney, that Mr Flash is now heir to half of the estate. Ms Hall dies 13 months later with the modified will to be executed. Ms Hall's daughter alleges that Mr Flash had undue influence over her mother and that the will should be invalidated.

Determining whether undue influence was present can be difficult because of the private nature of such relationships. The burden of proof falls on the individual who is challenging the validity of the will. The challenger may request assistance from mental health professionals to assist in the determination of whether various conditions in the testator and/or various characteristics of the alleged influencer may have contributed to a will created with undue influence. Mental health professionals should consider a wide variety of characteristics in the testator, which might increase susceptibility including their mental and physical health, their personality traits/disorders, and their overall intellectual function.

Redmond[10] has suggested some clues to the help evaluate the presence of undue influence:

1. The psychiatrist is assured by the person requesting the examination that a competency statement is routine because of the testator's age.
2. The appointment is made by someone other than the testator or his/her attorney.
3. The testator is brought to the appointment by someone who answers most of the questions for the testator and is reluctant to allow the testator to be interviewed alone.

Box 2
Fundamental elements of undue influence

1. A confidential relationship existed between the testator and the influencer

2. The influencer used that relationship to secure a change in how the testator distributed his estate

3. The change in the estate plan was unconscionable or did not reflect the true desires of the testator

4. The testator was susceptible to being influenced

Data from Frolik LA. The strange interplay of testamentary capacity and the doctrine of undue influence. Are we protecting older testators or overriding individual preferences? Int J Law Psychiatry 2001;24(2–3):253–66.

---

4. Specifics about the will are not given, or the testator seems unclear about specific items in the will.
5. There is reluctance to give information about potential heirs and their relationship with the testator.

CONDUCTING THE FORENSIC EVALUATION

Before conducting a forensic evaluation, the evaluator should clearly understand the questions to be answered by the court, attorney, or client. If there is concern over the content or scope of the questions or areas to be explored, clarification should be made before an evaluation. In addition, the evaluator should make clear to the requesting agency when limitations such as missing medical documents or an uncooperative or deceased testator may limit the accuracy of the provided opinions.

Records relevant to the testator's medical and psychiatric history should be reviewed when available. Additional records that may be of assistance include relevant financial records, accurate estimates of the person's financial worth, academic records, prior neuropsychological or IQ testing, work performance records, nursing home records, lists of current medications and medications taken at/about the time of the creation of the will, and statements and interviews with collateral informants such as family members. In addition, the evaluator should review the specific will in question as well as any other versions of the will. Being familiar with these records before the evaluation may better inform lines of questioning and potential areas to more carefully explore during the evaluation. Evaluators should not conclude a lack of testamentary capacity solely because another capacity (such as the ability to consent to medical treatment) is lacking. In fact, a person could lack the capacity to make medical decisions yet still retain testamentary capacity.

Evaluations may be requested for testators who are living or deceased and may therefore be contemporaneous or retrospective. Contemporaneous evaluations of the testator should ideally occur in environments providing an adequate level of privacy and a lack of distraction for both the interviewer and interviewee. Jurisdictions vary in their requirements to have attorneys present during court-ordered evaluations.[11] The evaluator should instruct the attorney that they should adopt a passive role during the interview, and deviations from such a role may result in an inaccurate or incomplete opinion regarding the questions posed. One-way mirrors may facilitate this arrangement. Another approach may be to have the interview recorded, though all parties should be aware of such an arrangement well in advance of the interview. Should the testator, or their attorney, wish to have the interview independently recorded, this should be agreed upon well before the evaluation.

Consider the following questions in your evaluation to determine the testator's understanding of their will and to rule out the presence of undue influence:

1. What is your current financial worth?
2. Describe your financial assets? (Property, valuable possessions, and so forth.)
3. What types of banking accounts do you hold and how much does each account contain? (Checking, savings, and so forth.)
4. What are your monthly expenses?
5. What is your monthly income?
6. Who are your relatives?
7. What is your relationship like with each of your relatives?
8. Have any of your relatives treated you unfairly? If yes, describe.
9. What is your understanding of a will?
10. Have you ever made a will before?

11. Have you made any changes in your will(s) over time? If yes, why?
12. Explain why you left the amounts you did to your various relatives.
13. Have you excluded relatives, or bequeathed to them lower amounts than might have been expected? If yes, why?
14. Do you intend to leave anything to individuals outside of your family? If yes, explain the history of your relationship with them and why you have made them a beneficiary.
15. Does anyone disagree with the content of your will? Do you anticipate anyone contesting your will? If yes, explain.

In addition, evaluators may consider presenting various hypothetical scenarios and having the evaluee complete tasks relevant to testamentary capacity. Examples include:

1. Have the evaluee describe how they would handle a philanthropic request for an amount greater than their current financial worth.
2. Have the evaluee describe how they might distribute 1 million dollars knowing that they could keep none of it themselves. Have them explain why they provided various amounts to various individuals.
3. Provide the evaluee a hypothetical example of undue influence to determine their response. An example might include creating a narrative involving an attorney who helps the testator create a will but suggests that a majority of the money be awarded to them because of "their friendship."

Common Cognitive Concerns

Common illnesses affecting testamentary capacity in older individuals may include delirium and dementia. The evaluator should carefully consider the presence of non-pathologic changes in memory related to normal gaining. Such changes are referred to as "benign senescence," "age-associated memory decline," or can be included in the term Age-Related Cognitive Decline in the *Diagnostic and Statistical Manual of Mental Disorders* (fourth edition, text revision) (DSM-IV-TR). Recently the Aging, Demographics, and Memory Study (ADAMS) found that 22.2% of Americans older than 71 years had cognitive impairment without dementia.[12] The Baltimore Longitudinal Study of Aging, the longest-running scientific study of human aging, indicates several significant findings in age-related alterations in cognition. Late-life cognitive changes may include a decreased ability to solve problems and to learn rapidly. In addition, visuospatial abilities, fluency of language, and general intelligence may also decline in late life. Typically there is a shortened attention span, slower incorporation of new ideas, increased sleep fragmentation and a decrease in brain weight. Moreover, frontal-lobe functioning may be increasingly impaired during aging.[13]

Dementia

Cognitive impairment without dementia is quite common, and 10% to 15% of those with cognitive impairment without dementia progress to dementia annually.[12] Dementia is characterized by cognitive defects caused by medical conditions, substances, or a combination of several conditions. The DSM-IV-TR lists several presumed causes that include: Alzheimer type, Dementia Due to Other General Medical Conditions, Substance-Induced Persisting Dementia, Multiple Etiologies, or Not Otherwise Specified if the etiology is indeterminate.[14] Several medical conditions, including heart disease, renal disease, congestive heart failure, thyroid dysfunction, and vitamin deficiencies, may present as manageable sources of dementia-type symptoms.

Medications or medical problems may induce what appears to be dementia or delirium. Scenarios whereby medications may cause such an effect include when a geriatric patient's dosage of medication is too high, the geriatric patient does not appropriately follow dosing directions, or the patient has an increased sensitivity to or impaired metabolism for a certain medication and/or drug-drug interactions. In an effort to educate medical providers about potentially inappropriate medications (PIMs) for older adults, Beers and colleagues initially published a list of PIMs in 1991 with revisions in 1991, 1997, 2003, and most recently in 2012. The most recent Beers Criteria update includes 53 medications, or medication classes, which qualify as PIMs for older adults.[15] The most common offending drug classes resulting in alteration of cognition are anticholinergics, antihypertensives, psychotropics, sedative-hypnotics, and narcotic analgesics.[16]

Alzheimer disease is the most frequent cause of dementia. It is estimated that 60% to 70% of dementia cases are of the Alzheimer type.[17] Studies have shown that Alzheimer disease has a cumulative incidence as high as 4.7% by age 70, 18.2% by age 80, and 49.6% by age 90 years.[18] The Alzheimer's Association estimates that 4.5 million Americans have Alzheimer disease.[17]

Testators in the early stages of Alzheimer may demonstrate a subtle loss of short-term memory. Anecdotes of becoming easily lost in their neighborhoods may be presented by collateral or the testator themselves. In addition, they may demonstrate problems with word finding and the naming of standard objects. Individuals in the early stages of Alzheimer disease may demonstrate apraxia (an inability to perform complex movements), or may have difficulty dressing or eating. During the late stages of Alzheimer disease, judgment often becomes impaired and personality changes may become apparent. Such personality changes may demonstrate increased apathy, hostility, or withdrawal toward peers or members of custody.[18] Alzheimer patients they may experience depression, anxiety, delusions, or hallucinations. If a will was created during the course of a dementing process, the evaluator should carefully explore the extent and content of cognitive impairment, psychiatric symptoms, and the impact of any delusions on the creation of a will.

Delirium

Abnormal changes in memory, judgment, and cognition may occur in both dementia and delirium; however, one of the best methods to differentiate the two is the presence or absence of a clouding of consciousness that fluctuates over the course of a short time (such as in a single day). This fluctuation is characteristic of delirium. In addition, an acute or subacute onset of symptoms more often indicates delirium as opposed to dementia.[19] Whereas delirium in a nonhospitalized older population is rare, in an inpatient hospital setting this population may have a prevalence of delirium as high as 80%.[20] The presence, severity, or timing of delirium may be of significant consequence during the contest of a will.[21]

Depression that resembles dementia has been termed pseudodementia or depression-related cognitive dysfunction.[19] Features indicating pseudodementia include the following: better premorbid functioning; a rapid onset of symptoms; a patient's detailed complaints of cognitive dysfunction; poor motivation to perform even simple tasks; negativistic answers to questions; and a personal or familial history of depression.[19]

Forensic Evaluation of Cognitive Status

A general psychiatric evaluation should be performed on the testator. In addition, the evaluator should consider the use of screening tools to detect the presence of cognitive disorders in the testator. Tools to detect cognitive dysfunction include the

Mini-Mental State Examination (MMSI), Cognitive Abilities Screening Instrument (CASI), and the Mini-Cog.

Mini-Cog

The Mini-Cog is a composite of a 3-item recall and a clock drawing to help determine the presence of a demented person. It has shown some advantage in comparison with other tools, in that it can be rapidly administered and can be used in individuals with a variety of educational levels and languages. To administer the Mini-Cog, the interviewer determines that they have the interviewee's attention and then asks the evaluee to repeat back 3 unrelated words. These words may be repeated up to 3 times if the interviewee has difficulty in repeating them back. The evaluee is told to remember these 3 words and informed that he or she will be asked to repeat them again later. Next, the evaluee is given a test of cognitive function, which also serves to temporarily distract them so that their memory can be later tested. The cognitive task involves having the person draw the face of a clock with specific times (such as 11:10 or 8:20). On completion of the clock task the interviewee is asked to repeat the previous 3 words. The Mini-Cog determines that the person to be "Demented" if no items are recalled or if the clock-drawing test is abnormal with 1 or 2 items recalled. An individual is "Nondemented" if he or she recalls all 3 items or if 1 to 2 items have been recalled with a normal clock test.[22]

Montreal Cognitive Assessment

The Montreal Cognitive Assessment (MoCA) is another cognitive screening test designed to assist health professionals detect mild cognitive impairment. The administration of the test takes approximately 10 minutes and evaluates different cognitive domains: attention and concentration; executive functions; memory, language; visuoconstructional skills; conceptual thinking; calculations; and orientation. The MoCA is offered free of charge and can be obtained at www.mocatest.org in a variety of languages.

Retrospective Evaluations

If the testator is deceased, the mental health evaluator must look toward collateral information and documentation to form an opinion regarding the testator's testamentary capacity. As previously stated, requests should be made for relevant records including copies of all wills, financial records, academic records, prior neuropsychological or IQ testing, work performance records, medical records, nursing home records, medical records, and lists of current medications and medications taken at/about the time of the creation of the will. In addition, relevant legal documents should be requested such as the petitioner's complaint, answer to the complaint, interrogatories, and relevant depositions. The evaluator should also request personal writings/correspondence with others for review when available. In addition, interviews with relevant collateral sources such as family members, close friends, and nursing home employees may be beneficial.

In looking for the possible presence of undue influence, the evaluator may find it helpful to create a timeline of the testator and to determine when changes in various versions of the will occurred. Liptzin and colleagues[21] suggest several questions to be asked in cases where persons change their will toward the end of their life. These questions are summarized in **Box 3**.

GUARDIANSHIP

Some individuals lack the ability to make important decisions about their medical care and/or other aspects of their personal lives owing to cognitive or mental impairment. In

---

Box 3
Areas to explore in late-life changes of a will

1. Was there consistency in the patient's wishes over time?

2. Were these wishes expressed during a "lucid interval" when the person was less confused?

3. Were the patient's wishes clearly expressed in response to open-ended questions?

4. Is there clear documentation of the patient's mental status at the time of the discussion?

Data from Liptzin B, Peisah C, Shulman K, et al. Testamentary capacity and delirium. Int Psychogeriatr 2010;22(6):950–6.

---

such situations the court may classify the individual as a "ward" of the court and appoint a "guardian" (or conservator) to make important life decisions for the ward. While establishing a guardian serves to protect the ward, careful consideration regarding its implementation should be made because of the potential reduction of the individual's rights. In particular, a person determined to be a ward of the state may lose many fundamental rights, including the following[23]:

- Consent or refusal of medical care
- Management of their finances
- Entry into contracts
- Ability to marry
- Self-determination of living arrangements

Mental health professionals may be asked to assist in a court's decision of whether guardianship should be initiated on an individual. Before performing an evaluation, the evaluator should be aware of the specific format and scope of the requested evaluation. A recent national review of guardianship laws found that 30 states require clinical evaluation before guardianship hearings, 15 states allow the individual court to decide, and 5 states have no specific rules. Less than half of the states include specific information to be considered/obtained by the evaluator in the opinion regarding possible guardianship.[24]

A recent review of 298 cases of adult guardianship in 3 states revealed concerning patterns of report writing by evaluators. Many reports were illegible, lacked a discussion of specific functional deficits, and made only general conclusions about decision-making abilities. This study indicated that more effective evaluations were correlated with those states that had more progressive reforms regarding guardianship.[25] Several progressive states have updated their guardianship statutes to be in line with the Uniform Guardianship and Protective Proceedings Act (UGPPA).[26] The UGPPA emphasizes due process, fair proceedings, and a limitation in the power of guardians and conservators. The Act states that powers of guardianships and conservatorships should be limited to specific deficiencies in the ward and should be the least restrictive possible.[26] Moye and colleagues[27] suggest a conceptual model of capacity evaluation in adult guardianship that addresses the following 6 areas:

1. What medical conditions are present that produce functional disability? What are the prognoses of the various medical conditions?

2. What is their cognitive functioning? (To include exploration of sensory acuity, motor skills, attention, working memory, short-term memory, long-term memory, understanding, communication, arithmetic, verbal reasoning, visual-spatial reasoning, and executive functioning.)

3. What is their ability to function daily? This should include a consideration of their capacity for self care and to care for their finances. Additional consideration should be given regarding their ability to make decisions regarding medical and legal decisions. Their functionality in home and community life should also be explored.
4. What are their individual values, preferences and patterns? The evaluator should consider the individual's desire to have a guardian, whether they prefer decisions be made alone or with others, where they would prefer to live, what are their goals, what general concerns are primary in their life, and what important religious or cultural beliefs should be taken into consideration that may affect decisions.
5. What is their risk of harm and what level of supervision is needed?
6. What, if any, methods can be used to enhance capacity?[27]

In addition, the evaluator should consider individuals' ADLs as well as their instrumental activities of daily living (IADLs). ADLs include routine behaviors frequently performed to facilitate self care such as bathing, eating, dressing, and moving throughout the living environment. IADLs are behaviors requiring the manipulation of various implements such as the management of money, taking medications, making phone calls or using a computer, maintenance of living environment, and shopping. Increasing limitation of both ADLs and IADLs is correlated with advancing age.[1]

When evaluating ADLs the investigator should investigate areas such as the ability to toilet, feed oneself, dress oneself, groom oneself, physically move throughout their living environment and the city, and to what extent they can bathe themselves. When exploring IADLs the evaluation should consider testators' ability to use a telephone, shop, prepare food, maintain their house, do laundry, use transportation, take their medications and handle their finances, and to what extent they require assistance from others.

Mental health professionals may be asked to perform subsequent evaluations on individuals who are already on guardianship status, as many states allow for subsequent hearings to determine whether competence to perform various functions has been restored. In such circumstances, the evaluator should review how the person's ADLs and IADLs have evolved since the establishment or previous renewal of the guardianship.

Finally, the evaluator should also screen for any potential abuse of the elderly evaluee. The National Center on Elder Abuse reports that 1 in 10 elders may experience some type of abuse, but only 1 in 5 cases of abuse are actually reported.[28] Evaluators should be aware of the laws in their state regarding the reporting of elder abuse and consider the inclusion of basic questions to assess for the presence of abuse. Such questions should include exploration of the following areas:

1. Physical abuse (eg, "Have you been struck, slapped or kicked?")
2. Emotional abuse (eg, "Have you been threatened with punishment, deprivation or institutionalization?")
3. Neglect (eg, "Have you been left alone for long periods?")
4. Financial abuse (eg, "Does your caregiver depend on you for shelter or financial support?")

SUMMARY

Mental health professionals play a fundamental role in assisting courts in areas of contested wills and the need for guardianship. The need for such evaluations will inevitably increase as our population grows in numbers and age. Mental health professionals involved in such matters must clearly understand the scope of the requested evaluation, prepare adequately for the evaluation, perform a thorough interview, consider relevant documentation and collateral sources, and prepare a clear, concise report addressing the requested areas.

REFERENCES

1. Administration on Aging, U.S. Department of Health and Human Services, 2011. A profile of older Americans: 2011. Available at: http://www.aoa.gov/aoaroot/aging_statistics/Profile/2011/docs/2011profile.pdf. Accessed May 05, 2012.
2. ARPP: Beyond 50: A report to the nation on trends in health security. Washington, DC, 2002. Available at: http://assets.aarp.org/rgcenter/econ/beyond_50_econ.pdf. Accessed May 05, 2012.
3. Black HC, Nolan JR. Black's law dictionary. 8th edition. St Paul (MN): West Publ; 2004.
4. Frolik LA. The strange interplay of testamentary capacity and the doctrine of undue influence. Are we protecting older testators or overriding individual preferences? Int J Law Psychiatry 2001;24(2–3):253–66.
5. Bove A. The complete book of wills, estates & trusts. 3rd edition. New York: Holt Paperbacks; 2005.
6. Rule S. Banks v Goodfellow: Delusions and testamentary freedom [Web log message]. 2011. Available at: http://rulelaw.blogspot.com/2011/08/banks-v-goodfellow-delusions-and.html. Accessed June 29, 2012.
7. Banks v Goodfellow, LR 5 QB 549 565 (1870).
8. Mutual Life Ins. Co. v Terry, 15 Wall. 580, 21 L. Ed. 236 (1873).
9. Hyatt v Wroten, 43 SW 2d 726 (Ark 1931).
10. Redmond FC. Testamentary capacity. Bull Am Acad Psychiatry Law 1987;15(3): 247–56.
11. Smith M. Quiet eyes: the need for defense counsel's presence at court-ordered psychiatric evaluations. Cap Def J 2004;16:421.
12. Plassman BL, Langa KM, Fisher GG, et al. Prevalence of cognitive impairment without dementia in the United States. Ann Intern Med 2008;148:427–34.
13. Ratcliff G, Saxton J. Age-associated memory impairment. In: Cummings JL, Coffey CE, editors. Textbook of geriatric neuropsychiatry. Washington, DC: American Psychiatric Press, Inc; 2000. p. 165–79.
14. American Psychiatric Association. Diagnostic and statistical manual of mental disorders, 4th edition, text revision. Washington, DC: American Psychiatric Association; 2000.
15. American Geriatrics Society 2012 Beers Criteria Update Expert Panel. American Geriatrics Society updated Beers criteria for potentially inappropriate medication use in older adults. J Am Geriatr Soc 2012;60(4):616–31.
16. Chutka DS, Takahashi PY, Hoel RW. Inappropriate medications for elderly patients. Mayo Clin Proc 2004;79:122–39.
17. Alzheimer's Association. Basics of Alzheimer's disease: What it is and what you can do. Edited by Alzheimer's Association. 2005. Available at: http://www.alz.org/national/documents/brochure_basicsofalz_low.pdf. Accessed March 6, 2012.
18. Santacruz KS, Swagerty D. Early diagnosis of dementia. Am Fam Physician 2001; 63:703–17.
19. Sadock BJ, Sadock VA. Delirium, dementia, and amnestic and other cognitive disorders and mental disorders due to a general medical condition. In: Cancro R, et al, editors. Kaplan and Sadock's synopsis of psychiatry. 9th edition. Philadelphia: Lippincott Williams & Wilkins; 2003. p. 319–70.

20. Liptzin B, Jacobson S. Delirium. In: Sadock BJ, Sadock VA, Ruiz P, editors. Comprehensive textbook of psychiatry. 9th edition. Philadelphia: Lippincott Williams & Wilkins; 2003. p. 4066–73.
21. Liptzin B, Peisah C, Shulman K, et al. Testamentary capacity and delirium. Int Psychogeriatr 2010;22(6):950–6.
22. Borson S, Scanlan J, Brush M, et al. The mini-cog: a cognitive 'vital signs' measure for dementia screening in multi-lingual elderly. Int J Geriatr Psychiatry 2000;15(11):1021–7.
23. Soliman S. Evaluating older adults' capacity and need for guardianship. 2012. Available at: http://www.currentpsychiatry.com/article_pages.asp?aid=10362. Accessed March 6, 2012.
24. Mayhew M. Survey of state guardianship laws: statutory provisions for clinical evaluations. Bifocal 2005;26:1–19.
25. Moye J, Wood S, Edelstein B, et al. Clinical evidence in guardianship of older adults is inadequate: findings from a tri-state study. Gerontologist 2007;47(5): 604–12.
26. Uniform Law Commission. Guardianship and Protective Proceedings Act Summary, 2012. Available at: http://uniformlaws.org/ActSummary.aspx?title=Guardianship and Protective Proceedings Act. Accessed July 18, 2012.
27. Moye J, Butz SW, Marson DC, et al. A conceptual model and assessment template for capacity evaluation in adult guardianship. Gerontologist 2007; 47(5):591–603.
28. National Center on Elder Abuse. Why should I care about elder abuse? 2010. Available at: https://www.google.com/url?q=http://www.ncea.aoa.gov/Main_Site/pdf/publication/NCEA_WhatIsAbuse-2010. Accessed June 30, 2010.

Forensic Mental Health Professionals in the Immigration Process

Maya Prabhu, MD, LLB*, Madelon Baranoski, PhD

KEYWORDS

- Forensic psychiatry • Refugees • Asylum-seekers • Immigration
- Cross-cultural psychiatry • Stress disorders • Posttraumatic stress disorder • Iraq

KEY POINTS

- Although the need for mental health expertise in immigration cases is clear and the number of diversity of refugees and asylum-seekers is increasing, the development of skills has lagged behind.
- At the crux of the asylum-seeker's or refugee's case is the need to show that the individual has been persecuted or has a well-founded fear that persecution will be inflicted on the basis of race, religion, nationality, political opinion, or membership in a particular social group if forced to return to the home country.
- Asylum and refugee cases often require analyses beyond a standard evaluation and case formulation. A person's response to trauma and stress can be described only through the detailed, integrated account of a human life from a psychiatric perspective.
- Cultural factors influence how asylum applicants and refugees define and respond to trauma, present symptoms of mental illness, respond to mental health treatment, and participate in the legal process.
- In asylum and refugee cases psychiatrists provide critical consultation to attorneys, asylum officers and the courts, and to other clinicians clarifying the effect of trauma on asylum-seekers' function in general and their ability to participate in the legal process.
- Community resource and referral networks, legal, clinical, and culture consultation and supervision are essential to sustain psychiatric services for the forensic assessment and clinical treatment of asylum-seekers and refugees.

Conflicts: None.

Previous presentation: Earlier versions of the contents of this article were presented at the 2011 American Academy of Psychiatry and Law Meeting, Boston, MA, October 29, 2011.

Department of Psychiatry, Yale University School of Medicine, 300 George Street, New Haven, CT 06519, USA

* Corresponding author. Law and Psychiatry Division, CMHC 34 Park Street, New Haven, CT 06519.

E-mail address: maya.prabhu@yale.edu

psych.theclinics.com

INTRODUCTION

The role for mental health professionals and in particular forensic psychiatrists in immigration cases has been growing in scope and complexity. According to the United Nations High Commissioner for Refugees (UNHCR), 2011 was a record year for forced displacement across borders[1]: there are currently 15 million refugees in the world and it is predicted that this number will only increase[2] as individuals are compelled to flee their home countries because of armed conflicts, famine, climate changes, and other complex humanitarian emergencies. The United States has had a long history of admitting individuals of special humanitarian concern, and for the past 6 years has been the largest resettler of refugees in the world.[3] As a result of this influx, the role of psychiatry, mental health, and medical services has expanded in the immigration and resettlement process.

Beyond providing services for displaced persons who come out of traumatic circumstances, there is a growing demand for mental health and forensic psychiatric input into the legal process itself. Legal questions, cross-cultural encounters, and stress reactions to past trauma and the resettlement process present unusual challenges and unique opportunities for mental health evaluators. For refugees and asylum-seekers, acceptance hinges on the testimony of the applicant. However, frequently, the very circumstances that led applicants to flee their home countries may cause mental health issues that may impair their ability to present their legal case credibly or to work with their legal counsel. Psychiatric professionals are in a position to assist attorneys, clients, and adjudicators in a variety of ways.

This article adds to the existing literature[4,5] on the role of mental health professionals in assisting attorneys in the asylum and refugee determination process in the United States. Briefly described are the legal context for asylum and refugee processing, challenges in conducting evaluations, diagnostic considerations, and specific competencies needed for mental health evaluators. The authors draw on the lessons learned from the Law and Psychiatry Division at Yale University, where a 12-year partnership between the Division and Yale Law School has evolved into a program of expertise in preparing forensic psychiatric evaluations in asylum proceedings with a new expansion into refugee law. Although the need for mental health expertise in these immigration cases is clear and the number and diversity of refugees and asylum-seekers is increasing, the development of skills has lagged behind. Various cases are used throughout the article to illustrate key points. These cases purposely do not include any identifying information of any specific client, yet they are representative of the range and scope of issues that arise in this context.

BACKGROUND
US Legal Framework

Mental health professionals and forensic psychiatrists who are involved in immigration cases will find it helpful to have an appreciation of the relevant law and standards. Although the acceptance of refugees and asylum seekers is sometimes portrayed as a purely discretionary impulse, immigration in this circumstance is a complex, multiparty and multistep process bounded by international and domestic legal regimes. Of the millions of refugees of concern to UNHCR around the world, only about 1% is submitted by the agency for resettlement, depending on the country of origin. However, resettlement is not a right and there is no obligation on "destination" countries to accept refugees. Moreover, even if a case is submitted to a potential resettlement state by UNHCR, whether an individual refugee is ultimately resettled depends on the admission criteria of the recipient country.

The cornerstone of the current US legal framework is the Refugee Act of 1980,[6] which amended the Immigration and Nationality Act of 1954.[7] Before the Refugee Act, refugees were defined and admitted on an ad hoc basis with references to their national origin.[8] For example, the earliest US refugee legislation, the Displaced Persons Act of 1948, made way for Europeans fleeing postwar Europe; later laws created provisions for persons escaping Communist regimes in Hungary, Yugoslavia, Poland, China, and Cuba. It was the experience of resettling Indochinese refugees in 1975 that led to the standardization of the process for all refugees admitted to the United States. The Refugee Act incorporated the international definition of refugees and asylees found in the 1951 international treaty, the Convention Relating to the Status of Refugees, to which the United States is a signatory.[9] The Convention also obligates the signatories to respect the principle of "non-refoulement," that a nation-state cannot forcibly return a person to a country where his or her life or freedom would be at risk for reasons of race, religion, nationality, membership of a particular social group, or political opinion.

Although they are sometimes used interchangeably, under US law the terms "asylum-seeker" and "refugee" are not synonymous: asylum seekers are those who claim to be refugees but whose claims have not yet been definitively evaluated and they are already in or are seeking admission at a port of entry to the United States. Refugees are outside the United States seeking to enter. US law defines refugees parallel to the definition provided by the United Nations Convention but makes several important additions. Being a refugee does not in itself automatically guarantee admission to the United States. To qualify under the US resettlement program, a refugee must also (1) be of a designated nationality and fall within the priority categories for that nationality in that region; or, (2) be referred by a US embassy, UNHCR, or a nongovernmental organization; and not be excludable or inadmissible on concerns (eg, health, security, or moral/criminal) listed in the Immigration and Naturalization Act.[7] As a practical consideration, refugees must also be able to access a US refugee processing post or US Department of Homeland Security/US Citizenship and Immigration Services (DHS/USCIS) officer and not be firmly resettled in any foreign country. Each year, a "refugee admissions ceiling" is set by the President in consultation with Congress, which establishes the number and groups of refugees eligible for admission. Multiple agencies then handle different aspects of the investigation, adjudication, and review of refugee and asylum claims including the Department of Homeland Security, the Justice Department's Executive Office for Immigration Review, and the State Department.

The Legal Burden on Applicants

Applicants have the burden of showing that they meet all of the required conditions to warrant the granting of asylum. At the crux of the asylum-seeker's or refugee's case is the need to show that the individual has been persecuted or has a well-founded fear that persecution will be inflicted if forced to return to the home country. Furthermore, there has to be a nexus between the persecutory act and the applicant's race, religion, nationality, political opinion, or membership in a particular social group. This means, essentially, that the person must be targeted, rather than simply being a victim of generalized violence. In the absence of clear evidence of past persecution, credible fear of future persecution must be established on subjective and objective grounds. Subjective grounds merely mean that the applicant is actually afraid of returning to the home country. Objective grounds are based on the situation of "similarly situated" individuals (ie, country conditions evidence indicates that many individuals in the same group as the applicant are also being persecuted). Many asylum-seekers and refugees face significant difficulties in meeting this bar. Rarely do refugees have adequate documentation of or witnesses to their experiences, nor do they have ready access to those materials. Their own oral testimony is usually the significant "proof" on which they make their case. This reliance on their self-report is challenging for applicants who have multiple interviews, sometimes ranging up to several hours in length. During these interviews, applicants may be asked to recall events, dates, and circumstances in painstaking detail, under what many applicants have reported to include aggressive questioning. The decision-maker must determine whether this testimony is sufficiently detailed and believable to justify a grant of asylum or refugee resettlement. Even if an applicant's story clearly meets all of the legal requirements of the refugee definition, if their credibility is called into question on even a minute issue, they may be rejected.

The stakes are very high for the asylum seeker and the United States as a potential receiving country. From the applicant's perspective, not only may their very life and safety depend on being able to make a credible case, under the Illegal Immigration Reform and Immigrant Responsibility Act of 1996 there are significant penalties for immigration violations. These penalties include expedited removal from the United States and a lifetime exclusion from admission to the United States. For their part, receiving countries wish to balance the identification and admission of bona fide asylum-seekers with the need to limit fraud and security concerns.

Representation by Counsel

In recent years, the complexity of the asylum and refugee application has focused attention on the applicants' access to counsel to assist in this process.[10] Asylum-seekers to the United States do not have a right to counsel but may be represented by attorneys at their own cost. Refugees situated abroad currently do not have this prerogative. Several recent studies have indicated that asylum-seekers were three times as likely to obtain asylum if they had legal representation.[11,12] Moreover, researchers have identified wide variations in asylum outcomes that were dependent on the immigration judge.[13,14] Disparities were also evident when immigration court decisions were analyzed by the asylum seeker's country of origin. The denial rates of Iraqi asylum-seekers were the lowest, spanning from 0% to 4%, and their variation was also the lowest at 4%. In contrast, the denial rates of Salvadoran asylum-seekers were the highest, spanning 90% to 98%, with only an 8% variation.[13]

Although there are limited systemic data indicating the impact of medical and psychiatric evaluations in asylum cases, the available literature suggests that these evaluations may be critical in adjudications, especially where maltreatment is alleged.[15] The physical consequences and psychological distress caused by displacement are well reported in the sociocultural and psychiatric literature.[16] According to the UNHCR Resettlement Handbook, posttraumatic stress disorder (PTSD) among refugee groups occurs at rates ranging from 39% to 100%, compared with 1% in the general population.[17] Adjudicative bodies also acknowledge that mental health issues may impair the testimony and credibility of applicants. The US Departmental of Homeland Security provides materials on PTSD and cross-cultural interviews in its training of adjudicators.[18,19] The Australian and Canadian refugee boards have also recognized that psychological trauma may have an adverse impact on refugees' abilities to participate in their own hearings and should be taken into account when evaluating behavior and credibility.[20,21] Thus, medical experts may play an important role in identifying and assisting traumatized refugees and helping adjudicators. The International Association of Refugee Law Judges recommends that medical experts should advise on the likely impact that a return to the country of origin could have on the claimant's mental health, the availability of medical and psychiatric services in the country of origin, and suggested prescribed treatment.[22] Evidence from domestic surveys indicates that the weight given to mental health expert reports rests on the appropriateness and scope of the testimony provided with descriptive clinical information, clear clinical diagnoses, data on diagnostic reliability, and interpretations of the legal standard being the most probative.[23] However, as with domestic criminal cases, immigration adjudicators may reject opinions as to credibility as being beyond the scope of the mental health evaluator.

THE YALE LAW AND PSYCHIATRY MODEL

Although empirical evidence of the impact of psychiatric assessments in immigration cases may be lacking, the experience of those involved in such consultations from the legal and psychiatric side has pointed to a productive if challenging collaboration. During the past 12 years, faculty and forensic psychiatry fellows from the Yale Law and Psychiatry Program have worked with the Jerome Frank Law Center's Immigration Clinic at Yale Law School. In 2010, this work expanded to include the Iraq Refugee Assistance Project, a student organization founded by two Yale Law School students in 2008 to assist Iraqi refugees. The engagement begins with attendance at the didactic courses in which immigration law is presented and clients are discussed. The forensic fellows and faculty then become part of the "firm" and understand and accept the responsibility for the confidentiality of information and records of the clients. As the legal teams develop the cases, law students seek guidance around interviewing techniques, management of clients' distress, and referrals for mental health assessment. The forensic psychiatry fellows also provide an audience for mock presentations and raise questions that point out strengths and weaknesses of the cases. Several of these cases can be referred for more intense assessments that may lead to a report or testimony.

ROLES FOR THE FORENSIC PSYCHIATRIST

The Yale experience has identified three different functions for the mental health professional in immigration cases: (1) consultation and education, (2) evaluation and case formulation, and (3) communication of an integrated narrative. These functions occur in different ways and stages of the case and usually overlap depending on the legal and psychiatric complexity of the case and the experience of the attorney and the court.

Consultation and Education

The psychiatrist's role as consultant and educator begins with the referring attorney and extends to the court and client. Attorneys often seek consultation from the psychiatrist early in the course of the legal case. An initial referral from the attorney may begin with the attorney presenting general concerns along with a request to assist in managing potential barriers. Consider the following example of Ms. Y, a 27-year-old woman who has left her abusive husband and four children in Ecuador. The attorney asks for a consultation: "Ms. Y changes her story. She adds detail or mixes up the sequence. She cries in every session and we can't get her to focus in time for preparing the affidavit. She often sounds angry and she misses appointments."

There are several questions embedded in this brief statement that a forensic psychiatrist can help clarify because of their unique position as a physician and expert. Important questions that are common to such referrals include the following:

- What are the effects of trauma on this individual?
- What cultural influences may play a role in this case?

- What is malingering and is there evidence of malingering psychiatric symptoms in this case?
- What are likely benefits of mental health care for this person?
- What are appropriate referrals for medical services that may assist this person?

In the case of this young Ecuadorian woman, the psychiatrist sat in on her evaluation and recognized symptoms of depression combined with self-condemnation related to her religious and cultural beliefs. Familiar with the woman's culture, the psychiatrist identified the woman's risk for suicide and referred her to treatment and other services.

Because persecution is at the heart of the legal definition of asylum and refugee, clients with traumatic histories are common. Even beyond their history of persecution, individuals are frequently in the midst of personal turmoil and loss, in a strange land cut off from a support system. In many ways they are in the midst of continued trauma, particularly if they have left their children or family behind. Moreover, an orderly and rapid discussion of the legally relevant historical details is needed to build a coherent case. However, the attorney's singular focus on the collection of information and detail with dates, places, names, and sequences can overwhelm clients, shutting down communication and jumbling the story. It is not unusual for the early impression in these cases to be that the client is fabricating a story because of difficulty giving an organized account. The following case example illustrates how psychiatric expertise can help clarify a client's presentation that may be mistakenly assumed to be false.

Psychiatric Expertise to Clarify a Client's Presentation

Faculty and fellows were consulted on a case that had been denied at the asylum office level on grounds of "malingering" and was being prepared for immigration court. The client was a woman from Zimbabwe. The asylum officer had judged the woman's claim of repeated rapes by members of an opposing tribe in the conflict in Zimbabwe to be false "because she was malingering since she was not showing the amount of upset that she should with that history."

In this case, the psychiatric evaluation concluded that the woman met criteria for PTSD. To help explain her limited emotionality during her interview, the psychiatric report and testimony presented research findings about the numbing effects of trauma. In addition, the psychiatrist explained how malingering presentations differed from this particular woman's history.

As illustrated, the forensic psychiatrist can educate the attorney about the effect of trauma on their client and develop goals for each interview. Attorneys may observe an interview and in certain circumstances even participate. Clarification and information that assist the immigration court and asylum officers are accomplished formally through the written report and testimony. Definitions, illustrative examples, and research citations demonstrate expertise and direct testimony can provide a foundation for understanding a case.

Evaluation and Case Formulation

The psychiatrist's diagnostic assessment plays a substantial role in formulating answers to legal questions specific to immigration cases. Immigration attorneys refer clients for psychiatric evaluations for different reasons. However, psychiatric evaluations, reports, and testimony are crucial even in factually strong cases when the PTSD symptoms, cognitive, memory, or other deficits interfere with the clients' ability to produce cogent accounts and credible account of their experiences. In these cases, the psychiatric report frames the difficulty as a symptom (when that is the case) and presents an alternative explanation to the idea that such problems indicate malingering. As an example, consider the following case:

Psychiatric Evaluation and Case Formulation

Mr Ole is a 34-year-old Chinese man who left China after persecution for his participation in an underground Christian church. While in China he sustained beatings from the police that resulted in head trauma. When interviewed, he is easily confused about dates and details, particularly when stressed. He has no personal documentation of his abuse in China. An attorney representing Mr Ole asks the following questions:

- Does Mr Ole display evidence of PTSD?
- If he has PTSD, could PTSD have been caused by the trauma he has reported experiencing in China?
- If he has PTSD, can you describe how PTSD symptoms are likely to manifest if and when he testifies?
- Are such symptoms likely to interfere with his testimony and if so how?

Mr Ole has genuine PTSD symptoms and the psychiatrist's case formulation can cogently address the above questions. In addition, the psychiatric report can also anticipate what the court and asylum officer might experience from the asylum-seeker during the legal proceedings. For example, in the psychiatrist's evaluation of Mr Ole, the psychiatrist may explain likely scenarios for Mr Ole as follows:

"When in a stressful or novel situation, Mr Ole may require questions to be repeated and may show long pauses before answering. He is more likely to forget details or have trouble with dates under these circumstances."

Articulation of an Integrated Narrative

Asylum and refugee cases often require analyses beyond a standard evaluation and case formulation. A person's response to trauma and stress can be described only through the detailed, integrated account of a human life from a psychiatric perspective. Many asylum seekers demonstrate remarkable resilience and psychological resources. These individuals have withstood the tortured and isolating losses that forced them to leave their country, families, and cultures. In some circumstances, the psychiatrist may play a unique role in explaining the absence of mental health symptoms in view of the overwhelming adversity experienced by the client.

Referrals in these cases often begin with the tautologic assumption that psychiatric symptoms are a measure of trauma (ie, PTSD must exist because the history of trauma is so dramatic). Attorneys often fear that good adjustment in their client may imply a false story about past events: if the trauma is true, then psychiatric illness must follow. In these cases, the psychiatrist offers a psychological and cultural explanation that highlights not only the trauma but also the sources of psychic strength and sense of purpose that inoculates against the more debilitating symptoms of trauma. In the example of the Zimbabwe client who endured horrific rapes yet outwardly maintained her composure, the psychiatric report explained the perceived inconsistency between the woman's demeanor and her alleged horrors. In particular, the report explained that some individuals, despite terrible traumas, experience a numbing dissociation that presents in a controlled calm manner. In addition, this woman was invested in rescuing her three children, who were in hiding with a relative, and this mission contributed to her determined resolve. In her report, the psychiatrist described the contribution of these factors to the client's presentation as follows:

"Her sense of purpose, her identity as a mother, and her commitment to the rescue of her children consumes her and successfully diverts her attention from her own past trauma. She does not grant herself the luxury of reflecting on her own plight.
This report included details of how sparsely the woman lived while working 'under-the-table' to send money home."

The integrated narrative may also be required when the converse is true, when the extent of trauma is not by asylum standards extensive, or even physical in nature, but the reaction is nevertheless severe. The psychiatric analysis of the asylum-seeker's vulnerability provides the foundation for explaining the subjective severity of the traumatic event. Although the client's past history may involve prior traumas not recognized in support of asylum, the narrative can demonstrate how a traumatic past may be synergistic with later events. For example, a young woman brutally and repeatedly raped by her uncle as an adolescent showed severe PTSD after a short detention by government forces as she tried to escape conflict in her town. The psychiatric assessment and narrative explained the inconsistency between her factual account of what happened and her reported psychic trauma. She sincerely described her captives as "kind" but described terror and certainty that she would be raped and killed. Without the psychiatric report, her account sounded exaggerated and self-serving. The following case illustrates the importance of taking a lifetime trauma history to search for pre-existing vulnerabilities that may play a role in emotional responses to subsequent immigration stressors.

Psychiatrist Role in Presenting Lifetime Trauma History

Mr G is a young man from Haiti who worked as a gardener for an unpopular political candidate. He ran off when demonstrators marched onto the grounds. He was neither captured nor hurt. His family feared that he would bring danger to them and encouraged him to flee. Having never before been away from home, he left Haiti, went to Mexico, and then crossed illegally into the United States, where he was then detained. He was distraught at the border, but still was released from custody, with a court date. The psychiatric evaluation diagnosed depression and PTSD, related to the synergistic trauma from a recent earthquake and the violent loss of his safe haven where he worked. Although he was not granted asylum, he was allowed to stay in the United States by another legal avenue.

Overall, the psychiatric report educates the legal community to the diathesis stress basis for psychiatric illness. It is the complex interaction of personal vulnerabilities, resources, and the extent and type of trauma that produces the reaction and symptomatology. The narrative also serves to communicate with those outside the profession; therefore, the report should avoid psychiatric jargon or shorthand notations of medical documents in order to clearly identify the connections between the person, the trauma, and the outcomes. Although clear communication of complex concepts is emphasized in of all of forensic psychiatry, this skill is especially compelling in asylum and refugee cases where culture, trauma, and disorders converge.

CONSIDERATIONS IN THE ASSESSMENT OF CREDIBILITY AND MALINGERING

Forensic evaluations commonly consider the possibility of malingering, particularly when there are clear secondary gains to appearing as if one has a psychiatric disorder. Asylum and refugee seekers have the established goal of avoiding deportation or return to a home state. Although this goal clearly qualifies as a potential secondary gain, attorneys may not specifically request that the possibility of malingering be evaluated. When detailing how malingering was assessed, the psychiatric report generally presents specific evidence for or against feigning. The assessment of malingering is complicated for several reasons: malingering and overall credibility of the case are often conflated, cultural differences exist in the expression of psychiatric symptoms, there are language and cultural barriers to the use of standardized measures, and there are factors in the flight experience itself that are unique complications in these assessments.

In asylum and refugee cases, the assessment of malingering may serve the attorney's purpose of establishing the credibility of the applicant's account of persecution and trauma. Because a credible account is the crux of an immigration case, much hangs on the establishment of "truthfulness." The attorney may use the absence of malingering to bolster the argument for credibility. Similarly, if a psychiatrist determines that the client is malingering, the attorney is unlikely to request a report, because feigning mental illness would undermine the client's credibility.

The forensic psychiatric report can make observations that may speak to the client's credibility. For example, the psychiatrist can outline how reported symptoms are or are not consistent with the presentation of genuine mental illness. However, the psychiatric opinion must stop short of declaring a story of trauma true or false. No psychiatric assessment, even augmented by psychological testing, can establish the truth or falsehood of a particular event. Rather, the opinion identifies the client's openness or defensiveness, the consistency in the detail or the lack of it, and the overall congruency between presentation and facts, in light of any cognitive limitations, culture, and psychiatric disorders. Furthermore, the attorney is responsible for providing documentation of the client's home country conditions and authenticity of documents.

Particularly useful is the psychiatric explanation for presentations that may raise suspicion about the client's account. The symptoms of numbing and avoidance after trauma can result in a story void of many details or told with a flat affect. The next case highlights the psychiatrist's role in assisting the court in evaluating the client's credibility.

Psychiatrist Role in Evaluating Client Credibility

A young man from Sierra Leone described an attack on his village in which his brother and parents were killed and he was injured. He quietly gave his account to the asylum officer with an absence of emotion. Each time he was asked about the number of rebels attacking the house he provided a different number (ie, 4, 7, and 12). His credibility was assessed as low, because he was "lying about the number of soldiers" and because he should have been far more upset about his loss. Moreover, he refused to show the asylum officer the scar he said he had on his chest from the attack. The forensic psychiatrist retained by the attorney diagnosed PTSD and depression. The psychiatrist recognized having a PTSD diagnosis did not necessarily validate his account of the traumatic event. The psychiatrist referred him for a physical examination through which his scar was documented. In addition, the evaluating physician noted that the scar was not a surgical scar, had healed poorly, and was consistent with the account of being cut by a machete. The psychiatrist referred the young man for treatment for depression and in her extended number of sessions, explored why the client had refused to show his scar, which was prominent and easily uncovered on his chest. His reasons reflected strong cultural and personal factors: a scar is a badge of courage, but in his case it was a mark of shame; he had survived while his family died. In her report to the court, the psychiatrist acknowledged that her evaluation could not directly determine the truth of the event. However, she provided explanations to address others' doubts, along with the psychiatric and physical evidence that made the man's account more likely true than false. In regards to the young man providing different numbers for the number of soldiers involved in the attacks, the psychiatrist clarified how PTSD symptoms could account for this seeming inconsistency. In particular, as a result if PTSD, he avoided thinking about the attack, and when experiencing minor flashbacks, he relived different parts of the traumatic event with different numbers of rebels involved. The psychiatric report noted, "Just as an actor can memorize lines and repeat them over and over, a liar can do the same. This young man was a university student studying engineering, familiar with memorization and accurate recall of numbers. There is no reason why he could not remember a simple number were he to lie to the court. In this case, his inability to give consistent answers each time and his lack of emotional display that one expects is evidence of the severity of the trauma and his response to it."

Although psychiatric assessments may assist in the evaluation of a client's credibility, the attorney is responsible for providing documentation of the client's home country conditions and authenticity of documents. Because such formal documentation is often lacking, especially in countries under siege of war or extended conflict, the psychiatric assessment may need to be completed without critical collateral data; conclusions may be more tentative, acknowledging limitations of the process.

In other cases, the psychiatric assessment and formulation can raise independent questions of credibility. In addition to the malingering of symptoms, the extensive psychiatric interview and assessment, complete with available collateral and supplemental medical and psychological evaluations, can identify gaps and inconsistencies that undermine the client's credibility. Faced with evidence of malingering or of a significantly false account, the psychiatrist's ethical and professional responsibility is to explore reasonable alternatives that could refute that opinion and then inform the attorney about the conclusion. In most cases, the attorney ends the psychiatrist's participation in the case and asks for no report. The psychiatrist is ethically barred from working for other parties on the same case. In general, the psychiatrist's opinion remains confidential, because the work was protected under attorney client privilege. However, if the psychiatrist encounters a situation that involves mandatory reporting in his jurisdiction (eg, child abuse or a threat to kill an identified person), then the psychiatrist must follow the law, even if confidentiality is violated. The following demonstrates how malingering of psychiatric symptoms may be uncovered during the psychiatric examination.

Psychiatrist Role in Questioning Possibility of Malingering

A man reported that he had been tortured as a Christian in a Muslim part of Nigeria and was seeking asylum. He had been in the United States as a student, returned to his country, and then fled after he and his family were attacked. He reported having severe flashbacks and other symptoms of PTSD and of depression. His account of the trauma he experienced was consistent with country conditions, and his story was consistent and well detailed. He had sought legal counsel to help him prepare his case before the asylum officer. The psychiatrist learned in the assessment that he had been in treatment in another state and asked him to sign a release for his records. Those documents included references to his having been in treatment for depression as a student and most recently in France where he was briefly hospitalized after his wife left him. His reported treatment in France was during the same time as the attack on his family. When the psychiatrist asked him to clarify, he became irate and reported to the attorney that he had been accused of lying and that he would no longer meet with that psychiatrist. The psychiatrist considered whether his response was related to a severe psychiatric illness, such as paranoia, or whether this was a defensive response to being caught in a lie. The psychiatrist raised these hypotheses with the attorney who thanked the psychiatrist but indicated that the psychiatrist's services were no longer needed.

Cultural Factors and Malingering Assessments

Cultural variation in the expression of symptoms, response to illness, and attitudes toward treatment is a consideration in all psychiatric assessments and formulations. In asylum and refugee cases, consideration of the client's culture is a critical and primary factor because most come from parts of the world with norms and traditions very different from the West. The forensic psychiatrist is often faced with the daunting task of overcoming language barriers when making a diagnosis and case formulation. In some cases, such as a person originating from a culture with a rare African tribal language, available interpreters may be virtually nonexistent. Furthermore, for many asylum seekers, the process of translation and interpretation is accomplished through a chaining of languages: going from the remote village language or a specific dialect to a national language, often in a dialect of a Western language, and then into English. The result is loss of precision, inconsistent detail, and misconstrued meaning. Consider the following case where language barriers and cultural misunderstandings could have resulted in a determination that the client seeking asylum was not credible.

A woman seeking asylum from Sierra Leone spoke a tribal dialect as her first language. She had learned French in school and then a different French dialect while in a Ghanan refugee camp. Three interpreters (one from France, one from Quebec, and one who mastered French in American schools) translated for the English-speaking lawyers and psychiatrists. Inconsistencies in the woman's account of her assault by rebels abounded and continued to raise the same credibility concerns identified by the asylum official. Clarity about the case came when a university student from Sierra Leone was engaged to interpret. Nuanced words related to the assault and what the woman experienced had been mistranslated. Of note, the word for rape in one French dialect does not translate to the same as in another. The distinction in meaning between the loss of dignity and respect and that of a physical sexual attack accounted for why her story seemed to vary and be at odds with other accounts. The communication with the woman had been at a level three times removed from her native language.

The interpretation of details of intimacy and social interactions, often relevant to the asylum claim, present challenges beyond language. Indeed, many cultural factors arise when conducting these assessments and, if not recognized, contribute to confusion and inconsistencies across reports. The cultural valence attached to types of violence, social interactions, and marital and child-rearing practices can influence the descriptions of events and make them seem at odds with the stark factual account. The following case highlights how a person's culture may impact what a client is willing to tell and not tell.

Psychiatrist Role in Eliciting Cultural Factors of Social Interactions

A woman from Guatemala sought asylum after being abused by her husband for taking contraception after having six children. Various records indicated that she had seven children, not six. The woman had not reported her first child, conceived as a result of her husband's father raping her when she was 13 years old and working as a laborer on his farm. She was ostracized by her family as an evil adultress, was pregnant out of wedlock, and became homeless. The father of the baby raised the male child as his and "gave" her (ie, a "damaged" woman) to his ne'er-do-well son for a wife. Her culture's judgment and resulting shame prevented her from making a disclosure of facts she believed would lead to rejection by her own attorneys. Without a meaningful psychiatric explanation, a lie that was irrelevant to her case evoked the threat that her entire case should not be believed.

Cultural variation also effects the reporting of symptoms, and indeed the experience of psychiatric disorders. In many cultures, somatic expressions of psychiatric disorders predominate. The neurovegetative symptoms common in the Western experience of depression are also present with the addition of culture-specific expressions. For example, people from New Guinea report feeling "a cloud behind the eyes," and Haitians often experience chest pains and rapid heart rate as symptoms related to depression.[24] Although expressions of depression vary across cultures, a characteristic many cultures share is a moral and characterologic judgment, related to the symptoms and the cause, directed against the individual. That is, the experience of depression in many cultures is attributed to failure, a fall from grace, weakness, and personal devaluation. Fear and public displays of emotion also have pejorative interpretations; some of the common hypervigilant and avoidant characteristics of PTSD fall into the same category. The negative valence of these symptoms influences how often they are reported and to what degree they are acknowledged. For some persons, answering a symptom checklist is experienced more as a forced confession than as the inquiry of a caring physician.

Culture also affects the most basic interpretations of the environment and understanding of oneself and others. For example, the Western measure of and adherence to time as a fundamental organizational framework is not universal. Some cultures view time as a concrete and variable concept rather than an abstract and fixed structure. When the concept of time is variable and imprecise, dates and even the idea of sequence can be unfamiliar. In some cultures, a person's birth date is far less important than a coming-of-age ritual. Years may not be as important as environmental occurrences, even those that happen on an irregular and unpredictable schedule.

When temporal orientation varies culturally, an orderly sequential report may be difficult to elicit. Such variability can give rise to apparent inconsistency. For example, one man reported that events happened "a year later" from each other. After struggling to explain an impossible time line, the psychiatrist guided the lawyers to draw a time line with intervals defined not in years or by date but by the births of the children and deaths of his parents. Although intervals were never precisely identified, the sequence of events was finally determined. Another variation in time that occurs across cultures is the concept of "backward" time or preordination; that is, what is so now was always so. An interesting case that illustrates this concept is provided next:

Psychiatrist Role in Elucidating Cultural Temporal Orientation

A man from Togo gave a confusing account of his being targeted, followed, and assaulted by government forces when he was a student protester. One source of confusion was his explanation that his wife, a fellow student, was also sought after by the government. Although he had married when he was 30 years old, he reported that the woman was his wife 4 years before when he was 26 years old and was first detained by police. That inconsistency, a major one by Western standards, was a main reason why the asylum office found his story to be not credible. Through the help of a cultural anthropologist, the lawyers were able to identify and explain that a wife or husband is preordained; the date of the marriage was irrelevant to him. His wife was always his wife, just not yet discovered.

What is remarkable about these cultural factors is that they are so elemental in experience that neither the North American nor the person from the other culture even considers the possibility that these fundamental ways of thinking might vary. Unfortunately, the most prevalent assumption when culture influences create confusion is that the story is false.

Barriers to Standard Measures of Malingering

In psychiatry and forensic work, standardized measures to assess feigning are often used as an adjunct to the psychiatric assessment. However, in asylum and refugee cases, language and cultural barriers may preclude use of these measures. Indeed, psychological testing, an important complement to forensic evaluations in most cases, requires significant modification if it can be used at all. For example, estimates of intellectual capacity in a client whose native language is not English or Spanish requires tools that use nonverbal tasks to prevent an underestimation of capacity. Similarly, the Minnesota Multiphasic Personality Inventory and other standard measures are not applicable for persons from a non-Western country even if they speak English. Although such measures can be used to assess the level of acculturation, the interpretation of such measures must be done cautiously with only tentative conclusions. Although their use may help to inform a clinical question, in forensic work the requirement of certainty and the consequences of overinterpretation are risks that counterbalance their use. Assessment with nonverbal measures may aid in identifying the psychomotor slowing in depression and signs of traumatic brain dysfunction and cognitive limitations. Generally, a referral for testing should be considered when there are unexplained difficulties in communication and evaluation. The use of psychological testing in an immigration evaluation is described next.

Psychiatrist Role in Psychological Testing in Immigration Evaluation

A 67-year-old man, who had escaped with his adult sons from Republic of Rwanda, had applied for asylum but was unable to answer even simple questions when challenged by the asylum officer about his case. His sons were no longer in the United States and he was living in a shelter. He reported that he had been a leader of the resistance to the oppressive government, and he had some documentation that made his case strong but his presentation was unconvincing. When interviewed, he seemed disinterested, reported no difficulties, and was generally distracted. Referred for a neuropsychological assessment to rule out brain trauma, he showed marked deficits in spatial organization and memory. The testing result suggested dementia. Because of his language and cultural experiences, confabulation was not easy to assess, and so nonverbal deficits were used as a partial substitute. He was referred for a brain scan, which showed evidence of deterioration. Collectively, culture, language, lack of collateral, and lack of local history made making a diagnosis difficult. However, the psychological testing provided another explanation for his questionable responses to questions.

SPECIAL CONSIDERATIONS WHEN CONDUCTING REFUGEE EVALUATIONS

There are unique and important considerations for psychiatrists who conduct refugee evaluations abroad. Although the mental health professional is examining the client at the request of the attorney, clinical questions and risk assessment responsibilities remain. Those responsibilities apply across all forensic work, but with asylum and refugee cases, the complexity of clinical issues is magnified. Most clients have little support, speak a language uncommon in the community, have not had medical care, and are unfamiliar with the concept of mental health services. Cultural issues complicate even a basic psychiatric assessment. The mental health professional needs a referral system that includes immigrant services in the community. When evaluating asylum seekers in the United States, it is good practice to ensure that "medical backup" is readily available should the client decompensate during the course of the evaluation or need subsequent care. Providing for the same kind of continuity of treatment abroad is more challenging but no less important. Provision of these services can be difficult because a refugee's legal status in his host countries is often precarious. It is necessary to consider all these issues with the legal team and make logistical arrangements well in advance. As with all foreign field work, the evaluator must be mindful that the evaluations not place undue burdens on limited health infrastructures or promise more than reasonably can be delivered. Some of those concerns are mitigated, however, because forensic evaluations are limited in scope and time and are not meant to replace long-term mental health services provided to this population.

A second consideration is the possibility that contact in any form (electronic, telephonic, or personal) with foreigners may place the client at heightened scrutiny and safety risk by the host government. Although experience has indicated that psychiatric evaluations can significantly improve the chances for success in having a case reevaluated, thus tipping the balance in favor of such evaluations, it is a decision that must be made in careful consultation with the client and the legal team.

Third, in conducting evaluations abroad, licensing and liability issues are important considerations. Although all countries regulate the provision of medical care and medical professionals, including recognition of foreign doctors' credentials, there is great variation in the context of emergencies.[25] Procedures are even less clear in situations that involve failed states or significant political conflict with a loss of the usual administrative and regulatory structures. Guidelines, such as the International Disaster Response Laws, may be helpful. Planning must be done in conjunction with the practice of other international aid groups in the area and the local collaborating partners on a country-by-country basis. A similar question is one of liability. There are limited malpractice options for overseas work. In the case of extended volunteer treatment provision, most aid organizations have physicians sign a liability waiver. One potential solution is to determine whether one's employer's malpractice insurance covers foreign evaluations, if the evaluations are done as part of official duties, such as fellowship training, supervision of fellows, or a Memorandum of Understanding with the legal organization.

COUNTERTRANSFERENCE IN ASYLUM WORK

The histories and trauma of asylum-seekers and refugees are different from those experienced in psychiatric clinics, and the effect on forensic psychiatrists merits reflection. The extent of trauma that amounts to persecution evokes many different responses. As expected with countertransference, one's own experiences contribute to the interpretation and the impact of the work. There are, however, several responses shared by faculty and the psychiatric fellows alike.

Denial and Disbelief

When the traumatic stories of the clients are presented during group supervision, a common tendency is to question the veracity of the accounts. Even among the more reflexively sympathetic clinicians, there is often more resistance to the acceptance of the story at face value. The questioning is effective in helping to identify the gaps in information and areas for further exploration. But utility aside, the response is often a protective one. As one forensic psychiatric fellow described and other agreed, "If I accept that account to be true then I have to change my belief in mankind as essentially good." Although history is filled with horrific atrocities, it is the encounter with one who bears witness that most threatens denial of such denigration and denial.

Judgment

Another common and related reaction is judgment of the asylum-seekers actions. Many of their accounts describe decisions that seem wrong and hard to understand when viewed through our cultural lens. For example, many women have had to leave their children behind; some have been out of contact with their children; and a few women even report that they do not know if their children are alive. The countertransference evoked by these circumstances can be strongly negative and can emerge in subtle ways. For example, in one report a psychiatrist repeatedly referred to a woman "abandoning her children" as she escaped her warring country. One of the most provocative experiences occurs when the client lies to the evaluating psychiatrist. As one forensic psychiatric fellow described, "It is a betrayal of trust. I felt deep sympathy for their plight; when they lied, I felt used."

Burden

The most common experience is one of frustration and tremendous responsibility. The evaluation is fraught with many barriers (language, culture, lack of information, lack of records), and many forensic psychiatrists experience their work as carrying the burden of outcome. This experience is evoked in part through the referral process when attorneys indicate that the psychiatric report is central to the success of the case. Certainly, in cases of the 1-year bar to asylum, the outcome does hinge on the psychiatric formulation making a convincing case for extraordinary circumstances. Such cases create a burden from the initial referral: an objective evaluation is needed, but without the right conclusion all is lost.

The burden is also experienced when legal barriers override the psychiatric merits of the case. In one case a woman suffered extreme abuse by her husband, but the abuse did not meet the legal requirements for asylum. The evaluating psychiatrist felt helpless and ineffective when the asylum case failed, even with the documentation of the woman's psychiatric response to trauma.

Over and Under Pathologizing

In response to the experience of burden and the other reactions, the assessments and formulations are at risk for overdiagnosis and underdiagnosis of psychiatric conditions. Many factors complicate these evaluations. Countertransference is one of them. The fear of being duped can lead to an overconservative approach to diagnosis. A client who does not meet all the criteria for PTSD or depression may be dismissed as meriting no psychiatric explanation. Indeed, the more creative approach is to recognize that for many asylum seekers, posttrauma does not apply because their traumatic episode continues in a different form: no longer physical torture but now isolation and displacement. However, there is a risk of being too liberal in diagnosing and espousing the tautology that the experience of severe trauma must lead to pathology even if unexpressed. Feeling compelled to offer a strong argument in favor of asylum will likely be encouraged by the referring attorney and by the evolving relationship with the client.

Addressing Countertransference

Countertransference is always more apparent to and first recognized by others. Supervision, particularly group discussion, has been critically useful in providing support and guidance for those new to asylum work. It is also necessary for veterans in the field. Peers can offer reflections and guidance from a shared platform. What is also critical is to use interdisciplinary resources to inform the process of the assessment and formulation. A university provides extensive resources not only from experts in the field but from students and faculty from different cultures.

As forensic psychiatric consultations increase in asylum cases, networks within psychiatry in general and within forensics can consolidate expertise, eventually set standards for these special cases, and offer opportunities for education for psychiatrists and attorneys. Eventually, such a critical mass of experts can engage in policy and legislative action to incorporate the critical psychiatric factors into asylum law.

SUMMARY

There are common experiences among refugees and asylum-seekers that extend beyond culture and ethnicity. They often come from countries where authority cannot protect them or has targeted them for harm. They use a variety of resources to get to the United States. Some have been provided false documentation; many are misinformed about what to do in America and how their lives will be; some have been instructed on what to say and what story to give. Most who have fled have a resiliency of spirit despite their suffering. Once here, or in a host country, they face tremendous obstacles without access to health care or mental health services. Even when services are available there is fear that discovery of their status would lead to arrest and deportation.

Against this background, the psychiatrist must attempt to forge an alliance to garner as much detail as possible to formulate an opinion. An effective forensic evaluation requires time to establish a working relationship that may begin with education of the client about the process itself. In asylum cases, the role of the evaluator is harder to maintain. The boundary between the assessment and therapy can quickly blur. If trust is established, the psychiatrist can become a primary support system and general referral source. Once the traumatic event is revealed, there is an expectation of help. For most the help needed is not primarily psychiatric but may include housing, a dentist, other health care, or employment. For others, a referral to a psychiatrist can be an affront that implies a characterologic flaw. The psychiatrist can explain the evaluation in a way that allays the client's humiliation.

An understanding of the asylum and refugee process and the culture of those seeking permanent resettlement is augmented through relationships with immigration attorneys who know the law and have experiences with cases and with asylum officers who have been willing to meet to explore the different roles and objectives. Community groups who serve immigrants are also critical resources and have access to networks of support. Knowledge of the asylum process from a legal and experiential perspective benefits the assessment and the formulation and delivery of the forensic opinion. The work is compelling, and the clients are deserving of expertise. Forensic psychiatry will also benefit from the expansion of its expertise into a challenging, worthy, and growing area of law. Moreover, what forensic psychiatry learns can benefit mental health services in general in our diverse culture.

ACKNOWLEDGMENTS

The authors acknowledge Howard Zonana, MD, Yale School of Medicine, Professors Jean Koh Peters and Steven Wizner, Yale Law School and Attorney Becca Heller, Iraqi Refugee Assistance Project, for their valuable collaboration and insights.

REFERENCES

1. UNHCR. Global Trends. 2011. Available at: http://www.unhcr.org/4fd6f87f9.html. Accessed August 13, 2012.
2. UNHCR. Global Report. 2011. Available at: http://www.unhcr.org/gr11/index.xml. Accessed August 13, 2012.
3. UNHCR. Asylum claims in industrialized countries up sharply in 2011. Available at: http://www.unhcr.org/4f7063116.html. Accessed August 13, 2012.
4. Meffert SM, Musalo K, McNiel DE, et al. The role of mental health professionals in political asylum processing. J Am Acad Psychiatry Law 2010;38:479–89.
5. De Jesús-Rentas G, Boehnlein J, Sparr L. Central American victims of gang violence as asylum seekers: the role of the forensic expert. J Am Acad Psychiatry Law 2010;38:490–8.
6. The Refugee Act of 1980, Public Law 96–212, approved March 17, 1980.
7. Immigration and Nationality Act, Public Law 414, approved June 27, 1952.
8. Inzunza R. The Refuge Act of 1980 ten years after—still the way to go. Int J Refug Law 1990;2:413–27.
9. UN General Assembly. Protocol Relating to the Status of Refugees, 31 January 1967, United Nations, Treaty Series, vol. 606, p. 267. Available at: http://www.unhcr.org/refworld/docid/3ae6b3ae4.html. Accessed 13 August 2012.
10. Ramji-Nogales N, Schoenholtz AI, Schrag PG. Refugee roulette: disparities in asylum adjudication. Stanford Law Rev 2007;60:295–412.
11. United States General Accounting Office. U.S. asylum system: significant variation existed in asylum outcomes across immigration courts and judges. Available at: http://www.gao.gov/assets/290/281794.pdf. Accessed August 13, 2012.
12. Wasem RE. United States Congressional Research Service. Asylum and "credible fear" issues in U.S. immigration policy. Available at: http://fpc.state.gov/documents/organization/168099.pdf. Accessed August 13, 2012.
13. Transactional Records Access Clearinghouse. Immigration judges: asylum seekers and the role of the immigration court. Available at: http://trac.syr.edu/immigration/reports/160/. Accessed August 13, 2012.
14. Transactional Records Access Clearinghouse. Asylum denial rate reaches all time low: FY 2010 results, a twenty-five year perspective. Available at: http://trac.syr.edu/immigration/reports/240/. Accessed August 13, 2012.
15. Lusting SL, Kureshi S, Delucchi KL, et al. Asylum grant rates following medical evaluations of maltreatment among political asylum applicants in the United States. J Immigr Minor Health 2008;10:7–15.
16. Savy P, Sawyer A. Risk, suffering and competing narratives in the psychiatric assessment of an Iraqi refugee. Cult Med Psychiatry 2008;32:84–101.
17. UNHCR. Resettlement Handbook. Available at: http://www.unhcr.org/4a2ccf4c6.html. Accessed August 13, 2012.
18. USCIS; Immigration Officer Academy. Asylum officer basic training, lesson plan overview, interviewing. Part V: Interviewing survivors. Available at: http://www.uscis.gov/USCIS/Humanitarian/Refugees%20&%20Asylum/Asylum/AOBTC%20Lesson%20Plans/Interview-Part5-Interviewing-Survivors31aug10.pdf. Accessed August 13, 2012.
19. USCIS; Immigration Officer Academy. Asylum officer basic training, interviewing. Part II: Eliciting testimony. Available at: http://www.uscis.gov/portal/site/uscis/menuitem.5af9bb95919f35e66f614176543f6d1a/?vgnextoid=2a1d1a877b4bc110VgnVCM1000004718190aRCRD&vgnextchannel=f39d3e4d77d73210VgnVCM100000082ca60aRCRD. Accessed August 13, 2012.

20. Australian Government, Migration Review Tribunal and Refugee Review Tribunal. Guidance on vulnerable persons. Available at: http://www.mrt-rrt.gov.au/Conduct-of-reviews/Conduct-of-reviews/default.aspx. Accessed August 13, 2012.

21. Canada Immigration and Refugee Board, Refugee Protection Division. Assessment of credibility in claims for refugee protection. Available at: http://www.irb-cisr.gc.ca/eng/brdcom/references/legjur/rpdspr/cred/Pages/index.aspx. Accessed August 13, 2012.

22. International Association of Refugee Law Judges. Guidelines on the judicial approach to expert medical evidence. Available at: http://www.iarlj.org/general/images/stories/working_parties/guidelines/medicalevidenceguidelinesfinaljun2010rw.pdf. Accessed August 13, 2012.

23. Redding RE, Floyd MY, Hawk G. What judges think about the testimony of mental health experts: a survey of the courts and bar. Behav Sci Law 2001;19(4):583–94.

24. Marsella AJ. Depressive experience and disorder across cultures. Handbook of Cross-Cul Psych Psychopath 1980;6:237–89.

25. Fisher D. Regulating the helping hand: improving legal preparedness for cross-border disaster medicine. Prehosp Disaster Med 2010;25(3):208–12.

Deposition Dos and Don'ts
Strategies for the Expert Witness

Thomas G. Gutheil, MD

KEYWORDS

- Deposition • Deponent • Deposing attorney • Dos and don'ts • Expert witness
- Qualifications as an expert • Retaining attorney • Tips and traps

KEY POINTS

- A deposition is serious business, even although it is not a trial, and the transcript may last the length of your career, always available for your possible impeachment.
- Depositions require special thought, special forms of answers to questions, constant alertness, appropriate breaks, and focus on the court reporter rather than on the deposing attorney.
- If you do not feel tired and drained by the end of the deposition, you have not been paying sufficiently close attention.
- Maintain your calm. If opposing attorneys get into a furious argument with each other, do nothing; just sit there until it is over.
- Getting you to guess or speculate is a favorite attorney tactic, which should be resisted; you should never fear to admit "I don't know."

OVERVIEW OF THE DEPOSITION PROCESS
Definitions True and False

To the average forensic practitioner, a deposition may seem adequately defined as an oral examination under oath, in the discovery phase of a case, usually involving an expert witness, a court reporter (or stenographer), and the attorneys in the case.[1–9] However, in practical terms, this definition falls short in an important way, because it focuses on the oral examination itself. A more accurate and relevant definition casts the deposition as the written transcript that emerges from the oral examination; it is that format that endures over time and is available for future impeachment of the expert, if later opinions seem to contradict viewpoints expressed in the present instance.

Disclosure: Dr Gutheil has authored or co-authored ca 300 publications, some of which generate income and some of which relate to the present topic.
This article derives from a presentation at the 2011 annual meeting of the American Academy of Psychiatry and Law and from this author's text, The Psychiatrist as Expert Witness.
Department of Psychiatry, Beth Israel-Deaconess Medical Center and the Massachusetts Mental Health Center, Harvard Medical School, 6 Wellman Street, Brookline, MA 02446, USA
E-mail address: gutheiltg@cs.com

Psychiatr Clin N Am 35 (2012) 947–956
http://dx.doi.org/10.1016/j.psc.2012.08.008
0193-953X/12/$ – see front matter © 2012 Elsevier Inc. All rights reserved.

This lasting availability derives from the fact that both the plaintiffs' bar and the defense bar (ie, organizations of attorneys that primarily take one side of the case or the other) maintain mainframe computers, on which those transcripts are stored. Thus, active expert witnesses are used to seeing a pile of that expert's past depositions on the opposing attorney's table, not just in deposition but also later in trial. This fact alone places a significant burden on the deponent to grasp that they are speaking for the ages, even when answering seemingly innocuous questions from the deposing attorney.

An immediate correlate of this last point is its implications for the audience of the deposition. Whereas during the trial the audience is the fact finder (judge or jury or both), the audience for the deposition is the court reporter. All answers to questions should be directed to that person, and every effort should be made to make the answers clear and unambiguous, so that a sound record can be made.

Saving Stenographer Sanity

Because the stenographer or court reporter, based on this reasoning, is the most important person in the deposition, certain principles should apply to optimize that person's functioning: some dos and don'ts.[1]

1. DO speak your answers to questions out loud; avoid nods, shakes, grunts ("uh-huh") and other gestures and noises that are acceptable in ordinary speech but might be unclear or unrecordable when rendered into typed format. Was that "uh-huh" meaning "yes" or "uh-unh" meaning "no"?
2. DON'T interrupt each other and speak in an overlapping fashion. The reporter cannot take down 2 or more simultaneous speakers. Let the deposing attorney finish the question completely, even if you think you can predict from the first 3 words what the question will be. The attorney may pull a switch in the final words of the question, so you may be wrong in your prediction.
3. DO make the effort to speak slower and more clearly than usual, even if this sounds artificial or stilted. Clarity is the desired effect.
4. DO spell odd words or names, such as medications. This is time-saving and promotes accuracy in the transcript.
5. DON'T discuss the case with the court reporter. Although the latter is in the thick of the action, they are not a friend, ally, or party in the case.
6. DO give your card to the reporter, both to aid in spelling your name and to provide contact information for any questions.
7. DO arrange to read and sign the deposition when the transcript is ready; this is a critical step, which is reviewed in more detail later.

In this discussion, some basic familiarity with the structure and concept of depositions is assumed; the guidelines herein aim at addressing the finer points of the task.

STAGES OF THE DEPOSITION
Preliminary Matters

Where will the deposition take place? Several possible sites afford different pros and cons.

1. Your office. The advantage of your own office is the comfort of home turf, where you spend much of your time; you can sit in your own chair at your own desk and feel in control of things. However, you may be subject to the same familiar interruptions that have always plagued you when you are working. In addition,

you may expose your own library, thus allowing the deposing attorney to pick books randomly off your shelf and grill you about them or get you to confess you have not read them.
2. The deposing attorney's office, if the case is local. This site exposes nothing but may feel uncomfortable to you as a foreign locale. A similar point may be made when the out-of-town lawyer borrows a local lawyer's office.
3. The court reporter's office. These sites are foreign to both attorneys and witnesses. Many of the larger court reporter firms have conference rooms and recording machinery, as well as teleconferencing facilities. The latter are probably the wave of the future, because they save considerable travel expenses, although posing problems of their own, addressed later.

When will the deposition take place? Scheduling 2 or more attorneys, a court reporter, and a clinician for the same time slot often takes a great deal of back and forth by phone or email to synchronize busy schedules for a single date and time. Flexibility is encouraged; every effort should be made not to reschedule, once the date is set. Make every effort as well to go into the deposition well rested.

What preparation is required? Knowing the case cold is the basic requirement, as is the critical importance of meeting with the retaining attorney before the deposition: no matter what the extent of your experience, insist on meeting, set aside sufficient time, and do not stint with this step. Feel free to rehearse your testimony; supply the attorney with questions you anticipate as potentially troublesome; and go over your CV together to ensure there are no errors or problems.[2]

A common deposition error is for the deponent to think that, because the deposition is not a trial, careful or extensive preparation is unnecessary, or that the oath sworn at the outset is not so binding; neither of these beliefs is accurate. The oath is just as binding and the risk of perjury, just as great. Moreover, the deposition often plays a pivotal role in later impeachment of the witness at trial.

For completeness, the converse (thinking a deposition is like a trial) is not strictly correct, either. As discussed later, deposition demeanor differs from trial demeanor in specific ways.

How long will it take? Most depositions taken by experienced, competent attorneys can be taken in a 2-hour to 3-hour time slot; however, because some attorneys cannot meet this level of efficiency, witnesses should clear a day or an afternoon at minimum. In addition, some attorneys replace skilled deposition strategy with brute force, prolonging the deposition interminably in the hope of wearing down the witness, so that the latter makes slips and errors because of fatigue.[1,2]

The Deposition Itself

After all the persons in the deposition are identified to the court reporter and the case caption is provided, the deposition proper begins. Some jurisdictions now require the witness to present picture identification to the court reporter. The reporter administers the oath; this is usually followed by questions aimed at identifying the witness and eliciting the latter's qualifications and identifying information, such as address, titles, training, and work history. This process is followed by the relevant (and irrelevant) questions that constitute the body of the deposition.

No matter what questions are asked, and no matter how obnoxious, hostile, demeaning, or contemptuous the attorney's demeanor may be, maintain your calm. At times, opposing attorneys may get into a furious argument with each other about some point of fact or law. You may be tempted to jump in or try to mediate. Do neither; just sit there until it is over. An angry or upset deponent cannot attain the necessary calm concentration to answer effectively. If seriously distressed, ask for a break and work to resume your calm.

ATTORNEY STRATEGIES IN DEPOSITION

Two legal scholars[3(p91)] gave this alphabetically influenced advice to the deposing attorney:

At a deposition [the attorney] should be assertive, bold, controlling, deferential, effective, fair, generous, hospitable, intelligent, just, kind, lucky, magnanimous, nurturing, original, professional, questioning, retentive, studious, thorough, unexcitable, versatile, wary, xenophobic, yielding, and zealous.

Although this advice had a facetious element, it does capture the broad range of behaviors that an attorney may show at deposition.

Attorneys have several goals in deposing the witness and several methods of achieving those goals. The most straightforward one is simply to get information and to elicit your opinions on the case at hand.

This elicitation and its record in the transcript have the added effect of freezing your opinion, under oath, at a particular time; if your opinion changes, that change requires recording, sometimes by means of interrogatories or even another deposition, and may be a basis for later impeachment.[2]

Getting you to guess or speculate is a favorite attorney tactic, which should be resisted; a deponent should never fear to admit "I don't know," although for some witnesses, that admission constitutes a narcissistic injury. In the 12th century, Maimonides is said to have pointed out: "Teach thy tongue to say 'I do not know' and thou shalt progress."

A related attorney strategy may be styled painting you into a corner by eliciting, through skilled questioning, an opinion that may be more speculative than the witness wishes to convey, more extreme, more inflexible, or excessively narrow. The success of this strategy usually depends on the care and alertness with which the witness responds to the questions.[1]

In addition, the deposing attorney may be attempting to obtain a variety of admissions about the limits of the witness's opinion, as well as concessions to the claims of the opposing side of the case. As a simple example of the former, in a malpractice case deriving from a patient's suicide, the deposing attorney usually has the deponent admit that the patient, being dead, was not interviewed, a situation precluding an independent diagnosis being made. As a simple example of the latter, the attorney may get the deponent to concede that different psychiatrists might disagree about a given patient's diagnosis. These admissions and concessions may or may not affect the way that a jury responds to the witness.

The deposing attorney may wish to see the witness in action, to see how the witness handles the challenges of the deposition, as a way of anticipating what the witness will do at trial. Decisions about settlement are sometimes made from the effectiveness of the witness in deposition. Knoll and Resnick[2(p26)] add the goal of probing the defendant (or deponent) for bias, arrogance, or hostility.

This last fact involves a subtlety about deposition approaches that does not apply in all instances. Some attorneys and some experts maintain a distinction between 2 kinds of depositions: poker and crusher. The poker deposition derives its name from the manner in which the poker player tries to avoid signaling or giving away any advantage to the other players, by holding the cards close to the vest; the witness here gives minimal answers, volunteers nothing, and insists on answering only highly specific and narrow questions. The crusher deposition has 1 goal: force a settlement by presenting an overwhelming case for the retaining side, by pulling out all stops, giving extended answers that make every possible point for the retaining side, and thus presenting a convincing case for settlement. The choice between these approaches should not be made by the expert but always by the retaining attorney, within whose vision of the case the approach must fit.

Some Attorney Tactics

1. "Let's have a conversation"

This tactic consists of attempting to distract the witness from the necessary focus and seriousness of the deposition by chatting beforehand to lull the expert into an informal attitude: "So, Doctor, what about those Red Sox, eh?" When the deposition begins, all chat should be put aside or ignored; only formal, relevant questions should be answered.

2. Scramble the order

As noted earlier, the beginning of the deposition proper usually follows a fairly standard format, consisting of administrative and demographic questions, before moving to the substance of the case and the opinion; however, this is not a requirement. The attorney may attempt to rattle the expert by scrambling the order of the subject matter involved. The following is an actual first question in a deposition (Clyde Bergstresser, personal communication, 2012):

Plaintiff's attorney: *"Doctor, when was the first time you sodomized my client on your analytic couch?"*

Defendant doctor: *"I think it was in February."*

One can readily imagine the deponent being rattled on that occasion. An expert may be similarly rattled by a first question such as "Give me all your opinions in this case" or "State every piece of evidence in the case materials that contradicts or seems to contradict your opinion." Such sweeping questions should probably be resisted as being too broad to answer without being broken down.

3. Keep up the speed and rhythm

The deposing attorney may have prepared a written list of questions in the order they will be asked; as a result, the questions may come at the witness quickly or in a steady rhythm. Because many of these questions are predictable, the witness may lapse into a comparably rapid mode of answering that matches the attorney's pace of questions, firing the answers back; this response interferes with the need for careful thought before answering any questions.

4. An end-run around objections

When inappropriate or badly worded questions are asked of the witness, the retaining attorney, also present, can lodge an objection for the record. The deposing attorney may seem to acknowledge the validity of the objection and attempt an acceptable rephrase; however, the rephrase may present the same objectionable content in an only slightly varied form (ie, attempting to do an end-run around the objection). The witness should wait to see if the retaining attorney wants to object to the new form before answering. In general, the witness should pay close attention to the objection, which may provide indirect advice on a useful answer.

5. The silent treatment

A common tactic for the deposing attorney is to ask a question, receive an answer, and then to gaze expectantly at the expert as if to encourage further comment. The less experienced expert is drawn into further discourse, despite the fact that there is no pending question. Into this conversational vacuum many inappropriate comments may flow, some potentially damaging. The witness should wait patiently for a question; if the silence grows intolerable, the witness may ask, "Are we finished, or do you have any further questions?" This strategy usually gets the ball rolling again.[1,2]

6. Lawyers' assumed personae

Knoll and Resnick[2(p39)] have identified 4 personae that deposing attorneys may adopt to get past the guard of the witness. The silent treatment has already been discussed. Another is "Mr/Ms Friendly," in which the attorney attempts to engage you in casual conversation outside the presence of the retaining attorney. This tactic is usually inappropriate. The "eager student" persona attempts to massage your ego and your possible function as a teacher to elicit extensive and excessive discourse. "Counselor Clueless" presents a persona of vast ignorance about the facts or the case, which may pull the witness into overly extensive educational efforts. In general, deponents should resist efforts to teach, no matter how greatly needed they may seem.

7. Massive distortion

The deponent is under oath; the deposing attorney is not. For a few attorneys, this discrepancy regrettably provides license to lie, distort your previous testimony, make up facts about the case, and misread documents, including your own writings. Therefore, do not assume that the attorney's quote or reading is correct; ask to see the cite, the document, or the transcript.

8. Who is your hero?

McElhaney[4] suggests asking the expert who is their professional hero:

Asking who the expert witness's professional hero is can be a natural road into what the witness reads. You may even go out and hire that person as your own expert witness (p. 23).

APPROACHES TO THE DEPOSITION BY THE EXPERT WITNESS

What was meant to be *mano a mano* (between deposing attorney and expert) turns out to be "quibble a quibble."[4(p22)]

Presentation and Demeanor

Like a trial, a deposition places strains on a deponent's ability to sustain concentration, attention, and focus for prolonged periods. It is especially important to watch out for a tendency to dissociate or space out late in the day or when long, boring questions are asked in a monotone. The moment concentration begins to fade, deponent witnesses should not hesitate to take frequent breaks, walk around, go outside, or splash cold water on their face, until their capacity to focus returns. If you are not tired and drained at the end of the deposition, it is possible that you have not been paying close enough attention.[1]

While in the deposition proper, the deponent should be awake and aware, functioning as an "active listener" (D Benjamin, personal communication, 2011); this term means to maintain a questioning attitude throughout: Where is this going? What is the attorney driving at? What is the subtext or hidden implication of this question?

The deponent should also avoid being shy about taking the time to think, to review documents that are alluded to in a question, to check medical records, to look at textbook entries if they arise, and so on. Attorney resistances ("Doctor, can't you answer the question without checking the records?") should be answered: "I am under oath, and I am checking because it is important to me to be truthful and accurate." If the deposing attorney mentions a document, ask to see it and take the time to read it; misquotation or distortion of document content is not unheard of among deposing attorneys.

The special way of speaking in deposition (slower, clearer, directed to the reporter) was noted earlier in this article. Novice deponents often note that this manner of speaking sounds dry, pedantic, pompous, stilted, and boring. In reality, that manner of speaking is just as it should be; it makes for a clean record. This mode of speech can be sharply distinguished from the hearer-friendly, informal, and interested manner of speaking to a jury or judge at trial, in which the manner of communication counts for a great deal of the effectiveness of the testimony.

When dealing with a younger or less experienced retaining attorney, it may be necessary to explain privately and reassuringly that this way of testifying is deliberate and is not the way you will communicate when it is time for trial testimony.

Because various video techniques are now being extensively used for depositions, some comments about the special problems associated with them may be in order. Given the current high costs of travel, more and more law firms are doing depositions by telephone, Skype, and teleconferencing; in addition, recording the deponent on video provides a means of preserving not only content but demeanor for the deposition; that recording can then be used in case of the deponent's absence at trial, as well as for study and critiquing by the attorney's firm.

Because that video may be shown to the jury at some point, for example, for impeachment of a different opinion given at trial, the deponent being videorecorded should regard the camera as the jury and speak to it directly, using the more hearer-friendly, informal language suitable to a trial. It is also important to avoid glancing about at other distractions in the recording site, because that may give the deponent on camera the appearance of a shifty-eyed look, associated in many lay minds as an indicator of deceptiveness and inauthenticity.

Deposition Language and Problem Questions

Was it you or your brother that was killed in the war?

—Actual deposition question

In addition to the mode of communication just mentioned, deposition language itself has certain important qualities. First, responses in deposition are generally governed by the rule of austerity: the answer contains just that minimum of information needed to answer the question. Deponents may get into trouble by attempting to cover every possible aspect of the topic asked about, by discoursing extensively, and by attempting to squeeze all the possible qualifiers into the answer. The short answer is always best. If more information is desired, the attorney will ask for it.

Second, it is often useful to include the question or its context within the deposition answer to give a complete response, an exception to the rule of austerity; this tactic tends to prevent quotation out of context in an impeachment attempt. Here is an example in which the attorney tried to pack multiple questions into one[1(p62)]:

Q: Now, are you seriously telling this court that that sentence [quoted from an article] is one which instructs the forensic witness and the medical health [sic] treater that, to determine competence, they have to enter into a dialog with their patient, that this is one of the ways in which you go about determining competence? Is that your testimony?

A: Well, let me answer all 3 components. First, yes, it is serious. I am serious. Second, the capacity to enter into a dialogue is considered by the Program in Psychiatry and the Law, which I co-direct, to be an appropriate way of determining competence in the clinical situation. And the third part of your question is, yes, this could be used to instruct both the forensic assessor and the treating clinician as to a means of determining the capacity to enter into informed consent.

Note that either a yes or no answer would fail to pin down the point and could easily be distorted later; note also that perfectly acceptable alternative answers would have been: "I could not follow that; could you rephrase?" or "Which of those several questions did you wish me to answer first?"

In addition, the deponent's answer can provide clarity to unfocused or deliberately vague questions, as here:

Q: Did you see Mr Jones again?

A: I next saw Mr Jones on his regular office visit on June 15th, 2010.

Q: And what happened? [This is a deliberately vague and broad question]

A: As usual, I performed an assessment of his condition. [The deponent provides the focus]

Again, the deponent could also request a more specific question. Here is another example of provided focus:

Q: Doctor, as a result of your examination, was the young lady pregnant?

A: The young lady was pregnant, but not as a result of my examination.

Third, it is important to listen carefully and alertly to the question, so that the answer given is fitted to the actual question asked. Some questions defeat the possibility of answering:

Q: Was that explanation amplified in any way with any details as to what that sexual abuse was supposedly to consist of during that conversation?

The only possible answer is "I do not understand the question."
Here is another classic:

Q: When he went, had you gone and she, if she wanted to and were able, for the time being excluding all the restraints on her not to go, gone also, would he have brought you, meaning you and she, with him to the station?

Other attorney present: Objection; that question should be taken out and shot.

These last 2 examples capture the tendency of some attorneys to believe that they can control the witness's answer by packing every subordinate qualifier into the question; the result is an incomprehensible question.

A more demanding response to a vague, rambling, or inexact question might be: "I understand you to be asking _____, and the answer to that question is _____."

Here the deponent takes over the question to reframe it for comprehensible answering; some attorneys may then snap back, "I will ask you the questions, Doctor, thank you very much."[1]

This next example involves a triple negative (bold italics used to identify the negatives):

> Q: Okay. And you believe that it is **not in**appropriate to **fail to** note that you've discussed with the patient the potential side effects of the medications that you are prescribing?

Once again, a "yes," "no," or even "maybe" would all make the answer, like the question, incomprehensible. Such confusing negatives can also infect the answer as here:

> Q: Okay, and I assume…you don't recall whether or not you used the term […] when you talked to Mr …., is that correct?

> A: No, Ma'am. That is correct.

> Q: No, you don't?

> A: Yes.

Is the answer to the question "yes" or "no"? Can anyone tell? Here is a perfect example of the need to include the question in the answer, such as "You are correct that I do not recall whether I used that term." Almost any other response would be meaningless.

Because deposition answers are the core of the deposition content, particular attention must be paid to their wording. To the surprise of some, deposition answers are drawn from a shallow pool.[1] They are: "Yes," "No," "I do not know," "I do not recall," and a brief narrative answer preferably containing the question, as explained earlier. Answers unreflected on can be surprising:

> A: There's clearly times after his death when he's saying things to his wife that sound like either his suicidality has returned or his suicidality, that never went away.

The reader will agree that a séance is not a typical part of an evaluation of suicidality.

The lesson here for the deponent is clear: listen to the entire question without interruption; make sure you understand it; pause briefly to allow the other attorney to object; plan your answer in your head and examine it for problems; then turn to the reporter and give your answer slowly and carefully.

Reading and Signing the Deposition

Most court reporters whom the author has encountered are competent, fast, and reliable performers of their challenging task. However, the witness should always read the deposition carefully for the subtle errors that can creep in. For example:

> Q: So you have been unable to locate some of your records on [patient]?

> A: I never tried to be honest with you. I was never told to try. I never had any reason to try.

This apparent frank and candid confession of perjury could have been avoided by noting the absent comma in the transcript, after the word "tried." That correction solves only part of the problem. A deposition under oath is no place to toss in informal comments, such as "to be honest with you," "to tell you the truth," "no, I tell you a lie," "if I said that, I'd be lying."[1]

Other ambiguities can arise if not checked:

Q: Do you agree that she had [MDD] at the time that you saw her on ___?

A: That was her diagnosis at the time.

Q: Was that your diagnosis also?

A: Yes.

This wording leaves unclear if that was also the diagnosis made by the deponent or the diagnosis suffered by the deponent, suggesting an impaired practitioner. Also note the possibility of simple mishearing:

Testified: It's an "us and them" situation.

Transcribed: It's an "S&M" situation.

SUMMARY

Depositions present many challenges for the deponent witness; although experience doubtless helps, this review, although it cannot be comprehensive, provides some guidance on how to approach the event. The importance of careful attention, both to questions and answers, is stressed throughout, because it is in those fundamentals that most errors occur. Armed by preparation, constant alertness, and knowledge of the pitfalls, the deponent can face the deposition with confidence.

REFERENCES

1. Gutheil TG. The psychiatrist as expert witness. 2nd edition. Washington, DC: American Psychiatric Press; 2009.
2. Knoll JL, Resnick PJ. Deposition dos and don'ts: how to answer eight tricky questions. Curr Psychiatr 2008;7:25–40.
3. Malone DM, Hoffman PT. The effective deposition: techniques and strategies that work. 2nd edition. South Bend (IN): NITA; 1996.
4. McElhaney J. Know what you're after: experts will tell you a lot in depositions if you ask the right questions. ABA J 2011;97:22–3.
5. Babitsky S, Mangraviti JJ. How to excel during depositions: techniques for experts that work. Falmouth (MA): SEAK; 1999.
6. Babitsky S, Mangraviti JJ. Depositions: the comprehensive guide for expert witnesses. Falmouth (MA): SEAK; 2007.
7. Gutheil TG, Dattilio FM. Practical approaches to forensic mental health testimony. Baltimore (MD): Wolters Kluwer/Lippincott Williams & Wilkins; 2008.
8. Brodsky SL. Coping with cross-examination and other pathways to effective testimony. Washington, DC: American Psychological Association; 2004.
9. Gutheil TG, Drogin EY. The mental health clinician in court: a survival guide. Washington, DC: American Psychiatric Press, in press.

Psychopharmacologic Management of Aggression

William J. Newman, MD

KEYWORDS

- Aggression • Psychopharmacologic • Violence • Assault • Aggressive
- Pharmacologic • Off-label

KEY POINTS

- There is no single strategy to pharmacologically manage aggression.
- There is currently no pharmacologic treatment for aggression approved by the Food and Drug Administration.
- Each year, approximately 1.6 million people lose their lives to violence worldwide.
- Aggression can be classified as impulsive, organized, or psychotic.
- Psychopharmacologic interventions should be guided by diagnoses.

INTRODUCTION

Many people use the terms aggression and violence interchangeably, despite these words not being synonymous. Aggression is generally defined as behaviors leading to nonaccidental harm. Violence is a subtype of aggression involving nonaccidental physical harm by one individual toward another. Violent behavior causes (or is likely to cause) death, physical injury, or psychological harm. Aggression encompasses violence, in addition to nonaccidental property destruction and verbal abuse during periods of agitation. Self-injurious behaviors and suicide are sometimes classified as forms of aggression, but this article focuses primarily on aggression toward others (physical and/or verbal).

Approximately 1.6 million people lose their lives to violence each year.[1] The financial impact of violence is also staggering. Annually, nations pay billions of dollars to cover costs associated with law enforcement, health care for victims, and lost productivity at work. Psychological manifestations of violence are difficult to quantify, but undoubtedly magnify the scope of the problem. Victims of single-incident or repeated violence (such as childhood abuse or domestic abuse) can experience psychological

Disclosures: None.

Division of Psychiatry and the Law, Department of Psychiatry and Behavioral Sciences, University of California, Davis Medical Center, 2230 Stockton Boulevard, 2nd Floor, Sacramento, CA 95817, USA
E-mail address: wjnewmanmd@gmail.com

Psychiatr Clin N Am 35 (2012) 957–972
http://dx.doi.org/10.1016/j.psc.2012.08.009
0193-953X/12/$ – see front matter © 2012 Elsevier Inc. All rights reserved.

manifestations for years, including additional lost productivity at work. Surviving victims' quality of life is often impacted, resulting in a range of potential problems.

Professionals from various disciplines have studied the antecedents and manifestations of violent behavior. Professions specifically interested in studying violence include mental health scholars, legal scholars, criminologists, sociologists, and biologists, to name a few. Each discipline brings unique perspectives to studying and assessing the issue. This article focuses on the medical management of aggression as it pertains to individuals with psychiatric diagnoses and therefore emphasizes the medical literature.

ASSESSMENT OF AGGRESSION

Aggression by individuals with psychiatric diagnoses presents in many forms. Providing a thorough assessment and accurate diagnoses is therefore the clinician's most important role. Aggressive behaviors displayed by two different patients can appear identical despite involving completely different contributing factors. Unique elements leading to the aggressive behaviors must be considered to formulate an appropriate treatment plan. Specific medications have shown varied results with different patient populations. There is no single approach that will be effective for every patient. Accurately determining aggressive patients' psychiatric diagnoses is the first important step in guiding pharmacologic management.

In addition to accurately determining the patient's diagnoses, analyzing the type of aggression displayed is another important step. One such system involves categorizing each aggressive act of psychiatric patients as impulsive, organized, or psychotic.[2] Impulsive acts are generally immediate responses to provocation or perceived provocation. The patient may seem agitated, out of control, hostile, and threatening. The aggressive act is typically not related to long-term goals or secondary gain. Organized acts generally involve planning, social motives, and/or secondary gain. The acts are premeditated and predatory in nature. Psychotic acts occur in response to delusional beliefs and do not have a clear rational alternative motive. Taking a patient's pattern of behavior into consideration helps guide management. Individual patients can display different types of aggression, even within short periods of time. Therefore, the evaluator should pay attention to overall patterns of an individual's aggressive behaviors when determining the best treatment approach.

Structured instruments can also be used to characterize aggression. Large-scale personality inventories, such as the Minnesota Multiphasic Personality Inventory (MMPI) and Personality Assessment Inventory (PAI), have been used for decades to infer patterns of responses consistent with aggressive tendencies. However, performing a lengthy and time-consuming personality inventory may not be practical or relevant in many circumstances. Other instruments have been developed that require less time to administer and are designed to specifically detect aggressive tendencies. These instruments include the Buss-Durkee Hostility Inventory[3] and the Brown-Goodwin Inventory.[4] These instruments were more commonly used for research purposes several decades ago, but are less often used in current studies.

Present-day investigators more commonly use instruments that rate individual aggressive acts. The most frequently used instrument in aggression studies is the Overt Aggression Scale (OAS).[5,6] The OAS guides evaluators to classify each aggressive act as one of the following: verbal aggression; physical aggression against self; physical aggression against objects; or physical aggression against other people. The evaluator also chooses from four defined degrees of severity within each scale. The final step in the OAS administration involves documenting interventions used by staff. Other researchers have created modified versions of this instrument that they use to evaluate specific outcomes.[7–10]

PHARMACOLOGIC MANAGEMENT OF AGGRESSION: GENERAL PRINCIPLES

There are currently no pharmacologic treatments for aggression approved by the Food and Drug Administration (FDA). Antiepileptic and antipsychotic medications are the classes most commonly used to address long-term aggression. However, research supporting this practice is limited. Some studies have addressed the benefits of individual agents in all psychiatric patients, whereas others have focused on patients with particular diagnoses. Based on the published data, no firm conclusions can be drawn about the use of medications to treat aggression. In the absence of FDA-approved interventions, psychiatrists use exclusively off-label interventions to manage aggression.

Prescribing medications off-label should be carefully considered. The informed consent process varies somewhat when recommending FDA-approved versus off-label prescriptions. In the United States, informed consent routinely involves several elements when starting medications for purposes approved by the FDA, as follows:

- Nature of the treatment
- Risks of the treatment
- Benefits of the treatment
- Alternative treatment options
- Risks associated with not receiving treatment

Although manufacturers are prevented from marketing medications for off-label purposes, physicians can legally prescribe FDA-approved medications to any patient for any purpose. As always, evidence-based prescribing is preferred, but physicians are free to prescribe based on their own experience and training. When starting an FDA-approved medication for off-label use, however, physicians should explain to the patient (or their substituted decision maker) that the use is off-label and document it. Physicians should also discuss FDA-approved alternatives and whether research supports the off-label use of the medication.[11] As mentioned, all pharmacologic treatments for long-term management of aggression are off-label, so no FDA-approved alternatives exist at this time. A risk-benefit analysis is also an important aspect of initiating an off-label prescription. For instance, with clozapine, which has an extensive side-effect profile with potentially fatal consequences, the anticipated benefits should be significant enough to outweigh the potential risks.

Most psychiatrists have experience managing acute agitation, and commonly use antipsychotic medications and benzodiazepines for this purpose. Benzodiazepines are both safe and effective for the treatment of acute agitation in most instances. Studies have shown that administering benzodiazepines alone can be very effective in treating acute agitation.[12,13] Antipsychotics and benzodiazepines can be administered together intramuscularly to provide rapid benefits. Antipsychotics should routinely be used in this situation when aggression is caused by, or exacerbated by, active psychotic symptoms. The most frequently used intramuscular antipsychotics are haloperidol, aripiprazole, olanzapine, and ziprasidone. Lorazepam is often used in conjunction with antipsychotics because it is the most reliably absorbed intramuscular benzodiazepine. The American Association for Emergency Psychiatry Project BETA Psychopharmacology Workgroup recently published an extensive protocol for the pharmacologic treatment of acute agitation.[14] The protocol provides a decision tree involving different known or presumed causes of agitation, and is reproduced in **Fig. 1**.

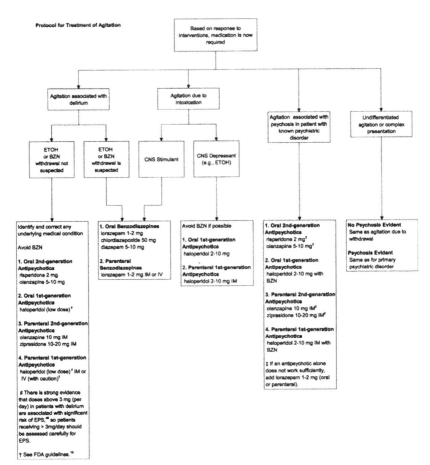

Fig. 1. Protocol for treatment of agitation. BZN, benzodiazepine; CNS, central nervous system; EPS, extrapyramidal side effects; ETOH, alcohol; FDA, Food and Drug Administration; IM, intramuscular; IV, intravenous. (*From* Wilson MP, Pepper D, Currier GW, et al. The psychopharmacology of agitation: consensus statement of the American Association for Emergency Psychiatry Project BETA Psychopharmacology Workgroup. West J Emerg Med 2012;13(1):26–34; with permission.)

In forensic psychiatric facilities and correctional environments, clinicians must pay particular attention to whether reported symptoms of acute agitation or anxiety are supported by objective observations. The purpose of this careful review is to minimize inappropriate prescriptions of commonly abused medications, such as benzodiazepines. Patients (even those with legitimate psychiatric symptoms) can collect medications for several reasons unrelated to therapeutic relief from anxiety or agitation. Such motivations include abuse of the prescribed substance, using the substance for bartering with others, and collecting medications for a suicide attempt. Limiting inappropriate prescriptions is also important in other inpatient and outpatient settings, especially when patients have a history of substance abuse.

In general, long-term strategies for managing recurrent aggression vary from medical approaches used for acute agitation. Fortunately, clinicians targeting recurrent aggression typically have the advantage of more extensive information about the individual. This information allows them to craft a focused pharmacologic intervention based on the patient's diagnoses and pattern of aggressive behaviors. For ease of use, this article focuses primarily on published data about patients with particular diagnoses, highlighting evidence for the long-term management of aggression.

PHARMACOLOGIC MANAGEMENT OF AGGRESSION: SPECIFIC CONDITIONS
Aggression Related to Primary Mental Illness

Patients with a primary mental illness such as major depressive disorder, bipolar disorder, schizophrenia, and schizoaffective disorder can behave aggressively. In their landmark 1990 study, Swanson and colleagues[15] illustrate the link between psychiatric disorders and violence. These investigators published evidence from the Epidemiologic Catchment Area Surveys.

The main objective for decreasing the risk of violence in patients with primary mood and psychotic disorders is to treat the underlying mental illness. The American Psychiatric Association (APA) Treatment Guidelines provide suggestions for treating primary mood and psychotic disorders.[16] Other groups have also published algorithms. The Texas Medication Algorithm Project (TMAP) provides one example of strategies for the treatment of schizophrenia, bipolar disorder, and major depressive disorder.[17–19] Algorithms like the TMAP provide standardized treatment guidelines that can increase the consistency of mental health treatment and help guide medication changes. After familiarizing themselves with the recommendations, clinicians can incorporate their own treatment preferences based on individual training and experience. However, it is beneficial for clinicians to at least be familiar with standardized treatment guidelines.

One important principle is that patients with psychotic symptoms should generally be treated with antipsychotic medications, at least initially, regardless of their primary diagnosis. Regarding the use of antipsychotics for depressed patients with psychosis, the APA Treatment Guidelines for Major Depressive Disorder note, "psychotic depression typically responds better to the combination of an antipsychotic and an antidepressant medication rather than treatment with either component alone, although some research has shown comparable responses for antidepressive treatment or antipsychotic treatment alone."[16] Regarding the use of antipsychotics for manic patients with psychosis, the APA Treatment Guidelines for Bipolar Disorder note that "the presence of psychotic features during a manic episode may not require an antipsychotic medication, although most clinicians prescribe them in addition to a maintenance agent."[16]

Depressed patients with psychotic symptoms typically respond more robustly when prescribed both an antidepressant and an antipsychotic medication until their mood stabilizes.[20–22] Manic patients with psychotic symptoms typically respond more robustly when prescribed both a mood stabilizer and an antipsychotic medication until their mood stabilizes.[23–26] Once the patient's mood stabilizes, antipsychotic medications can be discontinued in many instances. Depressed patients can then be managed with antidepressants alone and manic patients with mood stabilizers alone.

There has been some recent discussion in the literature about whether treatment with selective serotonin reuptake inhibitors (SSRIs) may actually promote violence.[27–29] Some of the cases discussed have involved extreme violence, including homicides or suicide-homicides. Other reports have contended that there is not an association between treatment with SSRIs and violent crime.[30,31] In perhaps the most extensive study on the subject published to date, Bouvy and Liem[32] describe results from a 15-year analysis using nationwide data from the Netherlands. These investigators report a negative association between lethal violence and prescription of antidepressants in the Netherlands. Based on the author's overall literature review, there does not appear to be a consistently established correlation between antidepressant use and aggression.

In patients with schizophrenia and schizoaffective disorder, a common cause of aggression is inadequate dosing of antipsychotic medications. Patients who do not respond to a particular antipsychotic medication should first have their dose optimized, based on treatment guidelines, as long as they tolerate the medication. If they still do not respond clinically, they should be switched to another antipsychotic medication. Once the primary symptoms are under control, clinicians can use additional strategies to target residual aggressive behaviors.

Psychiatrists have long debated the degree to which antipsychotic medications independently diminish aggression. Typical antipsychotics reduce aggression over the long term, but this effect seems to be directly related to dose-dependent sedation. Typical antipsychotics can also cause extrapyramidal side effects that indirectly limit the patient's ability to act aggressively. However, extrapyramidal side effects can cause other problems for the patient. Many clinicians have started using atypical antipsychotics for the long-term management of aggression. Despite this, based on the author's literature review, with the exception of clozapine the proven benefits of atypical antipsychotics for reducing aggression are equivocal.

Clozapine

Clozapine has been shown to reduce long-term aggression in patients with mental disorders in several studies.[33–37] These effects are not related strictly to sedation.[35,38] For those who are less familiar with initiating clozapine, the author has provided recommended steps for initiating the medication, based on the current guidelines, as outlined in **Fig. 2**.

However, the potential side effects and required laboratory monitoring associated with clozapine limit the number of patients who can tolerate this treatment. The laboratory monitoring begins at initiation of treatment with clozapine and must continue consistently. Over time, the frequency of required blood draws decreases. **Fig. 3** summarizes clozapine monitoring guidelines.

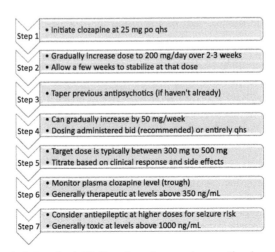

Step 1
- Initiate clozapine at 25 mg po qhs

Step 2
- Gradually increase dose to 200 mg/day over 2-3 weeks
- Allow a few weeks to stabilize at that dose

Step 3
- Taper previous antipsychotics (if haven't already)

Step 4
- Can gradually increase by 50 mg/week
- Dosing administered bid (recommended) or entirely qhs

Step 5
- Target dose is typically between 300 mg to 500 mg
- Titrate based on clinical response and side effects

Step 6
- Monitor plasma clozapine level (trough)
- Generally therapeutic at levels above 350 ng/mL

Step 7
- Consider antiepileptic at higher doses for seizure risk
- Generally toxic at levels above 1000 ng/mL

Fig. 2. Recommended steps for initiating clozapine. po, by mouth; qhs, nightly at bedtime.

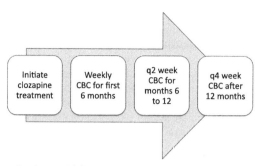

| Initiate clozapine treatment | Weekly CBC for first 6 months | q2 week CBC for months 6 to 12 | q4 week CBC after 12 months |

Fig. 3. Clozapine monitoring guidelines. CBC, complete blood count; q, every.

With respect to treating aggression, clozapine should primarily be reserved for chronically psychotic, recurrently aggressive patients who have failed other agents. Mood stabilizers such as lithium and lamotrigine can also be combined with clozapine for treating aggressive, refractory patients with schizophrenia.[39,40]

Mood stabilizers

Mood stabilizers are recommended as an adjunctive treatment for patients with schizophrenia who display residual aggressive behaviors while taking antipsychotic medications.[41] Valproate has been reported as beneficial in patients with schizophrenia who behave aggressively.[42] In a double-blind, placebo-controlled study, carbamazepine was found to decrease agitation and aggression in patients with schizophrenia.[43] Lithium has also been used for this purpose, but other than when used in combination with clozapine (as already mentioned), the benefits are not well supported in the literature.[44,45]

Benzodiazepines

Benzodiazepines, when used in conjunction with antipsychotic treatment, can also be useful for reducing aggressive behaviors in patients with schizophrenia. The long-term use of benzodiazepines is encouraged as a first-line or second-line treatment for patients with schizophrenia who do not have a history of substance abuse.[41]

Aggression Related to Substance-Use Disorders

Substance-use disorders are often comorbid with mood disorders, psychotic disorders, and certain personality disorders (particularly Cluster B). The presence of substance-use disorders complicates the pharmacologic management of aggression, especially when the substance use is unreported or underreported by patients. Focusing on the substance-use issues of individual patients and decreasing their substance use is a very important aspect of managing aggression over the long term. Addressing this issue may also help prevent patients from becoming the perpetrators or the victims of extreme acts of violence.

Alcohol

Alcohol has long been associated with aggression. In studies, perpetrators of violent crimes have higher blood alcohol levels than perpetrators of nonviolent crimes.[46,47] Alcohol is the substance of abuse most clearly shown to independently increase aggression.[48] Alcohol impairs several regions of the brain, most significantly the prefrontal cortex, which limits the individual's ability to resist impulses and make thoughtful decisions. Individuals who are intoxicated with alcohol are therefore more likely to commit violent acts and otherwise get themselves into dangerous situations.

Amphetamines and other substances of abuse

The evidence linking other substances of abuse directly to aggression is limited. There is some evidence that the following substances lead to increased aggression in humans: methamphetamine, cocaine, phencyclidine, and opioids (during with-drawal).[49] However, animal studies have shown different results. Other than animal studies involving alcohol, others do not reveal increased aggression with exposure to substances of abuse. One potential explanation for this discrepancy is that the aggression involving illicit substance users is often related to violent acts that occur while acquiring drugs, selling drugs, or obtaining money to pay for drugs.

Aggravation of primary mental illness

Despite the lack of clear evidence supporting direct associations between specific substances of abuse and aggression, substance use can aggravate primary mental illness. Several studies have shown increased aggression among individuals with comorbid substance abuse and primary mental illness.[15,50–52] Directly addressing a patient's substance use is the primary way to limit their risk of aggression. No phar-macologic intervention has been shown to independently decrease aggression in substance users.

Aggression Related to Personality Disorders

Patients diagnosed with personality disorders, particularly antisocial and borderline personality disorders, often behave aggressively. Aggression is so prevalent among these populations that it is an explicit criterion for both antisocial and borderline personality disorders.[53] Individuals with these personality disorders can exhibit impul-sive aggression, organized aggression, or both. Substance abuse, which is very common in individuals with antisocial and borderline personality disorders, can also exacerbate their aggressive behavior.

Cluster B personality disorders

There are published reports supporting the use of mood stabilizers, antipsychotics, antidepressants, and β-blockers in patients diagnosed with Cluster B personality disorders. Cluster B personality disorders include:

- Antisocial personality disorder
- Borderline personality disorder
- Histrionic personality disorder
- Narcissistic personality disorder

One double-blind, placebo-controlled study addresses the benefits of valproate for impulsive aggression in subjects with Cluster B personality disorders. The Cluster B patients in this study were treated with an average daily dose of approximately 1400 mg per day, with average valproate trough levels of 65.5 μg/mL.[54] One double-blind, placebo-controlled study shows the beneficial effects of lithium in inmates with "nonpsychotic personality disorders."[55] The plasma lithium levels of the subjects were generally lower than 1.0 mEq/L. Another double-blind, placebo-controlled study shows the long-term benefits of treating aggression with fluoxetine in patients with personality disorders.[56]

Borderline personality disorder

There are numerous studies that have examined the pharmacologic management of borderline personality disorder. Some medications have been demonstrated to signif-icantly decrease anger in this patient population. Aripiprazole is the antipsychotic medication that has proved to be most effective. A double-blind, placebo-controlled study shows decreased anger in subjects treated with 15 mg per day of aripiprazole.[57] Studies showing decreased anger have been published with mood stabilizers including lamotrigine, topiramate, and valproate.[58–62] Impulsivity itself contributes to aggressive behaviors. Aripiprazole, lamotrigine, topiramate, and valproate have also been shown to reduce impulsivity in patients with borderline personality disorder.[57–63]

Antisocial personality disorder

No medication has been proven to be beneficial for managing patients with antisocial personality disorder. Patients with antisocial personality disorder are very likely to display organized aggression, as described earlier. Pharmacologic treatments are not beneficial for managing organized aggression. Behavioral interventions and contingency management strategies are the most effective ways to manage organized aggression. However, patients with antisocial personality disorder can also display impulsive aggression. Some case reports have addressed the pharmacologic management of impulsive aggression in patients with antisocial personality disorder. One report discusses the benefits of quetiapine in four patients with antisocial personality disorder.[64] The investigators report improvements in impulsivity, hostility, aggression, and irritability. Since the publication of that report, the abuse of quetiapine has become much more prevalent in correctional settings and psychiatric hospitals. The use of quetiapine for this population and the risk of misuse should therefore be carefully considered. Another case report discusses the benefits of risperidone in one patient diagnosed with antisocial personality disorder.[65] A recently published case report, based on the author's own experience, describes the benefits of propranolol to address the impulsive aggression of a patient with antisocial personality disorder.[66]

Aggression Related to Mental Retardation and Acquired Brain Injury

Patients with mental retardation commonly display impulsive acts of aggression. Some medications have proved useful for managing aggression in this population. Controlled studies have shown the benefits of lithium in individuals with mental retardation.[67–69] The recommended lithium levels in these studies ranges from 0.5 to 1.0 mEq/L. Other controlled studies have shown valproate to decrease aggression in patients with mental retardation.[70] Atypical antipsychotics have demonstrated some benefits in this population.[71] Other than clozapine, risperidone is the atypical antipsychotic that has shown the most consistent benefits in treating individuals with mental retardation. Recommended doses in the literature range from 0.5 to 4 mg per day.[72] β-Blockers have also been proposed as a useful intervention for aggressive individuals with mental retardation.[73]

Aggression is often a frustrating component of managing patients with acquired brain injuries. Several medications have been used to target aggression in this population. β-Blockers seem to be most effective for managing aggression in patients with acquired brain injury. Some research has been encouraging, but published results are limited to relatively small studies. One group published three double-blind, placebo-controlled studies describing the beneficial effects of β-blockers in patients with organic brain disease.[74–76]

Propranolol and pindolol are the β-blockers that have been used in the majority of completed studies. The β-blocker doses used in early studies were actually higher than those commonly used for antihypertensive effects. These higher doses were sometimes associated with adverse effects related primarily to drops in pulse and blood pressure. However, a more recent study using pindolol to target aggression shows promising results with lower doses, 5 mg three times a day in this instance.[77] Pindolol is a very good alternative because it is generic, can be easily titrated, and displays partial agonism at the β-adrenergic receptor. This partial agonism helps prevent problematic drops in pulse and blood pressure. Pindolol can be started at 5 mg twice a day and titrated up to 10 mg twice a day within a week, as tolerated. Slightly higher doses can still be used, with careful observation and monitoring of the patient.

Other pharmacologic options for patients with acquired brain injuries have been published. There is one report of a patient with acquired brain injury who failed to respond to propranolol and haloperidol, but responded to lithium.[78] However, lower doses should be used in this population because of increased sensitivity to neurocognitive side effects with lithium.[79] There are other reports of patients with acquired brain injury who benefited from treatment with valproate.[80–82] One article discussed the benefits of carbamazepine in patients with acquired brain injuries.[83]

Aggression Related to Dementia

Patients with dementia sometimes behave aggressively, particularly as their level of functioning declines. If they display primarily psychotic aggression, antipsychotic medications should be prescribed. Haloperidol has been used for decades to treat agitation and aggression in patients with dementia. Low-dose haloperidol (1–5 mg daily) has been shown to reduce aggression in this population.[84,85] Low-dose risperidone (0.5–2 mg daily) has also been shown to reduce both aggression and psychosis.[84,86] However, the potential associated side effects (mortality, cerebrovascular events, and extrapyramidal side effects) limit the use of risperidone. In 2005, the FDA issued a black-box warning regarding the use of atypical antipsychotics in elderly patients with dementia. The warning is specifically for "cerebrovascular events, including stroke." The benefits associated with other atypical antipsychotics in aggressive patients with dementia have been equivocal.

There are several options other than antipsychotics to address primarily impulsive aggression in patients with dementia. Benzodiazepines, given alone or in combination with antipsychotics, are commonly used to treat aggression in patients with dementia, and have been shown to be useful in this population.[87] However, it is important to consider that elderly patients are at increased risk for paradoxic agitation, delirium, and side effects of benzodiazepines. β-Blockers, valproate, carbamazepine, and lithium have also been shown to provide some benefits when prescribed to patients with dementia.[88–90]

Aggression Related to Delirium

Delirium is a medical emergency and should be treated accordingly. The only definitive treatment for delirium is to address the underlying cause. Patients with delirium can display both purposeful and purposeless (arm flailing, kicking, and so forth) aggressive behaviors. These actions are typically related to the patient's disorientation and confusion. Low-dose typical and atypical antipsychotics are most effective at limiting these behaviors.[91–97] The American Association for Emergency Psychiatry Project BETA Psychopharmacology Workgroup recommends giving low-dose haloperidol or atypical antipsychotics, either by mouth or intramuscularly, for agitation and associated aggression related to delirium.[14]

If alcohol or benzodiazepine withdrawal is a consideration, appropriate doses of benzodiazepines should be administered immediately. Physiologic instability, such as hypertension and tachycardia, provides an indication that withdrawal is a potential cause of the delirium. In some instances, administering medications to target agitation can be harmful to this population. Unless alcohol or benzodiazepine withdrawal is being considered as a cause of the delirium, benzodiazepines should be avoided, as they can aggravate the patient's level of disorientation and worsen their delirium. This disorientation is particularly evident in instances of delirium in the intensive care unit.[98]

Antipsychotic medications should be viewed as a short-term intervention to target agitation while the cause of the delirium is being addressed. Delirium sometimes resolves naturally, and antipsychotics may prevent further neurologic injury during this period. Delirium is a potentially life-threatening condition and should be managed aggressively until the underlying cause has been discovered or the delirium resolves. Aggression is a secondary manifestation and will resolve along with the delirium. If the aggression persists after resolution of the delirium, other potential causes should be considered.

TREATMENT-RESISTANT PSYCHIATRIC PATIENTS

Some patients continue to display aggressive behaviors despite adequate pharmacologic trials. Medication changes can initially be tried after optimizing the dosing of the initial agent. The next agent should also be selected based on the patient's diagnoses and predominant type of aggression. When patients are not improving as expected, the clinician should consider that the patient may not be taking his or her medication as prescribed. When clinically indicated, this issue can be addressed by obtaining serum levels that are easily tracked. Examples of medications with available serum levels include lithium, valproate, and clozapine. Serum levels allow the prescriber to at least have knowledge about the patient's recent adherence and to make a fully informed decision regarding the next course of treatment.

Clozapine has most consistently decreased aggression in studies involving various populations of psychiatric patients. However, to be prescribed clozapine, the patient must be able and willing to perform regular blood draws beginning immediately after initiation, as shown in **Fig. 3**. The required monitoring eliminates several candidates from consideration for treatment with clozapine because of their unwillingness or inability to participate in the regular blood draws, including some patients with refractory psychosis related to schizophrenia.

Patients who fail to respond to multiple pharmacologic trials may benefit from having a more developed behavioral plan, this being particularly true for individuals who are long-term residents of psychiatric hospitals or other structured environments. Although behavioral plans are beyond the scope of this article, there is extensive literature about behaviorally managing aggression. Behavioral plans and pharmacologic interventions are frequently used in combination when managing aggressive patients.

SUMMARY

There is no single proven strategy to pharmacologically manage aggression. Existing evidence is limited and is largely based on small studies and case reports. There are several challenges to studying the pharmacologic management of aggression in a controlled manner. For example, encouraging a highly aggressive group of patients to comply with study parameters presents challenges for researchers. Furthermore, highly aggressive patients are often housed in correctional settings or forensic hospitals and are therefore classified as a protected population, making it difficult to obtain approval for controlled studies. Larger, controlled pharmacologic studies will likely be one important aspect of future aggression research. Another future goal is to integrate the research efforts of the various professions that study aggression and violence. There remains much to be learned about this topic.

REFERENCES

1. World Health Organization. violence and injury prevention. WHO Web site. Available at: http://www.who.int/violence_injury_prevention/violence/en. Accessed April 29, 2012.
2. Quanbeck CD, McDermott BE, Lam J, et al. Categorization of aggressive acts committed by chronically assaultive state hospital patients. Psychiatr Serv 2007;58:521–8.
3. Buss AH, Durkee A. An inventory for assessing different kinds of hostility. J Consult Psychol 1957;21:343–9.
4. Brown GL, Goodwin FK, Ballenger JC, et al. Aggression in humans correlates with cerebrospinal fluid amine metabolites. Psychiatry Res 1979;1:131–9.
5. Yudofsky SC, Silver JM, Jackson W, et al. The Overt Aggression Scale for the objective rating of verbal and physical aggression. Am J Psychiatry 1986;143: 35–9.
6. Silver JM, Yudofsky SC. The Overt Aggression Scale: overview and guiding principles. J Neuropsychiatry Clin Neurosci 1991;3:S22–9.
7. Kay SR, Wolkenfeld F, Murrill LM. Profiles of aggression among psychiatric patients. I. Nature and prevalence. J Nerv Ment Dis 1988;176:539–46.
8. Knoedler DW. The modified overt aggression scale. Am J Psychiatry 1989;146: 1081–2.
9. Ratey JJ, Gutheil CM. The measurement of aggressive behavior: reflections on the use of the Overt Aggression Scale and the Modified Overt Aggression Scale. J Neuropsychiatry Clin Neurosci 1991;3:S57–60.
10. De Benedictis L, Dumais A, Stafford MC, et al. Factor analysis of the French version of the shorter 12-item Perception of Aggression Scale (POAS) and of a new modified version of the Overt Aggression Scale (MOAS). J Psychiatr Ment Health Nurs 2012. [Epub ahead of print].
11. Wilkes M, Johns M. Informed consent and shared decision-making: a requirement to disclose to patients off-label prescriptions. PLoS Med 2008;5(11):1553–6.
12. Bick PA, Hannah AL. Intramuscular lorazepam to restrain violent patients. Lancet 1986;1:206.
13. Dorevitch A, Katz N, Zemishlany Z, et al. Intramuscular flunitrazepam versus intramuscular haloperidol in the emergency treatment of aggressive psychotic behavior. Am J Psychiatry 1998;156:142–4.
14. Wilson MP, Pepper D, Currier GW, et al. The psychopharmacology of agitation: consensus statement of the American Association for Emergency Psychiatry Project BETA Psychopharmacology Workgroup. West J Emerg Med 2012;13(1): 26–34.
15. Swanson JW, Holzer CE, Ganju VK, et al. Violence and psychiatric disorder in the community: evidence from the Epidemiologic Catchment Area surveys. Hosp Community Psychiatry 1990;41(7):761–70.
16. American Psychiatric Association. Clinical practice guidelines. APA Web site. Available at: http://www.psychiatry.org/practice/clinical-practice-guidelines. Accessed April 30, 2012.
17. Crismon ML, Trivedi M, Pigott TA, et al. The Texas Medication Algorithm Project: report of the Texas Consensus Conference Panel on medication treatment of major depressive disorder. J Clin Psychiatry 1999;60(3):142–56.
18. Suppes T, Rush AJ, Dennehy EB, et al. Texas Medication Algorithm Project, Phase 3 (TMAP-3): clinical results for patients with a history of mania. J Clin Psychiatry 2003;64:370–82.

19. Moore TA, Buchanan RW, Buckley PF, et al. The Texas Medication Algorithm Project antipsychotic algorithm for schizophrenia: 2006 update. J Clin Psychiatry 2007;68:1751–62.
20. Parker G, Roy K, Hadzi-Pavlovic D, et al. Psychotic (delusional) depression: a meta-analysis of physical treatments. J Affect Disord 1992;24:17–24.
21. Spiker DG, Weiss JC, Dealy RS, et al. The pharmacological treatment of delusional depression. Am J Psychiatry 1985;142:430–6.
22. Rothschild AJ, Williamson DJ, Tohen MF, et al. A double-blind, randomized study of olanzapine and olanzapine/fluoxetine combination for major depression with psychotic features. J Clin Psychopharmacol 2004;24:365–73.
23. McElroy SL, Keck PE, Strakowski SM. Mania, psychosis, and antipsychotics. J Clin Psychiatry 1996;57(Suppl 3):14–26.
24. Tohen M, Chengappa KN, Suppes T, et al. Relapse prevention in bipolar I disorder: 18-month comparison of olanzapine plus mood stabilizer v. mood stabilizer alone. Br J Psychiatry 2004;184:337–45.
25. Vieta E, Suppes T, Eggens I, et al. Efficacy and safety of quetiapine in combination with lithium or divalproex for maintenance of patients with bipolar I disorder. J Affect Disord 2008;109:251–63.
26. Marcus R, Khan A, Rollin L, et al. Efficacy of aripiprazole adjunctive to lithium or valproate in the long-term treatment of patients with bipolar I disorder with an inadequate response to lithium or valproate monotherapy: a multicenter, double-blind, randomized study. Bipolar Disord 2011;13(2):133–44.
27. Mason SE. Prozac and crime: who is the victim? Am J Orthopsychiatry 2002;72:445–55.
28. Healy D, Herxheimer A, Menkes DB. Antidepressants and violence: problems at the interface of medicine and law. PLoS Med 2006;3(9):1478–87.
29. Moore TJ, Glenmullen J, Furberg CD. Prescription drugs associated with reports of violence towards others. PLoS Med 2010;5(12):1–5.
30. Tardiff K, Marzuk PM, Leon AC. Role of antidepressants in murder and suicide. Am J Psychiatry 2002;159:1248–9.
31. Barber CW, Azrael D, Hemenway D, et al. Suicides and suicide attempts following homicide. Victim-suspect relationship, weapon type, and presence of antidepressants. Homicide Studies 2008;12:285–97.
32. Bouvy PF, Liem M. Antidepressants and lethal violence in the Netherlands 1994-2008. Psychopharmacology 2012;222(3):499–506.
33. Rabinowitz J, Avnon M, Rosenberg V. Effect of clozapine on physical and verbal aggression. Schizophr Res 1996;22:249–55.
34. Spivak B, Roitman S, Vered Y, et al. Diminished suicidal and aggressive behavior, high plasma norepinephrine levels, and serum triglyceride levels in chronic neuroleptic-resistant schizophrenic patients maintained on clozapine. Clin Neuropharmacol 1998;21:245–50.
35. Citrome L, Volavka J, Czobor P, et al. Effects of clozapine, olanzapine, risperidone, and haloperidol on hostility among patients with schizophrenia. Psychiatr Serv 2001;52:1510–4.
36. Volavka J, Czobor P, Nolan K, et al. Overt aggression and psychotic symptoms in patients with schizophrenia treated with clozapine, olanzapine, risperidone, or haloperidol. J Clin Psychopharmacol 2004;24(2):225–8.
37. Krakowski MI, Czobor P, Citrome L, et al. Atypical antipsychotic agents in the treatment of violent patients with schizophrenia and schizoaffective disorder. Arch Gen Psychiatry 2006;63(6):622–9.

38. Chiles JA, Davidson P, McBride D. Effects of clozapine on use of seclusion and restraint at a state hospital. Hosp Community Psychiatry 1994;45:269–71.

39. Bender S, Linka T, Wolstein J, et al. Safety and efficacy of combined clozapine-lithium pharmacotherapy. Int J Neuropsychopharmacol 2004;7(1):59–63.

40. Pavlovic ZM. Augmentation of clozapine's antiaggressive properties with lamotrigine in a patient with chronic disorganized schizophrenia. J Clin Psychopharmacol 2008;28(1):119–20.

41. McEvoy JP, Scheifler PL, Frances A. Treatment of schizophrenia 1999. The expert consensus guideline series. J Clin Psychiatry 1999;60:S3–80.

42. Dose M, Hellweg R, Yassouridis A, et al. Combined treatment of schizophrenic psychoses with haloperidol and valproate. Pharmacopsychiatry 1998;31:122–5.

43. Okuma T, Yamashita I, Takahashi R, et al. A double-blind study of adjunctive carbamazepine versus placebo on excited states of schizophrenic and schizoaffective disorders. Acta Psychiatr Scand 1989;80:250–9.

44. Collins PJ, Larkin EP, Shubsachs AP. Lithium carbonate in chronic schizophrenia—a brief trial of lithium carbonate added to neuroleptics for treatment of resistant schizophrenic patients. Acta Psychiatr Scand 1991;84:150–4.

45. Wilson WH. Addition of lithium to haloperidol in non-affective, antipsychotic non-responsive schizophrenia: a double-blind, placebo-controlled, parallel-design clinical trial. Psychopharmacology 1993;111:359–66.

46. Langevin R, Paitich D, Orchard B, et al. The role of alcohol, drugs, suicide, attempts and situational strains in homicide committed by offenders seen for psychiatric assessment. Acta Psychiatr Scand 1982;66:229–42.

47. Murdoch D, Pihl RO, Ross D. Alcohol and crimes of violence: present issues. Int J Addict 1990;25:1065–81.

48. Roth JA. Psychoactive substances and violence. In: Research in brief. United States Department of Justice; 1994. Available at: https://www.ncjrs.gov/txtfiles/psycho.txt. Accessed April 30, 2012.

49. Burbach R. Substance abuse disorders. In: Simon RI, Tardiff K, editors. Violence assessment and management. 1st edition. Washington, DC: American Psychiatric Publishing, Inc; 2008. p. 141–60.

50. Swanson JW, Borum R, Swartz M, et al. Psychotic symptoms and disorders and the risk of violent behavior in the community. Crim Behav Ment Health 1996;6:317–38.

51. Johns A. Substance misuse: a primary risk and a major problem of comorbidity. Int Rev Psychiatry 1997;9:233–41.

52. Steadman HJ, Mulvey EP, Monahan J, et al. Violence by people discharged from acute psychiatric inpatient facilities and by others in the same neighborhoods. Arch Gen Psychiatry 1998;55:393–401.

53. American Psychiatric Association. Diagnostic and statistical manual of mental disorders. 4th edition. Washington, DC: American Psychiatric Association; 1994.

54. Hollander E, Tracy KA, Swann AC, et al. Divalproex in the treatment of impulsive aggression: efficacy in cluster B personality disorders. Neuropsychopharmacology 2003;28(6):1186–97.

55. Sheard MH, Marini JL, Bridges CI, et al. The effect of lithium on impulsive aggressive behavior in man. Am J Psychiatry 1976;133:1409–13.

56. Coccaro EF, Kavoussi RJ. Fluoxetine and impulsive aggressive behavior in personality-disordered subjects. Arch Gen Psychiatry 1997;54:1081–8.

57. Nickel MK, Muehlbacher M, Nickel C, et al. Aripiprazole in the treatment of patients with borderline personality disorder: a double-blind, placebo-controlled study. Am J Psychiatry 2006;163:833–48.

58. Hollander E, Allen A, Lopez RP, et al. A preliminary double-blind, placebo-controlled trial of divalproex sodium in borderline personality disorder. J Clin Psychiatry 2001;62(3):199–203.
59. Nickel MK, Nickel C, Mitterlehner FO, et al. Topiramate treatment of aggression in female borderline personality disorder patients: a double-blind, placebo-controlled study. J Clin Psychiatry 2004;65(11):1515–9.
60. Tritt K, Nickel C, Lahmann C, et al. Lamotrigine treatment of aggression in female borderline patients: a randomized, double-blind, placebo-controlled study. J Clin Psychopharmacol 2005;9(3):287–91.
61. Loew TH, Nickel MK, Muchlbacher M, et al. Topiramate treatment for women with borderline personality disorder: a double-blind, placebo-controlled study. J Clin Psychopharmacol 2006;26(1):61–6.
62. Stoffers J, Völlm BA, Rücker G, et al. Pharmacological interventions for borderline personality disorder. Cochrane Database Syst Rev 2010;(6):CD005653.
63. Reich DB, Zanarini MC, Bieri KA. A preliminary study of lamotrigine in the treatment of affective instability in borderline personality disorder. Int Clin Psychopharmacol 2009;24(5):270–5.
64. Walker C, Thomas J, Allen TS. Treating impulsivity, irritability, and aggression of antisocial personality disorder with quetiapine. Int J Offender Ther Comp Criminol 2003;47(5):556–67.
65. Hirose S. Effective treatment of aggression and impulsivity in antisocial personality disorder with risperidone. Psychiatry Clin Neurosci 2001;55(2):161–2.
66. Newman WJ, McDermott BE. Beta blockers for violence prophylaxis—case reports. J Clin Psychopharmacol 2011;31(6):785–7.
67. Tyrer SP, Walsh A, Edwards DE, et al. Factors associated with a good response to lithium in aggressive mentally handicapped subjects. Prog Neuropsychopharmacol Biol Psychiatry 1984;8:751–5.
68. Craft M, Ismail IA, Krishnamurti D, et al. Lithium in the treatment of aggression in mentally handicapped patients. A double-blind trial. Br J Psychiatry 1987;150:685–9.
69. Spreat S, Behar D, Reneski B, et al. Lithium carbonate for aggression in mentally retarded persons. Compr Psychiatry 1989;30:505–11.
70. Mattes JA. Valproic acid for nonaffective aggression in the mentally retarded. J Nerv Ment Dis 1992;180:601–2.
71. Amore M, Bertelli M, Villani D, et al. Olanzapine vs. risperidone in treating aggressive behaviors in adults with intellectual disability: a single blind study. J Intellect Disabil Res 2011;55(2):210–8.
72. Hassler F, Reis O. Pharmacotherapy of disruptive behavior in mentally retarded subjects: a review of the current literature. Dev Disabil Res Rev 2010;16(3):265–72.
73. Ruedrich SL, Grush L, Wilson J. Beta adrenergic blocking medications for aggressive or self-injurious mentally retarded persons. Am J Ment Retard 1990; 95(1):110–9.
74. Greendyke RM, Kanter DR. Therapeutic effects of pindolol on behavioral disturbances associated with organic brain disease: a double-blind study. J Clin Psychiatry 1986;47:423–6.
75. Greendyke RM, Kanter DR, Schuster DB, et al. Propranolol treatment of assaultive patients with organic brain disease. J Nerv Ment Dis 1986;174:290–4.
76. Greendyke RM, Berkner JP, Webster JC, et al. Treatment of behavioral problems with pindolol. Psychosomatics 1989;30(2):161–5.
77. Caspi N, Modai I, Barak P, et al. Pindolol augmentation in aggressive schizophrenic patients: a double-blind crossover randomized study. Int Clin Psychopharmacol 2001;16(2):111–5.

78. Haas JF, Cope DN. Neuropharmacologic management of behavior sequelae in head injury: a case report. Arch Phys Med Rehabil 1985;66:472–4.

79. Hornstein A, Seliger G. Cognitive side effects of lithium in closed head injury. J Neuropsychiatry Clin Neurosci 1989;1:446–7.

80. Geracioti TD. Valproic acid treatment of episodic explosiveness related to brain injury. J Clin Psychiatry 1994;55:416–7.

81. Horne M, Lindley SE. Divalproex sodium in the treatment of aggressive behavior and dysphoria in patients with organic brain syndromes. J Clin Psychiatry 1995; 56:430–1.

82. Wroblewski BA, Joseph AB, Kupfer J, et al. Effectiveness of valproic acid on destructive and aggressive behaviors in patients with acquired brain injury. Brain Inj 1997;11:37–47.

83. Azouvi P, Jokic C, Attal N, et al. Carbamazepine in agitation and aggressive behavior following severe closed-head injury: results of an open trial. Brain Inj 1999;13:797–804.

84. De Deyn PP, Rabheru K, Rasmussen A, et al. A randomized trial of risperidone, placebo, and haloperidol for behavioral symptoms of dementia. Neurology 1999;53(5):946–55.

85. Allain H, Dauzenberg PH, Maurer K, et al. Double blind study of tiapride versus haloperidol and placebo in agitation and aggressiveness in elderly patients with cognitive impairment. Psychopharmacology 2000;148(4):361–6.

86. Katz IR, Jeste DV, Mintzer JE, et al. Comparison of risperidone and placebo for psychosis and behavioral disturbances associated with dementia: a randomized, double-blind trial. J Clin Psychiatry 1999;60(2):107–15.

87. Yudofsky SC, Silver JM, Hales RE. Pharmacologic management of aggression in the elderly. J Clin Psychiatry 1990;51:S22–8.

88. Mellow AM, Solano-Lopez C, Davis S. Sodium valproate in the treatment of behavioral disturbance in dementia. J Geriatr Psychiatry Neurol 1993;6:205–9.

89. Kunik ME, Yudofsky SC, Silver JM, et al. Pharmacologic approach to management of agitation associated with dementia. J Clin Psychiatry 1994;55:S13–7.

90. Lott AD, McElroy SL, Keys MA. Valproate in the treatment of behavioral agitation in elderly patients with dementia. J Neuropsychiatry Clin Neurosci 1995;7: 314–9.

91. Tune L. The role of antipsychotics in treating delirium. Curr Psychiatry Rep 2002; 4:209–12.

92. Foreman M, Milisen K, Marcantonia EM. Prevention and treatment strategies for delirium. Prim Psychiatr 2004;11:52–8.

93. Shrobik YK, Bergeron N, Dumont M, et al. Olanzapine vs haloperidol: treating delirium in a critical care setting. Intensive Care Med 2004;30(3):444–9.

94. Kalisvart KJ, de Jonghe JF, Bogaards MJ, et al. Haloperidol prophylaxis for elderly hip-surgery patients at risk for delirium: a randomized placebo-controlled study. J Am Geriatr Soc 2005;53:1658–66.

95. Milbrandt EB, Kersten A, Kong L, et al. Haloperidol use is associated with lower hospital mortality in mechanically ventilated patients. Crit Care Med 2005;33: 226–9.

96. Nordstrom K, Allen MH. Managing the acutely agitated and psychotic patient. CNS Spectr 2007;12:S5–11.

97. Lonergan E, Britton AM, Luxenberg J. Antipsychotics for delirium. Cochrane Database Syst Rev 2007;(2):CD005594.

98. Pun BT, Ely EW. The importance of diagnosing and managing ICU delirium. Chest 2007;132(2):624–36.

Index

Note: Page numbers of article titles are in **boldface** type.

Psychiatr Clin N Am 35 (2012) 973–981
http://dx.doi.org/10.1016/S0193-953X(12)00095-0
0193-953X/12/$ – see front matter © 2012 Elsevier Inc. All rights reserved.

United States Postal Service

Statement of Ownership, Management, and Circulation
(All Periodicals Publications Except Requestor Publications)

1. Publication Title	2. Publication Number	3. Filing Date
Psychiatric Clinics of North America	0 0 0 - 7 0 3	9/14/12

4. Issue Frequency	5. Number of Issues Published Annually	6. Annual Subscription Price
Mar, Jun, Sep, Dec	4	$286.00

7. Complete Mailing Address of Known Office of Publication *(Not printer)(Street, city, county, state, and ZIP+4®)*

Elsevier Inc.
360 Park Avenue South
New York, NY 10010-1710

Contact Person
Stephen R. Bushing
Telephone *(Include area code)*
215-239-3688

8. Complete Mailing Address of Headquarters or General Business Office of Publisher *(Not printer)*

Elsevier Inc., 360 Park Avenue South, New York, NY 10010-1710

9. Full Names and Complete Mailing Addresses of Publisher, Editor, and Managing Editor *(Do not leave blank)*

Publisher *(Name and complete mailing address)*

Kim Murphy, Elsevier, Inc., 1600 John F. Kennedy Blvd. Suite 1800, Philadelphia, PA 19103-2899

Editor *(Name and complete mailing address)*

Joanne Husovski, Elsevier, Inc., 1600 John F. Kennedy Blvd. Suite 1800, Philadelphia, PA 19103-2899

Managing Editor *(Name and complete mailing address)*

Barbara Cohen - Kligerman, Elsevier, Inc., 1600 John F. Kennedy Blvd. Suite 1800, Philadelphia, PA 19103-2899

10. Owner *(Do not leave blank. If the publication is owned by a corporation, give the name and address of the corporation immediately followed by the names and addresses of all stockholders owning or holding 1 percent or more of the total amount of stock. If not owned by a corporation, give the names and addresses of the individual owners. If owned by a partnership or other unincorporated firm, give its name and address as well as those of each individual owner. If the publication is published by a nonprofit organization, give its name and address.)*

Full Name	Complete Mailing Address
Wholly owned subsidiary of	1600 John F. Kennedy Blvd., Ste. 1800
Reed/Elsevier, US holdings	Philadelphia, PA 19103-2899

11. Known Bondholders, Mortgagees, and Other Security Holders Owning or Holding 1 Percent or More of Total Amount of Bonds, Mortgages, or Other Securities. If none, check box ☐ None

Full Name	Complete Mailing Address
N/A	

12. Tax Status *(For completion by nonprofit organizations authorized to mail at nonprofit rates)(Check one)*
The purpose, function, and nonprofit status of this organization and the exempt status for federal income tax purposes:
☐ Has Not Changed During Preceding 12 Months
☐ Has Changed During Preceding 12 Months *(Publisher must submit explanation of change with this statement)*

PS Form 3526, September 2007 (Page 1 of 3 (Instructions Page 3)) PSN 7530-01-000-9931 PRIVACY NOTICE: See our Privacy policy in www.usps.com

---

13. Publication Title	14. Issue Date for Circulation Data Below
Psychiatric Clinics of North America	September 2012

15. Extent and Nature of Circulation			Average No. Copies Each Issue During Preceding 12 Months	No. Copies of Single Issue Published Nearest to Filing Date
a. Total Number of Copies *(Net press run)*			934	869
b. Paid Circulation (By Mail and Outside the Mail)	(1)	Mailed Outside-County Paid Subscriptions Stated on PS Form 3541 *(Include paid distribution above nominal rate, advertiser's proof copies, and exchange copies)*	479	437
	(2)	Mailed In-County Paid Subscriptions Stated on PS Form 3541 *(Include paid distribution above nominal rate, advertiser's proof copies, and exchange copies)*		
	(3)	Paid Distribution Outside the Mails Including Sales Through Dealers and Carriers, Street Vendors, Counter Sales, and Other Paid Distribution Outside USPS®	192	206
	(4)	Paid Distribution by Other Classes Mailed Through the USPS (e.g. First-Class Mail®)		
c. Total Paid Distribution *(Sum of 15b (1), (2), (3), and (4))*		▲	671	643
d. Free or Nominal Rate Distribution (By Mail and Outside the Mail)	(1)	Free or Nominal Rate Outside-County Copies Included on PS Form 3541	64	61
	(2)	Free or Nominal Rate In-County Copies Included on PS Form 3541		
	(3)	Free or Nominal Rate Copies Mailed at Other Classes Through the USPS (e.g. First-Class Mail)		
	(4)	Free or Nominal Rate Distribution Outside the Mail (Carriers or other means)		
e. Total Free or Nominal Rate Distribution *(Sum of 15d (1), (2), (3) and (4))*		▲	64	61
f. Total Distribution *(Sum of 15c and 15e)*		▲	735	704
g. Copies not Distributed *(See instructions to publishers #4 (page #3))*		▲	199	165
h. Total *(Sum of 15f and g)*		▲	934	869
i. Percent Paid *(15c divided by 15f times 100)*		▲	91.29%	91.34%

16. Publication of Statement of Ownership

If the publication is a general publication, publication of this statement is required. Will be printed ☐ Publication not required
in the December 2012 issue of this publication.

17. Signature and Title of Editor, Publisher, Business Manager, or Owner

[signature] Stephen R. Bushing

Stephen R. Bushing –Inventory Distribution Coordinator

Date September 14, 2012

I certify that all information furnished on this form is true and complete. I understand that anyone who furnishes false or misleading information on this form or who omits material or information requested on the form may be subject to criminal sanctions (including fines and imprisonment) and/or civil sanctions (including civil penalties).

PS Form 3526, September 2007 (Page 2 of 3)

Printed and bound by CPI Group (UK) Ltd, Croydon, CR0 4YY

03/10/2024

01040461-0005